JOINT COMMISSION
RESOURCES

Timing is Everything

STRATEGIES FOR REDUCING DELAYS IN PATIENT CARE

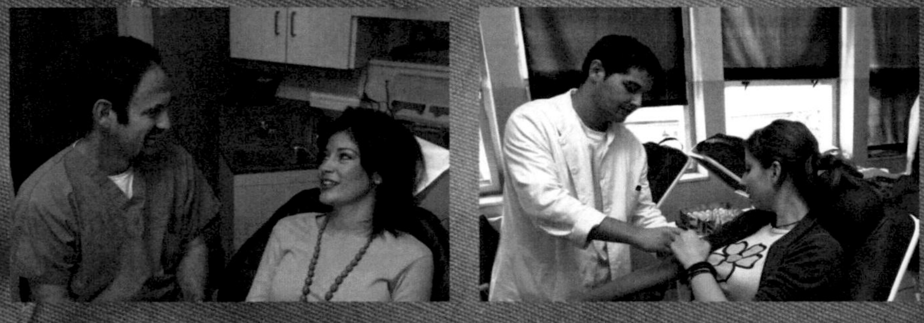

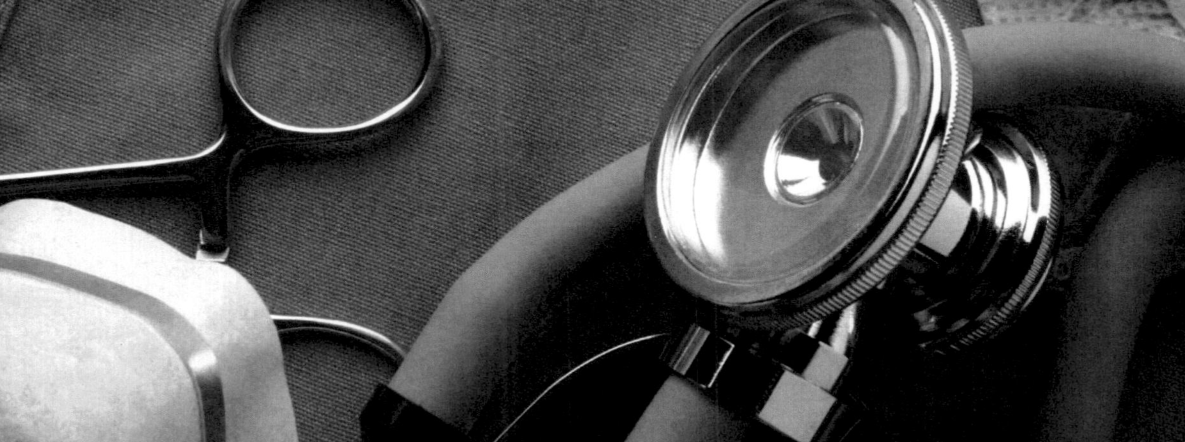

Senior Editor: Ilese J. Chatman
Senior Project Manager: Cheryl Firestone
Manager, Publications: Paul Reis
Associate Director: Johanna Harris
Associate Director: Cecily Pew
Executive Director: Catherine Chopp-Hinckley, Ph.D.
Joint Commission/JCR Reviewers: Richard Croteau, M.D., Patricia Adamski, R.N., M.S., M.B.A, Mark Schario, Robert Katzfey, Patricia McColl, R.N., M.S., Coleen Smith, R.N., M.B.A.

Joint Commission Resources Mission

The mission of Joint Commission Resources is to continuously improve the safety and quality of care in the United States and in the international community through the provision of education and consultation services and international accreditation.

Joint Commission Resources educational programs and publications support, but are separate from, the accreditation activities of The Joint Commission. Attendees at Joint Commission Resources educational programs and purchasers of Joint Commission Resources publications receive no special consideration or treatment in, or confidential information about, the accreditation process.

The inclusion of an organization name, a product, or a service in a Joint Commission publication should not be construed as an endorsement of such organization, product, or service, nor is failure to include an organization name, a product, or a service to be construed as disapproval.

This publication is designed to provide accurate and authoritative information in regard to the subject matter covered. Every attempt has been made to ensure accuracy at the time of publication; however, please note that laws, regulations, and standards are subject to change. Please also note that some of the examples in this publication are specific to the laws and regulations of the locality of the facility. The information and examples in this publication are provided with the understanding that the publisher is not engaged in providing medical, legal, or other professional advice. If any such assistance is desired, the services of a competent professional person should be sought.

Printed in the U.S.A. 5 4 3 2 1

Requests for permission to make copies of any part of this work should be mailed to
Permissions Editor
Department of Publications
Joint Commission Resources
One Renaissance Boulevard
Oakbrook Terrace, Illinois 60181
permissions@jcrinc.com

ISBN: 978-1-59940-111-9
Library of Congress Control Number: 2007927733

For more information about Joint Commission Resources, please visit http://www.jcrinc.com.

Contents

Introduction

A patient lies weak and helpless in a hospital emergency room, experiencing facial numbness and additional symptoms that are attacking the left arm and leg. The patient's symptoms are relative to a stroke.

A blood clot was found blocking a vessel that feeds the brain, and circulation worsened—circulation that is very much needed to keep brain cells functioning and alive. The blockage needed to be cleared.

As the symptoms continued to worsen, the patient granted permission to physicians to administer a drug that would unblock the vessel. Several days later, the patient was discharged from the hospital.

Stroke, the nation's third leading cause of death, is also the leading cause of long-term disability. Tackling root causes of delayed treatment, performing timely assessments, and introducing information technology strategies are just a few of the ways to help reduce delays in patient treatment and care. But problems such as delays by the patient or flaws in the health care system could have made the outcome of this fictitious story the exception rather than the norm.

Timing is everything.

Audience for This Book

Timing is Everything: Strategies for Reducing Delays in Patient Care is written for all members of the health care team who share responsibility and accountability for patients seeking medical attention in any health care setting or discipline, including, at a minimum, health care leaders, patient safety officers, and clinical leaders. The health care team will be interested in assessment issues of patients, clinical care responses, and resources to help reduce delays, which are the topic of this book.

Acknowledgments

We would like to thank all the Joint Commission reviewers who were involved in the development of this book. These individuals gave us information relevant to reducing delays in care, illustrating their high-quality expertise in the provision of care. A special thank-you to writer Ruth Carol.

Chapter 1
Diverse Root Causes of Treatment Delays—Where, How, and Why

A 54-year-old female presents to the emergency department (ED) complaining of nausea, light-headedness, and general aching in her upper body. Her condition is classified as non-urgent and it is flu season, so the patient is asked to take a seat. Because waiting times in the ED often vary based on patient acuity levels, she waits nearly an hour when she suddenly collapses. The patient is breathing abnormally and does not respond to gentle shaking. She is in sudden cardiac arrest due to ventricular fibrillation.

Delays in patient care, whether caused by an overcrowded ED as in the aforementioned case or a busy physician's office, are not just an inconvenience to patients—they can be deadly. In fact, treatment delays accounted for nearly 8% of all sentinel event cases involving patient death or permanent injury reported to The Joint Commission between January 1995 and December 2006.[1] In total, 303 sentinel events that involved delays in treatment were reported between January 1995 and December 31, 2006 (*see* Table 1-1, below).

Table 1-1. Sentinel Events Related to Delays in Treatment as of June 30, 2006		
Type of Sentinel Event	**Number of Events**	**Percentage**
Delay in Treatment	303	7.4%

Source: The Joint Commission: *Sentinel Event Statistics.* Dec. 31, 2006. http://www.jointcommission.org/SentinelEvents/Statistics/ (accessed Mar. 5, 2007).

Delays in Treatment in Other Units

Treatment delays are the source of more than one half of all reported sentinel event cases of patient death or permanent injury, according to Joint Commission sentinel event data.[2] Of the 303 reported cases of delays in treatment as of 2006, 94 were ED related.

But sentinel events can occur in other hospital and health care settings as well. Many cases have originated in the intensive care unit (ICU), medical/surgical unit, and operating room, not to mention inpatient psychiatric hospitals, freestanding and hospital-based ambulatory care services facilities, and home care settings.

In one of the first studies to examine the potential causes of medical errors in the outpatient setting, researchers from Brigham and Women's Hospital and the Harvard School of Public Health in Boston, found that more than half of the errors resulting in missed or late diagnoses caused serious harm to patients.[3] Of 307 closed malpractice claims reviewed retrospectively, 181 involved diagnostic errors that harmed patients. Of these errors, 59% were associated with serious harm, and 30% resulted in patient death. The most frequently cited delayed or missed diagnosis was for colorectal, breast, and skin cancer. Although most of these errors occurred in the physician's office, they also involved other nonhospital settings such as ambulatory surgery centers.

Reasons Cited for Treatment Delays

The reported reasons for treatment delays are multifactor. The most common factor is misdiagnosis (46%), according to Joint Commission sentinel event data. Other factors include delayed test results (15%), physician availability (13%), delayed administration of ordered care (15%), incomplete treatment (12%), delayed initial assessment (7%), patient left unattended (4%), paging system malfunction (2%), and inability to locate ED entrance (2%).

Of the 41 cases involving misdiagnoses, the most frequently missed diagnosis was meningitis; seven of the nine meningitis cases were in children. Other missed diagnoses included various forms of cardiac disease, pulmonary embolism, trauma, asthma, neurologic disorder, acute abdominal disorders, dehydration, sepsis, diabetes, vascular conditions, and four cases of unknown diagnosis due to the patient leaving without being evaluated. All of the nine cases that occurred in inpatient psychiatric hospitals were related to the delayed diagnosis or treatment of nonbehavioral medical conditions.

Root Causes of Treatment Delays

Just as several factors were responsible for treatment delays, multiple root causes contributed to each sentinel event, according to the Joint Commission's 2006 data.[4] The overwhelming majority of organizations (65%) cite a breakdown in communication, most often occurring with or between physicians. Organizations also cited problems with the patient assessment process (56%), continuum of care issues (35%) that most often relate to a lack of continuity of care across settings or shifts, staff orientation and training (27%), availability of critical patient information (31%), and insufficient staffing levels (17%). *See* Figure 1-1, page 3.

The Joint Commission has seen an increase in the average number of root causes identified for most types of sentinel events when comparing the root cause analysis results from the first 10 years of the sentinel event database, notes Richard J. Croteau, M.D., executive director for patient safety initiatives for the Joint Commission International Center for Patient Safety. In most cases, the difference is not significant. For example, an average of 4.5 root causes per event for delays in treatment rose to 5.0 root causes per event for delays in treatment. For the category of "orientation/training," the average number of root causes per event consistently decreased, although in other categories, such as "leadership and organization culture," the number consistently increased. Other categories remained the same. These fluctuations are all consistent with an increasing maturity of the root cause analysis process, says Croteau, as organizations are doing a better job at digging down and identifying more and deeper root causes.

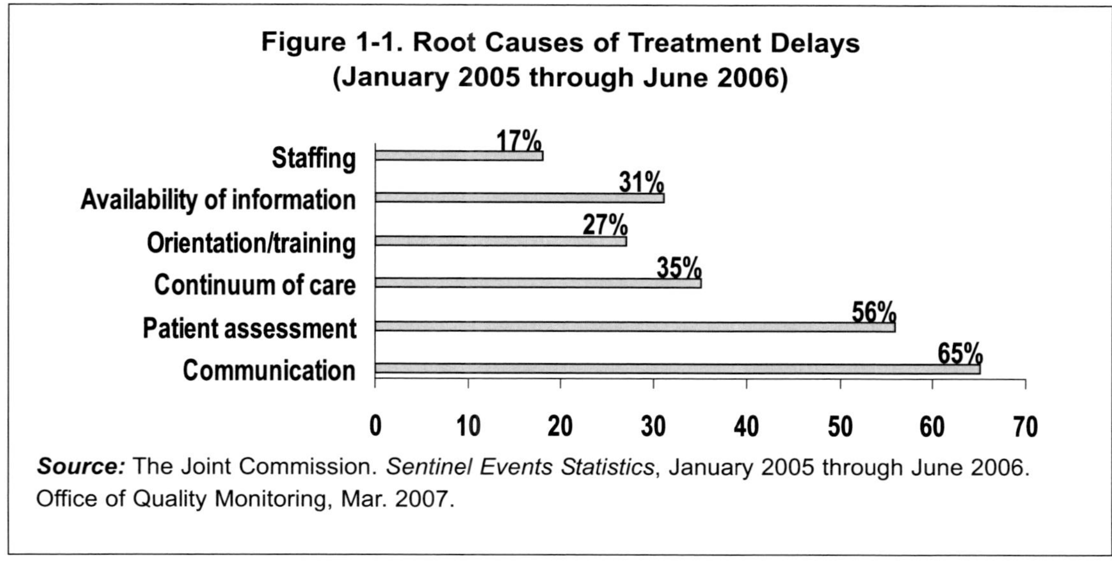

Source: The Joint Commission. *Sentinel Events Statistics*, January 2005 through June 2006. Office of Quality Monitoring, Mar. 2007.

Similarly, sentinel event cases due to delays in treatment have climbed steadily since The Joint Commission began tracking them in 1995 (*see* Figure 1-2, page 4). The increase in the number of cases regarding treatment delays is fairly consistent with the increase in reports for all types of events taken together, notes Croteau. The percentage of all reported sentinel events that involve delays in treatment has remained fairly constant over the years.

Delayed Diagnosis

A study reported in *Annals of Internal Medicine* analyzed malpractice claims that revealed poor internal communication as a root cause for common breakdowns in the diagnostic process.[5] For example, communication breakdown typically occurred during hand offs in care. Additionally, there was a failure to establish a clear line of responsibility and conflict. Gandhi et al.[3] note that diagnostic errors harmful to patients are rarely the result of one breakdown or one contributing factor, but rather the result of multiple root causes resulting from a combination of individual and system factors. (*See* risk reduction strategies that target multiple root causes in Sidebar 1-1, page 5.)

Timeliness: A Dimension of Quality

In light of numerous ongoing findings that suggest delays in treatment are not only a sign of poor-quality care but a real danger to individuals seeking treatment, timeliness has taken on a new importance in the health care community's efforts to improve the delivery of high-quality care.

In *Crossing the Quality Chasm: A New Health System for the 21st Century*, the Institute of Medicine's (IOM) Committee on Quality of Health Care in America identified timeliness as one of six key aims for improvement.[6] The committee suggests that a health care system that

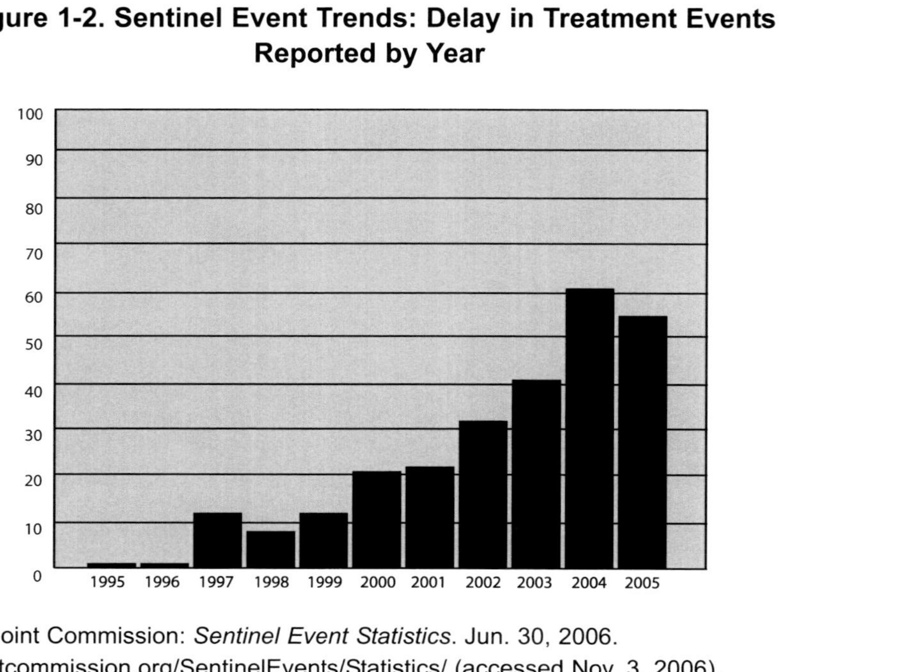

Figure 1-2. Sentinel Event Trends: Delay in Treatment Events Reported by Year

Source: The Joint Commission: *Sentinel Event Statistics*. Jun. 30, 2006. http://www.jointcommission.org/SentinelEvents/Statistics/ (accessed Nov. 3, 2006).

achieves major gains in the six identified areas would be far better at meeting patient needs. Patients would experience care that is safer, more reliable, more responsive to their needs, more integrated, and more available, and they could count on receiving the full array of preventive, acute, and chronic services that are likely to prove beneficial. *See* the IOM's Six Dimensions of Quality in Table 1-2, page 5.

In addition, timeliness is one of four dimensions of quality measured in the *2005 National Healthcare Quality Report* issued by the Agency for Healthcare Research and Quality (AHRQ). Timeliness is a key component in an organization's ability to provide the right care for every person every time, a concept that quality improvement organizations promote.

Quality Initiatives

Both governmental and nongovernmental agencies and organizations have developed quality initiatives to address the issues of high-quality care and patient safety. As noted in the afore-mentioned IOM and AHRQ reports, the issue of timeliness is one measure of quality care. Consequently, many efforts to improve the quality of care provided in hospital and outpatient settings incorporate the notion of reducing treatment delays even if timeliness is not the sole focus. For example, several initiatives to improve medical errors address reducing the time it takes to receive test results. Other initiatives look to improve the quality of care by ensuring that patients presenting to the ED or those attempting to make a primary care appointment are seen in a timely manner.

Sidebar 1-1. Risk Reduction Strategies Call for Redesign

Given that health care organizations cite multiple root causes for sentinel events arising from delays in treatment, implementing multiple risk reduction strategies in various areas can be beneficial. Redesigning the following areas is one strategy that organizations have implemented to reduce treatment delays:

- Orientation and training processes
- Transfer procedures
- Staffing plans
- On-call specialist contact procedures
- Triage procedures
- Physical space

Other strategies include the implementation of formal oral communication procedures and revised specialist on-call procedures. Additional procedures that have undergone a revision or redesign are initial assessment processes, patient information retrieval processes, credentialing and privileging processes, communication of abnormal laboratory or radiology results, and the implementation of voice recognition transcription software.

Table 1-2. The IOM's Six Dimensions of Quality

Safety	Avoid injuries to patients from the care that is intended to help them.
Effectiveness	Provide services based on scientific knowledge to all who could benefit; refrain from providing services to those unlikely to benefit.
Patient-centeredness	Provide care that is respectful of and responsive to individual patient preference, need, and values; ensure that patient values guide all clinical decisions.
Timeliness	Reduce waits and potentially harmful delays for both those who receive and those who give care.
Efficiency	Avoid waste, including waste of equipment, supplies, ideas, and energy.
Equity	Provide care that does not vary in quality because of personal characteristics such as gender, ethnicity, geography, or socioeconomic status.

Source: Adapted from Institute of Medicine: *Crossing the Quality Chasm: A New Health System for the 21st Century*. Washington, DC: National Academy Press, 2001.

The Leapfrog Group

The Leapfrog Group is most known for its four hospital quality and safety practices. The consortium of more than 170 Fortune 500 corporations and other large private- and public-sector health benefits purchasers, which represents more than 36 million enrollees, maintains that implementation of these evidence-based practices will significantly reduce preventable medical mistakes. Endorsed by the National Quality Forum (NQF), the four quality practices are as follows:

1. Computer prescriber order entry (CPOE): health care staff enter medication orders through computers linked to software that prevents prescription errors; this practice has been shown to reduce serious prescribing errors in hospitals by more than 50%.

2. Evidence-based hospital referral: the referral of patients requiring certain medical procedures to hospitals that offer the best survival odds based on scientifically valid criteria, which could reduce a patient's risk of dying by 40%.

3. ICU physician staffing: the use of "intensivists," physicians who have received special training in critical care medicine, whose use in the ICU has been shown to reduce the risk of patients dying in the ICU by 40%

4. The Leapfrog Safe Practices Score (added in 2004): the adoption of the NQF's 30 Safe Practices, which includes the original three Leapfrog leaps

In addition, the Leapfrog Group has a hospital quality and safety survey, a voluntary survey that nearly 1,300 hospitals nationwide responded to in 2006. Survey results are displayed on their Web site at http://www.leapfroggroup.org, which is accessible to the public.

The Leapfrog Group also operates the Leapfrog Hospital Rewards Program™ and Hospital Insights, the measures on which the rewards program is based. These measures are endorsed by NQF and are already being collected through the Joint Commission's ORYX® initiative and Leapfrog's own survey. The measures focus on the following five clinical areas:

- Coronary artery bypass graft
- Percutaneous coronary intervention
- Acute myocardial infarction
- Community-acquired pneumonia
- Deliveries/newborn care

As part of the program, hospitals are scored on the measures and rewarded for each of the five areas in which they demonstrate sustained excellence or improvement. Rewards are given as both financial incentives and increased market share.

Institute for Healthcare Improvement

Using the IOM's six dimensions of quality—safety, effectiveness, patient-centeredness, timeliness, efficiency, and equity—the Institute for Healthcare Improvement (IHI) created an initiative called "Transforming Care at the Bedside" (*see* Figure 1-3, page 8). In partnership with the Robert Wood Johnson Foundation, the IHI launched this initiative in 2003 to improve care specifically on hospital medical/surgical units. Beginning in 2004, models of care at the bedside were being tested, refined, and implemented at 13 pilot hospitals across the country. Many of the models, such as rapid response teams, can be used as strategies to reduce treatment delays (*see* Sidebar 1-2, page 9, for an example of a model). The IHI broadly disseminates progress on the resulting best practices on its Web site at http://www.ihi.org/ IHI/Programs/TransformingCareAtTheBedside/.

Where Do We Stand with Quality of Care?

With so many initiatives addressing quality of care, have these efforts improved the ability of the nation's health care organizations to provide care that is safe, effective, patient-centered, timely, efficient, and equitable? Hospitals and other health care settings have focused on improving patient safety and outcomes through implementing strategies ranging from the institution of new and modified processes and systems to the acquisition of new information technology. However, without valid outcome data, we cannot say with certainty that these efforts have improved the nation's health care.

It appears that hospitals might be safer today than when the IOM report was disclosed, according to a study identifying changes over time in two states that collaborated on a patient safety project funded by the AHRQ.[8] The study focused on patient safety systems that should be found in hospitals, especially in light of the IOM report and subsequent national patient safety efforts. The seven constructs studied were CPOE, computerized test results, and assessments of adverse events; specific patient safety policies; use of data in patient-safety programs; drug storage, administration, and safety procedures; manner of handling adverse event/error reporting; prevention policies; and root cause analysis.

Based on the study data, improvements occurred in five of the seven patient safety constructs. The overwhelming majority of hospitals had a patient safety committee and routinely conducted trend analyses on incidents, the study found. Among those hospitals that required root cause analysis following a near miss, almost all reported that actions were taken based on an analysis of findings. During the study period, there was an increase in the percentage of hospitals that implemented a written patient safety plan (55% to 74.4%) and in those that used standardized formats and methods to disseminate data (40.8% to 55.2%).

But not all the news is good. Although 74.4% of hospitals reported full implementation of a written patient safety plan, nearly 9% reported no plan. A substantial percentage of hospitals reported having medication safety systems, but only 34.1% implemented CPOEs.

This humble improvement leads the study authors to conclude that quality systems are

Figure 1-3. The IHI's Initiative for "Transforming Care at the Bedside" Created in Partnership with the Robert Wood Johnson Foundation

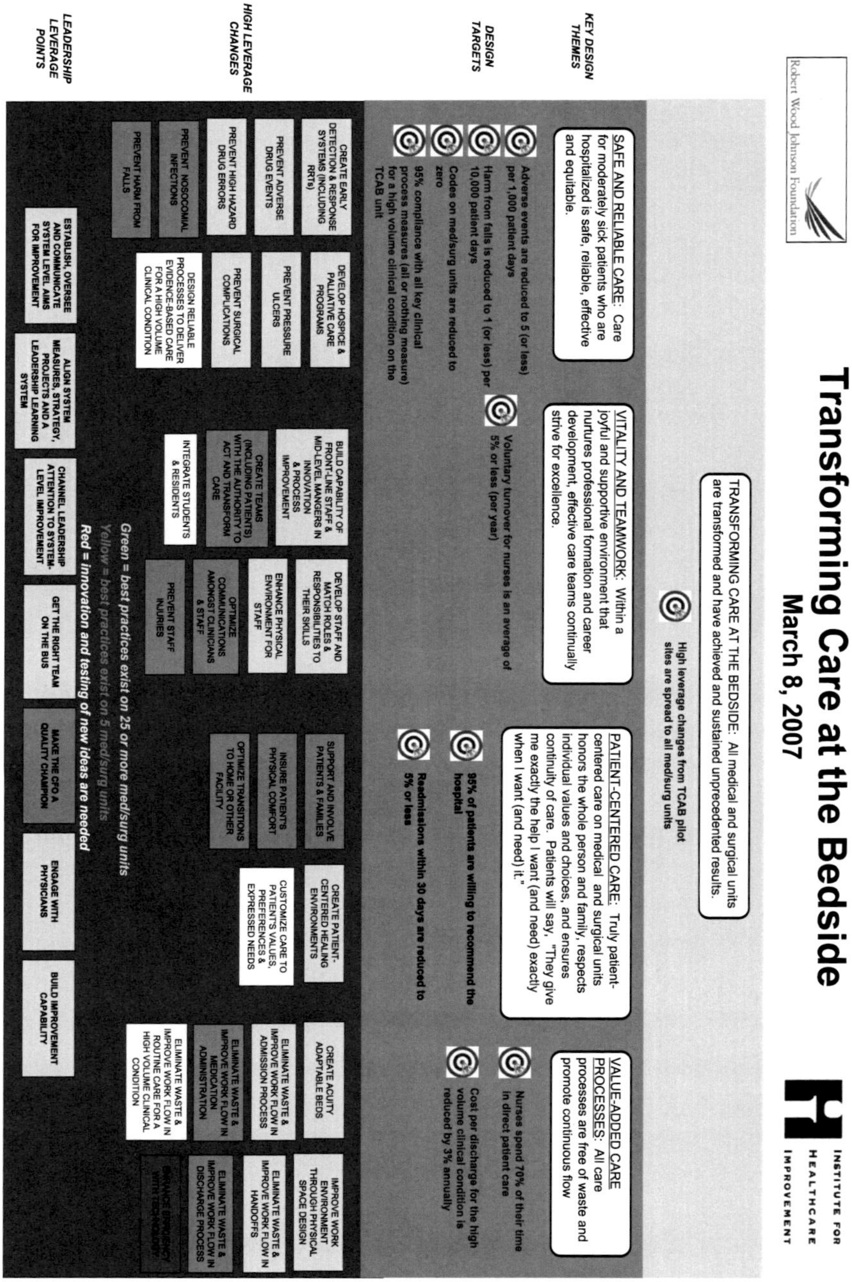

Source: Institute for Healthcare Improvement: *Transforming Care at the Bedside.* Mar. 8, 2007. http://www.ihi.org/NR/rdonlyres/37FDB5E8-52ED-4CC2-8E43-E2C22DA53AFE/0/VisioTCABFramework11107.pdf (accessed Apr. 7, 2007).

Sidebar 1-2. Rapid Response Teams

The use of rapid response teams (RRT) can help reduce treatment delays by empowering staff to call upon the team at the first sign of concern.

The use of RRTs is one of many methods being used by hospitals involved in the Institue for Healthcare Improvement's (IHI) initiative to transform care at the bedside. The deployment of RRTs also is one of 12 interventions endorsed in the 5 Million Lives Campaign launched by the IHI in 2006, designed to reduce medical harm in U.S. hospitals.

RRTs are small groups of providers who have experience at assessing patient symptoms and anticipating the trajectory of medical conditions. Typically, these teams include a critical-care-trained nurse, a respiratory therapist, and/or an intensivist. The RRT avails itself to all hospital providers, but mainly to medical/surgical nurses who want a second opinion. Bedside providers can summon the RRT because of a measurable change in a patient's vital sign or simply because of a "gut feeling" that the patient's health might be deteriorating.

Although U.S. hospitals are just beginning to use RRTs, their Australian counterparts already have had positive outcomes as a result of their use. The use of an RRT at an Australian medical center resulted in a 65% reduction in cardiac arrests, a 56% decrease in deaths from cardiac arrests, and an 88% decrease in inpatient days following cardiac arrests.[1] Similarly, the introduction of an RRT reduced the incidence of unexpected cardiac arrest by 50%.[2] The introduction of an RRT in an Australian teaching hospital was associated with reduced incidence of postoperative adverse outcomes, mortality rate, and mean duration of hospital stay.[3] One of the first published reports documenting RRTs in a U.S. hospital found a 17% decrease in the incidence of cardiopulmonary arrests.[4]

Although the use of RRTs is gaining strong support, some experts question the scientific grounds for advocating their use, citing equivocal evidence coupled with a lack of cost-effectiveness data.[5]

References

1. Bellomo R., et al.: A prospective before-and-after trial of a medical emergency team. *Med J Aust* 179(6):283–287, 2003.

2. Buist M.D., et al.: Effects of a medical emergency team on reduction of incidence of and mortality from unexpected cardiac arrests in hospitals: Preliminary study. *BMJ* 324:387–390, 2002.

3. Bellomo R., et al.: Prospective controlled trial of effect of medical emergency team on postoperative morbidity and mortality rates. *Crit Care Med* 32(4):916–921, 2004.

4. DeVito M.A., et al.: Use of medical emergency team responses to reduce hospital cardiopulmonary arrests. *Qual Saf Health Care* 13:251–254, 2004.

5. Winters B.D., Pham J., Pronovost P.J.: Rapid response teams—Walk, don't run. *JAMA* 296:1645–1647, Oct. 4, 2006.

improving, but that such change takes time, and that the gap between the best possible care and actual care remains large.[8]

The Leapfrog Group's *2006 Hospital Quality and Safety Survey* shows similarly mixed results. Of the hospitals surveyed, 9 out of 10 have implemented procedures to avoid wrong-site surgeries, and 8 out of 10 require a pharmacist to review all medication orders before drugs are dispensed.

But other findings indicate that many hospitals still have significant progress to make. The following findings are notable:

- More than 9 in 10 hospitals have not implemented CPOEs.
- Nine in 10 hospitals fail to meet the standards for performing two high-risk procedures:
  –Coronary artery bypass graft surgery (90%)
  –Abdominal aortic aneurysm repair (96%)
- Seven in 10 hospitals do not enlist intensivists to oversee patient care in the ICU.
- Five in 10 hospitals do not have an explicit protocol to ensure adequate nursing staff or a policy to check with patients to make sure they understand the risks of their procedures.
- Three in 10 hospitals lack procedures for preventing malnutrition in patients, and do not vaccinate their health care workers against the flu.

The *2005 National Healthcare Quality Report* also recognizes that health care quality continues to improve, though at a modest pace. The third of such reports, it analyzed 179 measures assembled across four dimensions of quality: effectiveness, patient safety, timeliness, and patient-centeredness. Overall, most measures of quality improved over the previous year. Specific improvements were seen in the following areas:

- Of the 44 core report measures with trend data, 23 showed significant* improvement, 2 showed significant deterioration, and 19 stayed the same.
- Measures that improved significantly outnumbered those that deteriorated significantly by a large margin: over 10 to 1.[8]
- A sizable percentage of the measures (43%) showed no significant change (*see* Figure 1-4, page 11).

Timeliness: Where Do We Stand?

With regard to timeliness, the *2005 National Healthcare Quality Report* focused on three core measures related to timeliness of primary, emergency, and hospital care. Measures of timeli-

---

* **Significance** is defined as a statistical difference with a *p* value less than .05 and with an average change of 1% or more per year over a period of two or more years, depending on the measure.

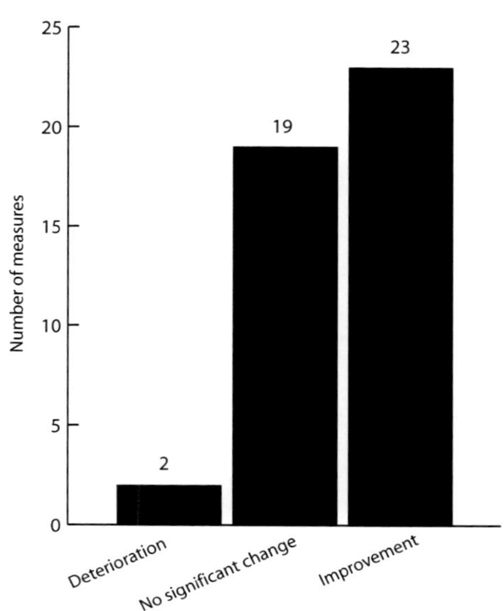

Figure 1-4. *2005 National Healthcare Quality Report* Core Measures

Number of *2005 National Healthcare Quality Report* core measures showing significant improvement, no significant change, or deterioration over multiple years (n = 44). The median rate of annual change for the 44 core measures is a 2.8% improvement, the same rate reported in the 2004 report.

Source: Agency for Healthcare Research and Quality (AHRQ): *2005 National Healthcare Quality Report,* Pub. no. 06-0018. Rockville, MD: AHRQ, Dec. 2005.

ness include waiting time spent in physicians' offices and EDs, and the interval between identifying a need for specific tests and/or treatments and actually receiving those services. The core measures are getting care for illness or injury as soon as wanted, ED visits in which the patient left without being seen, and time to initiation of thrombolytic therapy for heart attack patients. The report findings are as follows:

- Approximately 15% of adults report that they sometimes or never get care for illness or injury as soon as wanted.
- Between 2001 and 2002, the overall percentage of ED visits in which the patient left before being seen was 1.7%, an increase from the 1.2% reported between 1997 and 1998.
- Among heart attack patients with Medicare coverage, the median time from hospital arrival to the initiation of thrombolytic agents was 46 minutes in 2003.

Providing timely treatment and avoiding delays is a constant challenge. Causes of delays tend to be multifactor and occur throughout the hospital and other health care settings. The aforementioned findings reveal a health care system that is improving but has a long way to go to achieve optimal quality. Consequently, the question posed by the IOM authors of *To Err Is Human* remains relevant today: "Must we wait another decade to be safer in our health systems?"[6]

References

1. The Joint Commission: *Sentinel Event Statistics.* June 30, 2006. http://www.jointcommission.org/SentinelEvents/Statistics/ (accessed Nov. 3, 2006).

2. The Joint Commission: *Sentinel Event Alert* 26. Jun. 17, 2002. http://www.jointcommission.org/SentinelEvents/SentinelEventAlert/sea_26.htm (accessed Nov. 3, 2006).

3. Gandhi T.K., et al.: Missed and delayed diagnoses in the ambulatory setting: A study of closed malpractice claims. *Ann Intern Med* 145(7):488–496, 2006.

4. The Joint Commission: *Root causes of delays in treatment:* 1995–2004.2005. http://www.jointcommission.org/NR/rdonlyres/276AFB5C-0224-4B66-ABD7-EC4B78C9FB2A/0/se_rc_delays_treatment.jpg (accessed Oct. 6, 2006).

5. Institute of Medicine: *Crossing the Quality Chasm: A New Health System for the 21st Century.* Washington, DC: National Academy Press, 2001.

6. Institute of Medicine: *To Err Is Human: Building a Safer Health System.* Washington, D.C.: National Academy Press, 1999.

7. Leape L.L., Berwick D.M.: Five years after *To Err is Human*: What have we learned? *JAMA* 293(19):2384–2390, 2005.

8. Agency for Healthcare Research and Quality: *2005 National Healthcare Quality Report*, Pub. no. 06-0018. Dec. 2005. http://www.ahrq.gov/qual/nhqr05/nhqr05.pdf (accessed Oct. 26, 2006).

Chapter 2
Strategies for Timely Patient Assessment

"We have to bring the science [of management] back into health care in a way that we haven't in a very long time."

Source: Donald Berwick, president of the Institute for Healthcare Improvement. Allen S.: Emergency room recovery. *Boston Globe* p. A1, Jul. 8, 2004.

Typically, patients present to the emergency department (ED) to receive emergency care. A patient injures a wrist, which turns out to be fractured; a patient experiences severe abdominal cramps, which are diagnosed as appendicitis; or a patient complains of chest pains, which are indicative of a heart attack. Whatever their symptoms, patients could require immediate care and attention. What they might get instead are longer and longer waits to be seen by an emergency physician. It is a common tale being told through the growing occurrence of overcrowded EDs, longer reported wait times, patients leaving before being seen, and/or ambulance diversions.

Problems in the ED Lead to Problems with Timely Assessment

The American College of Emergency Physicians (ACEP) defines ED overcrowding as "a situation in which the identified need for emergency services outstrips available resources in the emergency department. This situation occurs in hospital EDs when there are more patients than staffed ED treatment beds and wait times exceed a reasonable period."[1]

In 2002 the majority of hospital EDs, 62%, reported operating at or over capacity, according to an American Hospital Association (AHA) study.[2] Although Level 1 trauma centers and large hospitals with 300-plus beds were hardest hit—90% reported that their EDs are filled to capacity and cannot easily accommodate more patients—they were by no means alone. The same was true for 79% of urban, 45% of rural, 81% of teaching, and 56% of nonteaching hospitals.

The situation has not improved in recent years. Approximately 45% of EDs—and nearly 64% of those in metropolitan areas—experienced overcrowding at some point during 2003 and 2004, based on figures from the National Center for Health Statistics.[3] The criteria used to make this determination were ambulance diversion hours, average waiting time greater than or equal to 60 minutes for urgent cases, or percentage of visits in which the patient left before being seen greater than or equal to 3%.

Several factors have contributed to ED overcrowding. Patients presenting to the ED are increasingly experiencing high acuity levels and more complex conditions. As the U.S. population ages, increasing numbers of elderly patients are seeking care, treatment, and services in the ED. Generally, elderly patients have a higher proportion of emergent visits compared with all other age groups.[4] They also tend to have comorbidities that require more complicated evaluations.

Patients who lack access to health care show up at the ED because it is the only place they can receive care, either because they are uninsured, underinsured, or cannot schedule a timely appointment with their primary care physicians (PCPs). In 2005 a record 46.6 million Americans were uninsured, according to the U.S. Census Bureau.[5] This figure accounts for nearly 16% of all Americans and represents an increase of 1.3 million from the number of uninsured in 2004. Access to primary care is limited because so many PCPs are booked several weeks in advance. Consequently, patients—and in particular health maintenance organization enrollees—are seeking care in the ED because of their inability to schedule timely appointments.[6]

When hospitals become overcrowded, patients are often "boarded" until inpatient beds are made available for their use. Such patients require treatment space (often found in nontreatment areas), equipment, and staff time, further shrinking hospital resources. In a point-in-time survey of nearly 90 EDs across the country on a typical Monday evening, 73% of the surveyed hospitals reported boarding two or more inpatients.[7] Moreover, 59% of the EDs reported routine use of corridors for treatment, 38% reported admitting more patients than available beds, and 47% reported using nonclinical spaces for patient care. The latter included offices, storerooms, conference rooms, and even showers.

Overcrowding might also involve an inability of staff to appropriately triage patients or reassess them, forcing such patients to wait longer in the ED waiting area—a delay that can lead to adverse outcomes.

Five Strategies to Prevent Overcrowding and Provide Safe, Timely Care

Emergency room overcrowding typically involves patients being monitored in nontreatment areas, such as hallways, while waiting for ED treatment or inpatient beds.

Managing patient flow is one method that can be used to eliminate factors that can lead to ED crowding. The following strategies can be used to increase your hospital's efforts to monitor and improve patient flow, the latter of which increases patient safety and reduces treatment delays:

1. **Appoint a "bed czar."** Assign a physician responsibility for discharges or an advanced practice nurse primary responsibility for accounting for beds and working with housekeeping to quickly turn them over. Give this person the authority to do the following:

   a. Make decisions on inpatient bed transfers and discharges

    b. Notify relevant medical staff of an impending patient overload

    c. Cancel elective admissions, elective surgeries, and scheduled diagnostic procedures

    d. Initiate ambulance diversion after consulting with others

2. **Form a "bed briefing group."** This group should discuss what admissions are scheduled for the day, how many patients need to be placed from the ED, and the types of inpatient beds expected to become available. This group should meet daily, either in the morning or a few times throughout the day. The group should include representatives from the ED, inpatient units (for example, critical care, medical/surgical), nursing management, administration, and environmental services. If your hospital has individuals designated to address such issues as patient placement, care management, and bed coordination, they should also be involved. Examples might also include a postanesthesia care unit for surgery schedule information (impacting postoperation bed availability), cath lab information, and infection control.

3. **Use a computerized patient tracking system.** These systems can be used to keep tabs on a patient's movement throughout the ED, including how long he or she waits to get registered, seen by a physician, treated and tested, and either discharged or admitted. Tracking systems can provide real-time access to accurately determine ED occupancy and capacity monitoring. The data gleaned from these systems can be evaluated as frequently as necessary. Although many such systems use bar codes to track patients, new technology using radio frequency identification (RFID) is making its way into this arena. RFID tags can be worn by patients on ankle bracelets.

4. **Implement the use of a unit assessment tool.** The purpose of a unit assessment tool is to determine current capacity in units throughout the hospital, not just the ED. More important, this tool uses real-time data to identify when the unit lacks any capacity to accept additional patients without risking safety for patients or burnout for staff. The idea is to smooth the variances in supply and demand by redistributing valuable resources when bottlenecks are detected in various parts of the hospital. In other words, the bottlenecks are addressed *before* the unit becomes overloaded. The information from the tool can be displayed on a grid so that all inpatient units will know each other's status. When a unit is experiencing an excessive work load, then the charge nurse, in consultation with the medical director, can make the call to cap the unit, similar to the bed czar.

5. **Use capacity-monitored measures to improve patient flow.** The Agency for Healthcare Research and Quality recently developed capacity-monitored measures to be used to assist in the management and prevention of ED overcrowd-

Case at Hand

According to the 2002 AHA survey of ED and hospital capacity, a majority of hospital EDs perceive they are "at" or "over" operating capacity (62% of all hospitals surveyed). Hospitals reporting time on diversion at 20% or more had an average R.N. vacancy rate of 16%.

Strategy: Work with community services to better coordinate the flow of emergency cases into and out of the ER and inpatient areas from paramedic and ambulance services to long term care and home care agencies. If discharges from inpatient areas are expedited, the ED is able to admit more patients.

STRATEGY

Instead of "boarding" patients in offices, storerooms, and conference rooms, scope out "overflow areas" in the hospital where patients can wait in comfort for an inpatient bed. A good option is a department with a large recovery area that might be busy during the day but not in the evening when the ED census is higher.

ing. The 38 measures focus on seven areas: patient demand, ED capacity, patient complexity, ED efficiency, ED work load, hospital efficiency, and hospital capacity. The measures were published in the December 2003 issue of the *Annals of Emergency Medicine*. Additionally, the Institute for Healthcare Improvement (IHI) recommends tracking three types of measures—outcome, process, and balancing measures—when working to improve the flow of patients through the hospital. The measures can be found on the IHI Web site at http://www.ihi.org/IHI/Topics/Flow/PatientFlow/Measures/.

Waiting Times Grow

Patients presenting to the ED are waiting longer and longer to be seen by a physician.

In 2004, an estimated 110 million visits were made to the ED, up 18% from approximately 93 million visits a decade earlier, according to the National Center for Health Statistics. The rise represents an average increase of more than 1.5 million visits per year.

At the same time, the number of hospital EDs has decreased by approximately 12%. Between 1993 and 2003, the total number of hospitals in the United States declined by 703 and the number of EDs fell by 425, states the Institute of Medicine (IOM) in its report entitled *The Future of Emergency Care in the United States Health System*.[8] During 2003 and 2004, there was an average of 4,500 EDs operating in this country.

The amount of time a patient spent waiting to be seen in the ED was 47 minutes in 2004. On average, patients spent a total of 3.3 hours in the ED.

In nearly 13% of ED visits, patients' conditions were classified as emergent. Almost 38% were classified as urgent, nearly 22% as semiurgent, and approximately 12% as nonurgent (*see* Figure 2-1 on page 17).

This classification is important because the ratio of waiting time to treatment time varied based on patient acuity level. Patients in need of more urgent care spent less time waiting to see a physician and more time in treatment (*see* Figure 2-2 on page 18).

Waiting times were the longest in EDs located in metropolitan areas, based on the National Center for Health Statistics' report *Staffing, Capacity, and Ambulance Diversion in EDs for 2003–2004.* One fifth of patients in metropolitan EDs waited more than an hour to see a physician. Approximately 13% of metropolitan EDs had average waiting times greater than 60 minutes for urgent cases, which are defined during triage as cases that should be seen between 15 and 60 minutes after arrival.

According to one recent study, approximately 8% of the estimated 26.6 million adults who sought care in a hospital ED during 2000 reported a delay in receiving care, reported having difficulty receiving care, or reported being unable to receive care.[9] Of the 2.8 million adults who reported ED access problems, more than half cited long waiting times as the cause.

STRATEGY

At one for-profit health care organization, a new patient assessment process was implemented to ease ED overcrowding. When a patient presents to the ED, the patient is initially seen by a nurse who assesses for illness or injury. Next, a physician examines the patient. If the physician determines that the patient's condition is not an emergency, the patient has one of three options: (1) stay and be treated in the ED after paying for the care up front; (2) schedule an appointment with a family physician at a later date; or (3) seek medical care at a community clinic.

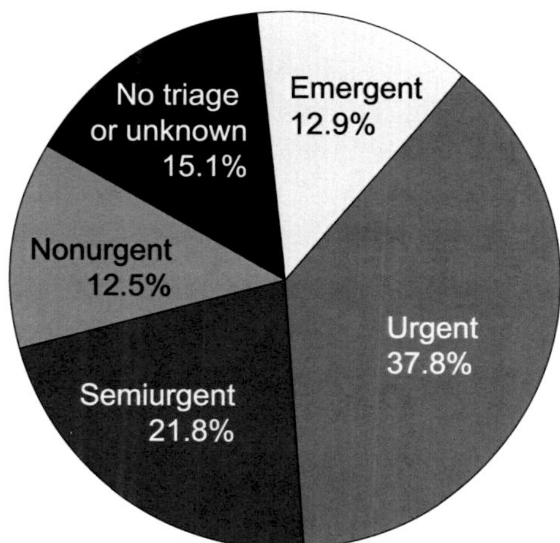

Figure 2-1. Patient Classification for 2004 ED Visits

Source: McCaig L.F., Nawar E.N.: *National Hospital Ambulatory Medical Care Survey: 2004 Emergency Department Summary. Advance Data from Vital and Health Statistics,* Pub. no. 372. Hyattsville, MD: National Center for Health Statistics, Jun. 23, 2006.

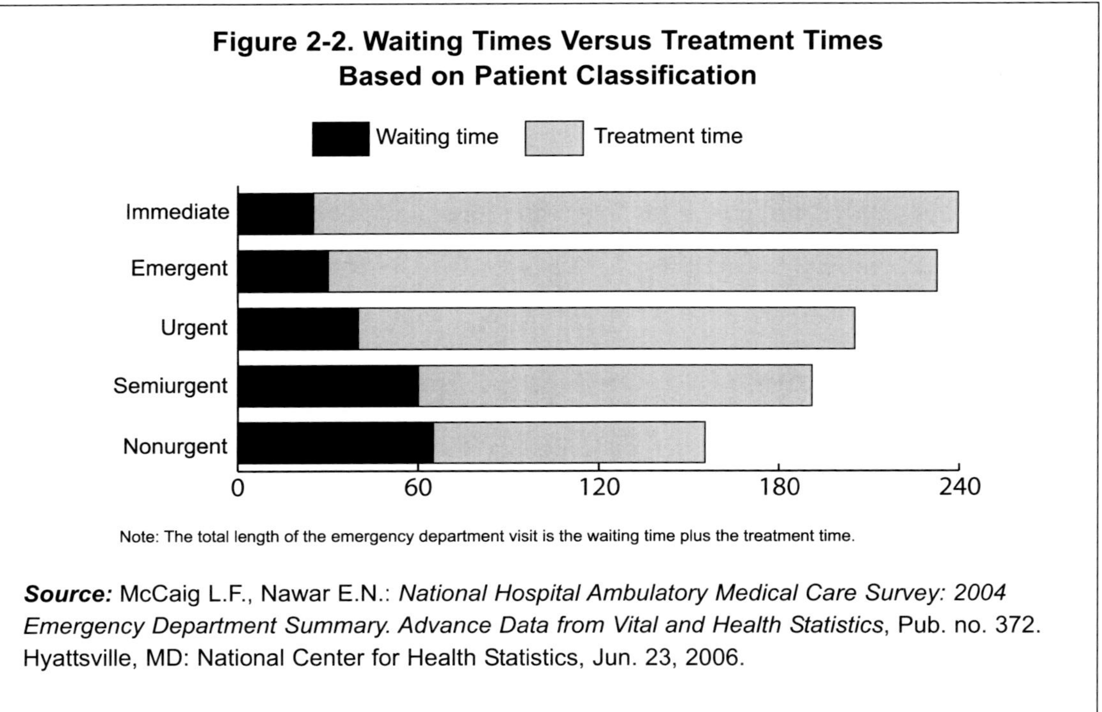

Figure 2-2. Waiting Times Versus Treatment Times Based on Patient Classification

Note: The total length of the emergency department visit is the waiting time plus the treatment time.

Source: McCaig L.F., Nawar E.N.: *National Hospital Ambulatory Medical Care Survey: 2004 Emergency Department Summary. Advance Data from Vital and Health Statistics*, Pub. no. 372. Hyattsville, MD: National Center for Health Statistics, Jun. 23, 2006.

Test Results and Consultation Add to Wait

Test results and consultation with a specialist can make the wait even longer. Diagnostic and screening services were ordered or provided at nearly 90% of the ED visits in 2004. Among the most frequently ordered tests were imaging, complete blood count, and urinalysis. The percentage for diagnostic and screening services is up from approximately 85% in 2001, at which time the average visit length for patients who received an MRI or CAT scan was 4.9 hours.[10]

Case at Hand

Difficulty communicating critical test results directly to the responsible provider is the cause of many treatment delays, which are common even when such results are reported promptly.

Strategy: Reevaluate and revise the process for informing providers about critical test results as part of the hospital's performance improvement activities.

In a 2001 ACEP survey designed to provide a snapshot of the dimensions of overcrowding in EDs across the country, approximately 8% of patients presenting to the unit were waiting for specialty consultation by on-call physicians. ACEP is informing health care consumers that individuals with a minor illness or injury can expect a one- to two-hour ED visit, provided that the ED is not overcrowded.[11] If the visit requires extensive diagnostic tests, individuals can expect to wait longer for test results. If the emergency physician must consult with a specialist, the wait also will be extended.

Even when test results are returned promptly, they are not necessarily acted upon in a timely manner. In a study conducted in a large academic tertiary-care hospital, even when critical laboratory results were reported quickly by the lab, treatment delays were still common.[12] Among the 99 critical lab results, the median time it took to order an appropriate treatment was 2.5 hours. For 27% of the critical lab results, an appropriate treatment was ordered only after 5 or more hours. The median time until the patient's condition resolved was 14.3 hours. Not only are there implications when treatment is delayed, but it also takes longer for the condition to resolve. Difficulty communicating critical results directly to the responsible caregiver is the likely cause of at least some of the treatment delays.

Patients Leaving Before Being Seen

During the past few years, patients left before being seen in approximately 2% of ED visits.

In its 2003 report *Hospital Emergency Departments: Crowded Conditions Vary Among Hospitals and Communities,* the General Accounting Office reports that between 1% and 3% of patients leave after triage but before medical evaluation.[13]

Based on recent numbers from the National Center for Health Statistics, patients left before being seen by a health care provider for 1.9% of the ED visits in 2004.

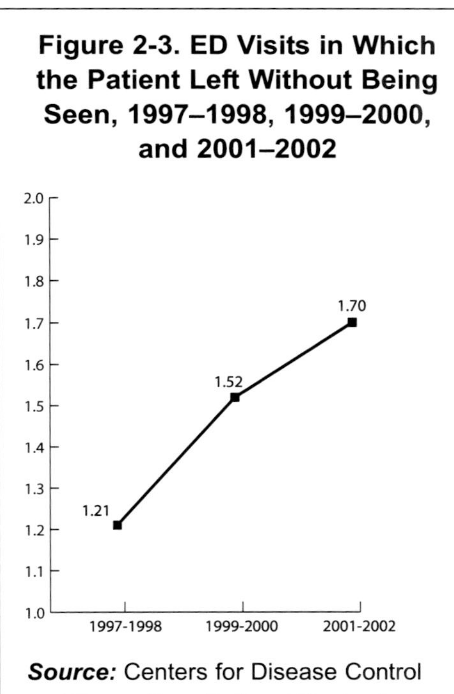

Figure 2-3. ED Visits in Which the Patient Left Without Being Seen, 1997–1998, 1999–2000, and 2001–2002

Source: Centers for Disease Control and Prevention, National Center for Health Statistics, National Hospital Ambulatory Medical Care Survey, 1997–1998, 1999–2000, 2001–2002.

The *2005 National Healthcare Quality Report* says that between 2001 and 2002, 1.7% of patients presenting to the ED left without being seen.[14] This percentage is up from 1.2% in 1997–1998 (*see* Figure 2-3, left). Many reasons might lead a patient to leave without being seen, but long waits clearly exacerbate the problem.

Why Patients Leave

The primary reason people leave is the length of the wait.[15,16] Long waits in the ED not only prompt them to leave without being seen, but also discourage them from using the facility for future health care needs.

Not surprisingly, the percentage of patients who leave without being seen is significantly higher at EDs with longer waiting times.[17] In one study, patients who left without being seen would have waited 52 minutes longer than patients who were seen, had they stayed to see a physician.[18] Patients who left without being seen reported that they had waited an average of 3 hours and 30 minutes before leav-

> # Case at Hand
>
> In approximately 2% of all ED visits, patients leave before being seen. Studies show that even patients triaged as urgent are walking out of EDs because of long wait times.
>
> **Strategy:** Implement a program to streamline the registration process, improve triage efficiency, and begin tests and interventions of patients before they are placed in ED beds. An ED in an urban hospital that implemented an ED rapid-entry and accelerated-care-at-triage program reduced the frequency of patients who left without being seen by nearly 50%, despite an increase in ED census. In addition, average monthly patient wait times decreased by 24 minutes, and overall ED length of stay dropped 31 minutes.[22]

ing. Only 5% of patients who left without being seen waited less than 30 minutes before leaving. Of the patients who left without being seen, 86% did so simply because the wait was "too long."

Some studies suggest that individuals reach a certain threshold and decide to leave when ED capacity has gone beyond it. For example, one study noted that the most powerful predictor of patients leaving without being seen was the total number of patients treated in the ED.[19] The saturation point was reached when the average daily census reached 100 patients in the ED. Similarly, another study found that when ED capacity was exceeded by 140%, patients began leaving at greater rates.[20] In fact, 1.8% of the visits resulted in patients leaving without being seen over the four-month study period, in which there were a total of 11,652 ED visits.

Even Urgent Patients Walk Out

A substantial number of patients who leave before they are seen by an ED provider are classified as urgent at presentation. In one study, half of the patients who left without being seen had urgent care needs as determined by the triage nurse. Although many patients who left without being seen were better within a week or two, the health and safety of some patients might have been jeopardized by the long delay. Specifically, half of the patients who left saw a physician within a week of leaving the ED, and 27% returned to an ED. In a similar prospective study, 46% of patients who left before being seen by an ED provider were considered in need of immediate medical attention, and 29% were assessed as needing care within 24 to 48 hours.[21] Of those who left, 11% were hospitalized within the next week, and three persons required emergency surgery. Even after implementing improvements at one hospital that significantly reduced the number of patients leaving without being seen, 16 out of 51 patients who left without being seen, 31%, were considered urgent.

If seriously ill patients leave before receiving appropriate care, they might be leaving the ED untreated.

Ambulances Being Diverted

Half a million times each year, an ambulance carrying an emergency patient is diverted from an ED that is full and sent to one that is farther away, according to the IOM's report.[8] That translates into an ambulance being diverted, on average, once every minute.

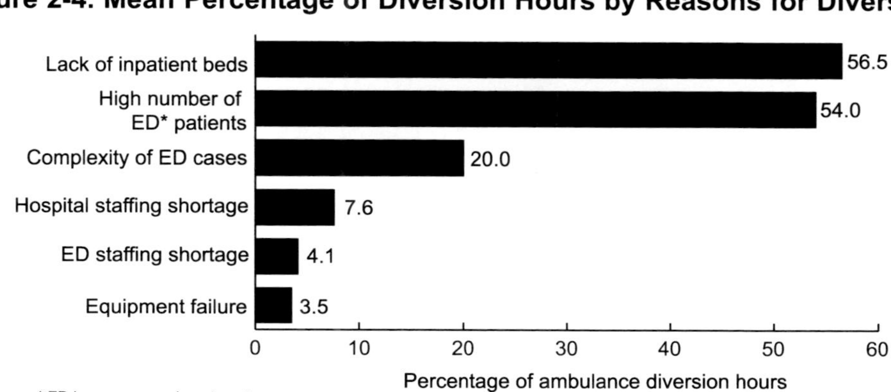

Source: Burt C.W., McCaig L.F.: *Staffing, Capacity, and Ambulance Diversion in Emergency Departments: United States, 2003–2004. Advance Data from Vital and Health Statistics.* Pub. no. 376. Hyattsville, MD: National Center for Health Statistics, Sep. 27, 2006.

Approximately one third (34%) of U.S. hospitals reported going on ambulance diversion sometime during 2002. Hospitals located in metropolitan areas were more likely to be on diversion compared with hospitals located in nonmetropolitan areas. In fact, half of the metropolitan hospitals were on diversion compared with approximately 9% of others. Approximately 12% of hospitals in metropolitan areas reported having spent between 5% and 19% of their operating time in diversion status. Although the duration of diversion time periods varied widely, the most frequently reported duration ranged between three and four hours. Lack of inpatient beds and ED crowding were the most frequent reasons cited for going on diversion (*see* Figure 2-4, above). The incidence of ambulance diversions seems to be growing.

> ## Case at Hand
>
> Half a million times each year—or, on average, once every minute—an ambulance is diverted.
>
> **Strategy:** Implement plans to efficiently move patients through a health care facility without going on ambulance diversion.

Assessment

At approximately 10:30 P.M., a woman presented at a local community hospital complaining of chest pains. The patient was evaluated and then waited for more than two hours to be seen by a physician. By the time the doctor reached the patient, she lacked a pulse. The patient was pronounced dead at 2:00 A.M. The autopsy showed that she died of a heart attack.

This scenario not only highlights the deadly consequences of delays in treatment, but the importance of conducting a timely assessment and reassessment of all patients presenting to the ED.

Patients presenting to an ED should undergo an initial assessment, which comprises three distinct stages: triage, a nurse's assessment, and the medical screening examination.

In most EDs, a triage nurse assesses the severity of a patient's condition upon arrival based on symptoms, personal and medical history, and vital signs. Based on this assessment, the nurse must quickly determine if the patient is emergent, urgent, semiurgent, or nonurgent.

During a screening examination, the patient's immediate and emerging needs are evaluated, and his or her physiological, psychological, and social statuses are assessed.

The information gathered at the first patient contact might indicate that the patient requires a more detailed examination. This more comprehensive examination will depend, at least in part, on the following:

- Patient's diagnosis
- The care he or she is seeking
- Care setting
- Patient's response to any previous care
- Patient's consent to treatment

The medical screening examination can be performed by a physician, a physician's assistant, or a staff nurse as defined in the scope of services for the ED. This more thorough assessment actually comprises a variety of assessments that include a more in-depth medical, family, and social history. The social history delves into the patient's use of nicotine, social drugs, and alcohol, as well as sleep patterns and living arrangements. The medical screening examination should assess the patient's pain, functional status, nutritional status, and mental health. When a patient is identified as being at risk for nutritional problems, for example, the patient is referred to a dietitian for further assessment.

The Medical Screening Examination

After the nurse's assessment is complete, the patient will undergo a medical screening examination. At this time, the triage nurse will determine if the patient has an emergency medical condition. As part of this assessment, the triage nurse obtains a more detailed medical history about the patient's present illness or condition. Then the triage nurse performs a focused examination targeting the organ system that is the source of the patient's complaint. If the findings of this exam are grossly abnormal, the patient is deemed to be at risk for an emergency medical condition. The patient must then be treated and stabilized in the ED. At a minimum, the medical screening examination should assess the following:

- Chief complaint
- Present illness
- Medical history
- Psychosocial or personal history
- Family history

Depending on the patient's complaint, one or more of the following organ systems should be assessed:

- Skin, head, eyes, ears, nose, mouth, and throat
- Respiratory
- Neurological
- Musculoskeletal
- Cardiovascular
- Gastrointestinal
- Urinary
- Genito-reproductive
- Endocrine
- Hematologic
- Psychological

Ordering Diagnostic Tests. Emergency physicians typically order a progression of tests for a patient presenting to the ED to exclude an emergency medical condition. For instance, a patient who presents with abdominal pain and distention, nausea, vomiting, and a low-grade fever will undergo a careful physical examination to include an exam of the abdomen. The physician will likely order blood work to check for signs of infection. A urinalysis will be used to rule out a urinary tract infection. A radiograph might be ordered to show signs of obstruction, perforation, and foreign bodies. An ultrasound might be ordered to rule out appendiceal inflammation, gall bladder disease, and pregnancy. If the clinical impression is still in doubt, the physician might order a CAT scan to facilitate diagnosis.

Typically, diagnostic tests ordered for an ED patient include both invasive and noninvasive procedures. Laboratory, radiologic, electrodiagnostic, and other functional tests and imaging technologies also fall under the category of diagnostic tests.

In 2004, diagnostic and screening services were provided at nearly 90% of all ED visits. These services included imaging tests (nearly 44%), complete blood counts (33%), and urinalyses (19%).

Goal of Patient Assessment

The goal of patient assessment in the ED is to determine the kind of care required to meet the patient's initial needs and those that occur in response to care. Related activities include collecting and analyzing data. Staff in the ED not only collect data about each patient's physical and psychosocial status and health history, but they analyze data to determine information about each patient's care needs and to identify any additional necessary information. As a result of these two activities, ED staff make care decisions.

Individualization of Assessment

Each patient must receive an individualized assessment according to his or her needs. The following are assessed and documented as appropriate to the patient's age and needs:

Case at Hand

In 2004 abdominal and chest pain were the leading patient complaints for all ED visits.

Strategy: Make sure pain assessments include a question about the location of pain. You might want to include check boxes to address locations such as the abdomen, chest, or back.

■ Emotional, cognitive, communication, educational, social, and daily activity needs
■ The effect of the family or guardian on the patient's condition and the effect of the patient's condition on the family or guardian
■ The patient's immunization status
■ The family's or guardian's expectations for and involvement in the patient's assessment, initial treatment, and continuing care

A pediatric patient's developmental age, height, head circumference, and weight are also documented. Problems related to a child's development can also be identified through assessment; growth failure is an example. Some of this information, such as immunization status, can be obtained from a third party, including a family physician or school records.

Pain Assessment

As part of the initial assessment, the ED staff must screen for pain and assess the level of pain. The intensity and quality of pain are measured by asking the patient to describe the pain's character, frequency, location, and duration. These attributes must be assessed in a manner that is appropriate to the patient's age. Pain scales are often used for the patient to self-report pain.

Results of the pain assessment should be recorded to facilitate regular reassessment and follow-up.

Reassessing Pain in Nonurgent Patients. Patients who are categorized as nonurgent must be reassessed for pain as exemplified by the following case:

A 43-year-old woman presented to a crowded ED complaining of a headache. Her vital signs were normal except for a temperature of 101.2°F (38.4°C). Because the triage nurse had seen many patients that day whose symptoms included headache and this patient seemed no worse than the others, the nurse sent the patient to the waiting room. Four hours later, another patient came to the triage desk to report that the woman, who was still in the waiting room, was having a seizure. Five hours after initial presentation, her temperature escalated to 104.5°F (41.4°C), and the patient was admitted to the hospital with a diagnosis of meningitis.[23]

If patients who are kept waiting are not routinely reassessed, their conditions can become life-threatening. This includes patients who are triaged as nonurgent cases. To ensure that patients are re-assessed, the following steps should be implemented as part of repeat assessments[24]:

■ Check in with the patient regularly. It is important to conduct a repeat assessment, especially if the wait in the ED is long. A repeat assessment could include obtaining repeat vital signs, getting updated pain scores, providing medications, refilling an ice bag, or even comforting a patient.

- Ask patients to report changes in symptoms, particularly if they are worsening.
- Perform procedures while patients are waiting. Implement a "quick triage process" to obtain the patient's name, complaint, vital signs, allergies, and level of pain. If a treatment room is unavailable, send the patient to a "quick registration" that generates a patient number. Order any necessary lab tests, an ECG, or x-ray while the patient is waiting. Use the ordering of diagnostic testing as an opportunity to reassess the patient.
- Assign a specific nurse to conduct reassessments. Designate a "waiting room" nurse to document hourly reassessment of patients.

This includes checking lab results and starting standing orders. When diagnostic test results are abnormal, this nurse would be responsible for speeding up the intervention as needed.

> **S T R A T E G Y**
>
> How often a nurse should conduct a pain reassessment will depend on the patient's condition, presenting complaint, and comorbidities. For example, if the ED uses a five-scale triage system, a patient with an acuity level of three should be reassessed every one to two hours. A patient with an acuity level of four to five should be reassessed with any change in symptoms.

Providing Timely Laboratory Results

The ED must have a system for providing laboratory services required by its patient population, services, and licensed independent practitioners. Lab services, including those required for emergencies, could be provided within the hospital, by agreement with another organization, or both. Initial tests, such as cultures, require follow-up, as their results can take longer to process.

Technology can be used to resolve difficulties associated with communicating critical test results directly to the responsible provider, which have been cited as the likely cause of treatment delays.[25] Such delays for patients awaiting critical care test results could result in organ damage or death.

Delays in Providing Timely Results. Waiting for test results can make the ED wait even longer. In 2001 patients waiting for results from MRIs and CAT scans waited, on average, 4.9 hours—1.9 hours longer than patients waiting to be seen by a physician.

If the ED is not providing diagnostic and screening test results in a timely fashion, then it should develop policies and procedures to make that happen. Lab turnaround times for routine tests and other more complex tests should be addressed in department policy. The latter should be monitored to ensure that it is being followed.

> **S T R A T E G Y**
>
> Post a sign in the ED waiting area informing all patients to "Contact a nurse immediately if your symptoms worsen" in languages appropriate to the patient populations served.

One hospital cut delays in lab turnaround time to the ED by revising the process.[26] After examining all the steps in the process, the hospital focused on the step between when the order is written and when the specimen is collected. The new process involved the ED nurse determining if the patient meets preapproved criteria for blood work during the initial assessment. If the patient meets the criteria, the nurse pages the lab phlebotomist to do a blood draw, obtain a sample, and log it into the computerized lab analysis system. All of this is done from the patient's bedside. When the physician orders specific tests, the blood sample is already in the lab, and the technician can begin the analysis. To ensure that the nurses were identifying patients who met the criteria for a blood draw, the hospital tracked the percentage of times the nurses initiated criteria-based blood draws. Their performance was categorized as either above department average, consistent with it, or below it. After the individual profiling was instituted, there was an approximate 42% criteria-based blood draw rate, up from 31%. Also, approximately 72% of the "lab order to draw" occurred in less than 12 minutes. The new process cut the length of stay for ED patients by 30 minutes.

S T R A T E G Y

If your lab turnaround times
are too long, consider
streamlining systems to speed
specimens to the lab and
developing alternative systems
for processing lab tests.

Another hospital reduced ED patients' length of stay by 25 minutes by identifying lab specimens to distinguish them from specimens sent from other parts of the hospital. The ED uses a pneumatic tube system only for specimens transferred between the ED and lab. The tubes also have different labels. For stroke patients, a sticker is put on the specimen indicating it is a "priority." Also, when a trauma patient is on the way to the ED, the department receives a call and activates trauma pagers, which are also in the lab. Technicians come to the ED to draw blood, often arriving even before the patient.

Other hospitals are turning to point-of-care testing (POCT). One hospital used POCT for strep, urinalysis, guiacs, and urine human chorionic gonadotrophin testing to cut the ED patients' stay by 25 minutes. Having a designated competent person to perform POCT might help smooth the process.

Results from critical lab tests are especially important because they can show problems in key physiologic systems. Treatment delays for such patients could result in organ damage or death. Studies have shown that difficulty communicating critical results directly to the responsible provider is the likely cause for such delays. When that process is improved, the time until an appropriate treatment is ordered can be reduced.

In one study, the use of an automatic alerting system reduced the time for an appropriate treatment to be ordered for patients with critical lab results.[27] The computer system, which was used to detect critical conditions and automatically notify the responsible physician via the hospital's paging system, looked for 12 conditions involving lab results and medications. During the two-month study period, 192 alerting situations (94 interventions, 98 controls) were analyzed. In the intervention group, it took 1 hour (median time) before an appropriate treatment was ordered compared with the control group, which took 1.6 hours. That represents a 38% shorter median time interval. The mean time was 4.1 hours versus 4.6 hours, respectively. The time until the condition was resolved was slightly less in the intervention group, 8.4 hours versus 8.9 hours (median). The mean time was 14.4 hours versus 20.2 hours, respectively. Consequently, communicating critical lab results directly to the responsible caregiver not only decreased the amount of time in which an appropriate treatment was ordered, but there was also a trend toward a decreased duration of the life-threatening condition.

> ## Case at Hand
>
> Lab turnaround times for routine tests and more complex tests should be addressed in department policy.
>
> **Strategy:** Simplify and standardize screening and assessment processes that correlate to peaks of activity, not averages.

The study authors believe that the intervention was successful because the key clinician received the information directly, with the pertinent data highlighted and in a context that made ordering the correct treatment easier.

Massachusetts hospitals participated in a statewide patient safety initiative aimed at improving communication of critical test results in a timely and reliable way to clinicians.[28] Convened by the Massachusetts Coalition for the Prevention of Medical Errors and the Massachusetts Hospital Association, a consensus group developed Safe Practice Recommendations (*see* Table 2-1, pages 28–36). The recommendations address the following:

- Who should receive the results
- Who should receive the results when the ordering provider is unavailable
- Which results require timely and reliable communication
- When the results should be actively reported to the ordering provider within explicit time frames
- How to notify the responsible provider
- How to design, support, and maintain the systems involved

Performing Nutritional Screenings When Warranted

A nutritional assessment helps determine whether or not a patient is at nutritional risk. Among the factors that contribute to such a risk are living alone and taking multiple medications. Patients who live alone, and thus eat alone, tend to eat less healthily than individuals who eat meals with others. The more medicine a person takes, the higher the chance of side effects that could affect the appetite.

Hospital ED staff sometimes fail to perform nutritional screenings even when they are warranted. Staff might be unaware of symptoms of malnutrition or ignore them. Failure to screen the condition, however, thwarts an opportunity to arrange for further assessment by an appropriate professional and could increase the need for readmission.

Establishing Criteria for Identifying High-Risk Patients. Because few, if any, EDs can afford to hire a full-time dietitian, nutritional screening triggers can be added to the initial assessment

Table 2-1. Safe Practice Recommendations for Communicating Critical Test Results

Safe Practice Recommendation	Implementation Context
1. Identify *who* should receive the results.	
■ The primary responsibility for receiving and following up on test results lies with the ordering provider or the responsible provider as appropriate.	■ The ordering provider should receive and follow up on the results of all ordered tests. ■ The ordering provider has the responsibility to communicate outstanding diagnostic tests and assign responsibility for follow-up to a covering provider.
■ Test results must be reported directly to a provider who can take action, not an intermediary. *For "red" category values/interpretations, notify the nurse caring for a patient on the inpatient unit simultaneously.*	■ Notify the PCP and the ordering physician of all "yellow" category test results to ensure follow-up. ■ Institutions can make institution-specific additional recommendations for notification of clinicians who serve as the "end point" for taking clinical action (e.g., nurse-run Coumadin clinics). ■ Identify situations when other members of the clinical team should also be notified (e.g., pharmacy).
2. Identify *who* should receive the results when the ordering provider is not available	
■ Develop a procedure to link each patient with either a provider or a service at the time of admission. *A patient should be linked at all times with a provider (or practice) who is responsible for his or her care.*	■ Identify and/or validate a PCP or practice for each patient at the time of admission.
■ Create a call schedule/system that works to identify whom the results should go to when the ordering provider is not available. *Clinical team members should always be able to easily identify which provider is responsible for each patient at any given point in time.* *"Role-based" coverage models have proven more reliable than traditional call systems.* *"Role-based" models link each patient with a position/service designated at admission and then have an on-call system tied to that position; traditional call systems create a chain for each physician rather than work from the patient.*	Elements of a successful call system ■ Simple to understand ■ Easily available to all stakeholders ■ The procedures for changes to the call schedule are explicitly clear to all users. ■ Supports reporting clinicians in identifying and reaching responsible provider ■ Supports automatic forwarding of calls to the covering provider/service if ordering provider not available Effective implementation strategies ■ *Simplify:* Call systems that use a "role-based" ("coverage list") model are patient focused, e.g., patient is linked to role (position) and the role is linked to various responsible individuals, depending on coverage, shift changes, etc. ■ *Improve Access:* Place call schedule information on the hospital intranet; integrate technology solutions (e.g., auto-paging, auto-forwarding).

(continued)

Table 2-1. Safe Practice Recommendations for Communicating Critical Test Results (continued)	
Safe Practice Recommendation	**Implementation Context**

■ Centralize and empower the hospital or practice call (communication) center to serve as the centralized repository of all call schedule and notification operations.
 	
A centralized hospital call system under the management of the communication center is a demonstrated strategy to promote reliability.
 	
Practice call centers should be linked to the hospital call center.
	Effective Implementation Strategies
	Build reliability
	■ The hospital has the responsibility to know who is on call in every service, every day; the call center should serve as the primary source for all services, including reference laboratories; ancillary departments may maintain separate lists in addition.
	■ Practice call centers should be coordinated for the practice—i.e., who is on call for every physician, every day; practice call systems should be linked to the hospital call center.
	■ Assign accountability and responsibility for the accuracy and administrative control of call schedules to the call center and the medical staff executive team.
	  — Medical staff executive team defines rules to ensure the safety of the patient.
	  — Empower only the communications center with the authority to make edits/changes to call schedules.
	  — Provide authority to activate the "fail-safe" system if necessary.
	  — Maintain a database and ensure that the call center has an up-to-date personal notification plan for all providers.
	■ In a centralized system, call schedules should be
	  — Sent to the call center
	  — Input by the call center only
	  — Typed, legible
	  — Complete, using full names of providers
	  — Coordinated with answering services to validate accuracy
	Monitoring effectiveness of systems
	■ Validate that the call center has the most current call schedule list and that users assign coverage 100% of the time.
	  — Conduct periodic tests to validate "accepting coverage" process (e.g. beeper/pager check or acknowledgment process).
	■ Validate the accuracy of provider access information as part of existing hospital systems (e.g., credentialing process).
	■ Validate accuracy of contact information with physicians' answering services.
	■ Gather data about delays in notification process.
	
	(continued)

Table 2-1. Safe Practice Recommendations for Communicating Critical Test Results (continued)

Safe Practice Recommendation	Implementation Context
3. Identify *what* test results require timely and reliable communication.	
■ Maintain a prioritized list of critical test values/interpretations that require accelerated notification systems. *Define a set of "high alert" results that get special precedence; set priorities to focus energies, limited resources on what really matters.* ■ Limit the number of tests categorized as highest priority ("red").	Ensure that your institution's list ■ Is segmented into categories that correspond to differentiated notification time requirements ■ Introduces institutionwide standardized terminology for naming each category (e.g., "red," "orange," "yellow" categories) ■ Focuses primarily on the Consensus Group set of "starter set" of results identified for the "red" category ■ References existing standards and evidence on criticality ■ Addresses all practice areas: inpatient, outpatient, and ED ■ Addresses all test types: laboratory, cardiology, radiology, etc. ■ Is reviewed and verified at least annually and includes a process for adding/dropping tests from each list
4. Identify *when* test results should be actively reported to the ordering provider and establish explicit time frames for this process.	
■ Define appropriate notification time parameters for communicating critical test results according to urgency (e.g. within 1 hour, within the shift [target 6–8 hours], within 3 days). *For "orange" categories, the guiding principles for decision making are* ■ *Maximize efficiencies of workflow issues.* ■ *Avoid unnecessary calls late at night.* ■ *Synchronize calls with other existing systems (e.g., change of shifts, etc.)* ■ *Describe explicit steps in notification system; describe when reporters should initiate and follow up on notifying the ordering provider about critical test results.*	Example (all categories require acknowledgement) ■ "Red" category—requires stat page, immediate clinical decision required ■ "Orange" category—results should be called; clinical decision required within hours ■ "Yellow" category—results can be sent passively; clinical decision required within days

(continued)

Table 2-1. Safe Practice Recommendations for Communicating Critical Test Results (continued)

Safe Practice Recommendation	Implementation Context

■ Describe explicit steps in notification system; describe when reporters should initiate and follow up on notifying the ordering provider about critical test results.	An example of a sequential notification system for "red" category values/interpretations would include the following:
	■ First call to M.D. #1 (ordering or covering)
	■ Coincident call to R.N. (inpatient), pharmacy, and/or PCP under specific circumstances
	■ If no response after 15 minutes, call M.D. #1 again.
	■ After 30 minutes, escalate to M.D. #2; identified by call center.
	■ After 45 minutes, call M.D. #2 again.
	■ After 60 minutes, activate "fail-safe" plan; notification of "fail-safe" clinical provider, examples below.
	
	Note: An example of a more accelerated follow-up would be 3 calls within the first 10 minutes.
	
	■ Implement a reporting strategy that is clinically useful to the physician but does not overburden the laboratory; aim to reduce the number of alerts to clinicians about conditions of which they are aware.
	  — To determine whether a particular test result deserves urgent communication, consider the degree of change from historical results; the time span in which the change occurred; the direction of change (worsening vs improving); and the patient's medical history.
	  — The reporting strategy, in order of preference, follows:
	    • Identify a trend and report critical values if trend criteria are met.
	    • Calculate delta changes and report only when criteria are met.
	    • If reporting absolute values only, strongly consider use of "first instance of" (as described in operating definitions).
	
	If unable to easily implement manual or programmed logic into laboratory systems, continue to call all "orange" values "red."

(continued)

Table 2-1. Safe Practice Recommendations for Communicating Critical Test Results (continued)

Safe Practice Recommendation	Implementation Context

■ Develop a fail-safe plan for communicating critical test results when the ordering or covering provider cannot be contacted within the designated time frame.
 	
Hospitals should have "fail-safe" plans in place for reporting critical findings and to ensure that the patient will receive timely clinical attention.
	■ Key elements of a "fail-safe" plan include
	— Utilized when clinical decision is required ("red" category)
	— Provides a schedule to identify a clinical provider who:
	  • Is able to assume responsibility for patient
	  • Can take clinical action
	  • Available 24/7/365
	  • Has access to the medical record
	■ Examples of "fail-safe" provider would be
	— Inpatient areas
	— ED physician
	— Senior medical resident
	— Medical officer of the month/day
	— A member of the medical emergency team
	— A member of a mini-code team
	— Lab director
	Outpatient areas
	— PCP or covering physician, lab directors, or clinic directors who could call the EMTs or direct the patient to the ED

5. Identify *how* to notify the responsible provider(s).	
■ Identify and utilize the communication techniques that are most appropriate for the particular clinical situation (e.g., active "push" system for results requiring a prompt clinical response).	■ "Red" category results should be called to the responsible provider; provider response to a page necessary. ■ Results should not be left with secretary or answering machine.
■ Ensure acknowledgement of receipt of test results by a provider who can take action for all categories ("red," "yellow," "orange") of critical test values/interpretations. *Although the time frames for notification in the "orange" and "yellow" categories are extended, systems should reliably ensure that the handoff to the responsible clinician is complete—i.e., systems should verify that a responsible provider is aware of the communication and has accepted the handoff. The responsibility for follow-up should be clear to all parties.*	■ When communicating test results, senders should document — Name and credentials of sender — Name and credentials of receiver — Test name — Test value/interpretation — Date and time ■ Guidelines for acceptable acknowledgment systems — Sender must receive confirmation from the receiving provider that he or she has accepted the responsibility for follow-up (e.g., phone call, confirmation of receipt of list, change of shift report, call back from page).

(continued)

Table 2-1. Safe Practice Recommendations for Communicating Critical Test Results (continued)

Safe Practice Recommendation	Implementation Context
	— Acknowledgment must occur within time frames for each category of test. — Communication of these test results/interpretations must occur between responsible providers, not an intermediary. ■ Examples of unacceptable acknowledgement systems include answering machines and all e-mails, including those with read-receipt.
6. Establish a shared policy for uniform communication of all types of test results (laboratory, cardiology, radiology, and other diagnostic tests) to all recipients.	
■ Make the notification system explicitly clear to all stakeholders.	■ Develop a consistent standardized communication technique for the sender to identify (flag) "red" category values/interpretations to alert the receiver that this is a "red" category finding. ■ All stakeholders should share the same understanding of the clinical urgency categories and the steps to take when escalation is necessary ■ Use "read back" techniques in the process of acknowledging receipt of results. ■ Develop a shared policy with the key elements of — Definitions of all categories of values — Lists of all values from each diagnostic area as appendixes — Time parameters and procedures for notification for all categories — A description of the "fail-safe" plan — Description of the responsibilities of all team members — Documentation requirements — Quality improvement monitoring plan — Plan for annual review and validation — References
■ Encourage and foster shared accountability and teamwork across and between clinical disciplines.	■ Implement face-to-face interdisciplinary change-of-shift debriefings for the hand off of laboratory, cardiology, radiology, and other relevant clinical information (e.g., problem lists, allergies, medications, a "to do" list). ■ Describe relative responsibilities of the laboratory, cardiology, radiology, ordering provider, covering provider, and nurse. ■ Address the importance of shared responsibility and partnering when facing a "red" category finding.

(continued)

Table 2-1. Safe Practice Recommendations for Communicating Critical Test Results (continued)	
Safe Practice Recommendation	**Implementation Context**
	■ Develop action plans/protocols for the R.N. jointly by medicine and nursing and other related disciplines; clearly describe criteria for use (e.g., insulin, heparin, solution changes, glucose for hypoglycemia, monitoring expectations). ■ The clinical team should provide sufficient information to the responsible or backup provider to support action. — In many situations the R.N. will be central in providing access to this information. — The laboratory will provide results information and recent previous results when available.
■ Decide what information should be included as a minimal data set to be communicated to the responsible person.	■ Examples of a minimal data set should include — This is a "red" ("orange") category finding — Significant comorbidities — Prior test results, if available — Related medication(s) — Other relevant clinical information
7. Design reliability into the system.	
■ Utilize forcing functions at the point of test ordering to identify the ordering provider with complete contact information with pager or beeper number. ■ Utilize forcing functions at the point of test ordering to include a minimal data set of clinical information to support the interpretation of diagnostic tests.	■ Use manual or computer systems. ■ Expand information at point of test ordering regarding call-back instructions (e.g., alternative contact providers, identify PCP, patient contact information, location). ■ Expand information at point of test ordering (for cardiology, radiology, and other diagnostic tests) to include — Diagnosis — Reason for requesting this test — What the clinician wants to assess or rule out
■ Create tracking systems to assure timely and reliable communication of test results.	■ Develop special procedures for situations where delays typically occur. — After discharge — Ambulatory (cross border) — Late arriving — Other predictable relevant situations (shift changes, after-hours, surgeon in OR, etc.) ■ The responsibility for tracking and follow-up on positive findings lies with the individual physician practice.

(continued)

Table 2-1. Safe Practice Recommendations for Communicating Critical Test Results (continued)

Safe Practice Recommendation	Implementation Context
	■ Develop or utilize existing tracking systems in ambulatory areas to prevent test results from falling through the cracks (e.g., automated or manual tickler systems). ■ Design reliable follow-up systems for high-risk situations (e.g. certified letters with return receipt requested). ■ Explore possibility that laboratory, cardiology, and radiology would monitor the receipt (acknowledgement) and document hand off of findings.
8. Support and maintain systems.	
■ Partner with patients in the communication about test results. *Include family as appropriate, given consideration to confidentiality and regulatory compliance.*	■ "Nothing about me, without me" ■ Provide patients access to their test results (whenever medically reasonable). ■ Develop strategies to assist clinicians in assessing when and how to notify patients, especially in cases when patient is no longer at the hospital. ■ Develop strategies to educate patients/families to participate in monitoring prompt turnaround of critical test results (e.g., Joint Commission Speak Up™ program).
■ Provide orientation and ongoing education on procedures for communicating critical test results to all health care providers.	Provide orientation and continuing education on ■ How to communicate critical test results ■ How to respond to critical test results in the "red" category ■ Principles of communication and teamwork for clinical emergencies ■ Core curriculum on patient safety
■ Provide ongoing monitoring of the effectiveness of systems (e.g., weekly failure rates, tests of call systems, response times).	■ Monitor effectiveness of — Call schedule — Existing notification system — Feedback loops/tracking systems
9. Support infrastructure development.	
■ Adopt advanced communication technologies.	Upgrade call center/communication capabilities: ■ Intranet access ■ Automatic page forwarding and other automated notification systems ■ E-mail to patients with attention to confidentiality issues

(continued)

Table 2-1. Safe Practice Recommendations for Communicating Critical Test Results (continued)

Safe Practice Recommendation	Implementation Context
■ Improve laboratory and other test system capabilities.	Upgrade call center/communication capabilities: ■ Intranet access ■ Automatic page forwarding and other automated notification systems ■ E-mail to patients with attention to confidentiality issues ■ Plan for integrated medical record solutions to link clinical information with laboratory results, as in the following: — Drug-drug interactions — Previous test results — Enable reporting of complex threshold criteria such as renal and pediatric dosing. — Track trends in patient conditions. — Link to medical record to identify first diagnosis of cancer or diabetes. ■ Distribute tracking system reports to responsible clinicians. ■ Link documentation of acknowledgement fields to tracking reports to monitor feedback loop. ■ Evaluate the use of POC testing in critical and ambulatory areas carefully with consideration of emerging evidence-based studies; integrate POC test results with other test results and make them available to other providers.

PCP, primary care provider; ED, emergency department; M.D., physician; R.N., registered nurse; EMT, emergency medical technician; OR, operating room; POC, point-of-care.

Source: Hanna D., et al.: Communicating critical test results: Safe practice recommendations. *Jt Comm J Qual Patient Saf* 31(2):68–80, 2005.

form. For example, ED staff can ask the patient about an unplanned weight loss of 15 pounds during a three-month period and nausea or vomiting for more than three days. Asking the following questions, for example, can help identify nutritional problems:

■ What is your height and weight?
■ Do you have problems swallowing?
■ How is your appetite?
■ Have you lost weight?
■ Are you well?
■ Do you drink milk and/or a supplemental drink?

Reviewing the patient's medication regimen, including herbal supplements, can help identify

> **2007 National Patient Safety Goal 2**
> Improve the effectiveness of communication among caregivers.
>
> **Requirement 2A**
> For verbal or telephone orders or for telephonic reporting of critical test results, verify the complete order or test result by having the person receiving the information record and read back the complete order or test result.
>
> **Rationale for Requirement 2A**
> Ineffective communication is the most frequently cited category of root causes of sentinel events. Effective communication, which is timely, accurate, complete, unambiguous, and understood by the recipient, reduces error and results in improved patient safety.
>
> **Implementation Expectation for Requirement 2A**
> 1. The receiver of the information writes down the complete order or test result or enters it into a computer.
> 2. The receiver of the information reads back the order or test result.
> 3. The receiver of the information receives confirmation from the individual who gave the order or test result.

possible drug-food and drug-drug interactions. For patients who cannot remember all their medications, support staff can contact their PCPs or the pharmacies where they have their prescriptions refilled.

In addition to the elderly being at risk for malnutrition, younger patients (primarily adolescent females) can suffer from eating disorders such as anorexia nervosa or bulimia.

A Look at Life-Threatening Conditions

Patients come to the ED with a variety of life-threatening ailments and conditions. Managing such patients requires ongoing assessment followed by appropriate treatment and care. When these activities do not happen or happen in a delayed manner, they can have devastating consequences.

The following sections explore the importance of conducting an appropriate assessment for two patient populations that routinely present to hospital EDs and the consequences that occur when these activities are delayed. The populations discussed are psychiatric and cardiac patients.

Desirable Outcomes Through Early Psychotic Detection

Patients with psychiatric-related disorders represent a substantial number of ED visits that continues to grow each year. Approximately 4.3 million psychiatric-related ED visits occurred in the United States in 2000, which translates into an annual rate of 21 visits per 1,000 adults.[29] This represents a 15% increase of such cases between 1992 and 2000, accounting for 5.4% of all ED visits. The most common psychiatric conditions seen in ED visits were sub-

S T R A T E G Y

The Massachusetts Coalition for the Prevention of Medical Errors and its collaborative members have developed example tools, including forms and policies, as well as staff and patient education materials, to support the adoption of its Safe Practice Recommendations for communicating critical test results. The toolkit is available online at http://www.macoalition.org/Initiatives/CCTRToolkit.shtml.

stance abuse (27%), neuroses (26%), and psychoses (21%).

The increase in psychiatric-related ED visits is occurring largely because EDs have become the safety net for a fragmented mental health infrastructure. As a result, ED staff members are increasingly finding themselves managing patients or victims with a myriad of psychiatric conditions such as the aforementioned ones, as well as suicidal ideation as a result of domestic violence, sexual assault and abuse, and alcohol/drug abuse.

There is convincing evidence that the longer the duration of untreated psychosis, the poorer the prognosis.[30] Specifically, a longer duration between the time the first psychotic symptom appears to the initiation of adequate treatment, the worse the outcome in terms of the patient's total symptoms, overall functioning, positive symptoms, and quality of life. Moreover, patients with a long duration of untreated psychosis are significantly less likely to achieve remission. Reducing the duration of untreated psychosis through earlier detection and treatment should have a positive effect on patient outcome.

Consequently, ED staff should know how to address psychiatric patients' physical needs, as well as how to assess their mental health needs, to ensure that they are on their way to receiving appropriate treatment.

Assessing Patients at Risk for Suicide. The majority of life-threatening and medically severe suicide attempts are treated in the ED (*see* Sidebar 2-1 and Sidebar 2-2, page 39). However, ED staff can be so focused on treating the physical aspects of critically ill patients that they might overlook the patient's state of mental health and consequently fail to diagnosis a patient's risk of suicide. This oversight can have serious consequences. According to one study, the suicide mortality rates for patients seen and subsequently discharged from the ED for a suicide-related complaint were higher than those for other ED patients.[31] The study suggests that a single ED visit for overdose, suicidal ideation, or self-harm is strongly associated with increased suicide risk. Consequently, ED staff should be trained to recognize behavioral patterns that place individuals at risk for suicide and should become adept at assessing such patients.

A situation in which staff are informed that a patient has suicidal tendencies either by the patient or someone accompanying the patient to the ED would warrant an assessment of the patient's mental health.

Using a suicide risk assessment tool developed specifically for use in the ED might be beneficial. A risk stratification model used to assess ED patients after self-harm was found to be highly sensitive in discriminating between patients at higher and lower risk of repetitive self-harm or suicide.[32] The four-question model had a sensitivity of 94% and a specificity of 25%

Sidebar 2-1. Hot Topic: ED Visits for Suicide on the Rise

ED visits for attempted suicide and self-inflicted injury are relatively common and are on the rise.

In 2004 the number of ED visits for attempted suicide and self-inflicted injury was approximately 535,000. That number has jumped more than 100,000 in less than three years.

Between 1997 and 2001, approximately 412,000 annual ED visits were for attempted suicide and self-inflicted injury. The annual visit rate was 1.5 visits per 1,000 American citizens.

ED visit rates were higher among female patients than male patients and higher among African Americans than Caucasians. Although the mean patient age was 31 years, ED visits were more common among patients aged 15 to 19 years, at a rate of 3.3 visits per 1,000 U.S. citizens.

The most common method of injury was poisoning, followed by cutting or piercing.

A psychiatric disorder was coded for 55% of ED visits, with depressive disorder accounting for 34% of these visits, and alcohol abuse for 16%.[4,35]

Source: Doshi A., et al.: National study of U.S. emergency department visits for attempted suicide and self-inflicted injury, 1997–2001. *Ann Emerg Med* 46(4):369–375, 2005. Used with permission.

Sidebar 2-2. Hot Topic: Management of Suicidal Patients in California Hospital EDs

Although evaluation of patients with suicidal ideation by a mental health professional is the usual practice in California hospital EDs, according to a survey of 253 ED directors in the state, no such professional was available in more than half of the respondent EDs. That means there was no psychiatrist, social worker, county or private psychiatric evaluation team, psychiatric nurse, or psychologist available for evaluating these patients.

Moreover, 23% of the respondents reported that they occasionally send these patients home without an evaluation, and nearly 9% report that this was done more than 10% of the time.

In the majority of EDs, psychiatric evaluations were performed by either mobile county or private psychiatric evaluation teams, or by social workers on call to the ED. Psychiatrists evaluated the majority of suicidal patients in only 10% of the EDs.

Only 27% of respondents were able to admit patients to a psychiatric service at their hospitals. When patients needed to be transferred, they waited seven hours, on average.

Overall, the estimated proportion of ED visits by suicidal patients was 1.7%, which is similar to national figures.

Source: Baraff L.J., Janowicz N., Asarnow J.R.: Survey of California emergency departments about practices for management of suicidal patients and resources available for their care. *Ann Emerg Med* 48(4):452–458, 2006. Used with permission.

<table>
<tr><td>

Case at Hand

Every year, 30,000 Americans take their lives by suicide, with 650,000 receiving emergency care only after attempting suicide, according to the National Council for Suicide Prevention.

Strategy: Ensure that ED staff are trained to recognize behavioral patterns that place individuals at risk for suicide.

</td></tr>
</table>

in a study that used data from 9,086 patients who presented with self-harm at five EDs between 1997 and 2001.

Some suicide risk assessment tools are geared to specific patient populations. Given the increasing treatment encounters with pediatric patients who have mental health problems, having a screening tool that can guide ED staff in the rapid and accurate detection of suicide risk for this patient population is advantageous. A 14-item screening survey administered by a triage nurse to 144 pediatric mental health patients on admission to a pediatric ED in an urban teaching hospital accurately detected suicidality in children and adolescents with a mean age of 13.6 years.[33] The tool designed for non–mental health clinicians inquired about suicidal behavior, past suicidal ideation, past self-destructive behavior, and current stressors, yielding a sensitivity of 98%.

The Geriatric Suicide Ideation Scale is a 10-item scale that differentiates psychiatric patients from nonpsychiatric patients.[34] It assesses suicide ideation, death ideation, loss of personal and social worth, and perceived meaning of life. When used on 107 adults 65 years or older, the scale was found to be a sound measure of late-life suicide risk and psychological resilience.

Sidebar 2-3, page 41, provides a list of possible suicidal signs to look for when a patient presents to the ED.

In addition, ED staff should be aware of local or national suicide prevention hotlines and should pass that information along to the patient's family members and/or friends for referral.

Assessing Patients at Risk for Domestic Abuse and Sexual Assault. Routine screening of all patients who have experienced domestic violence is integral to the prevention of further violence and to the safety of those who are victimized. Studies have shown that when ED nurses directly ask questions about domestic violence during their assessments, more victims of abuse are identified.[35] Moreover, failure to identify victims of abuse can result in a continuation of the abuse, frequent returns with vague medical complaints, severe injury, rape, and even death.

Abuse should be suspected when the injuries sustained do not fit the history and when patients seem ashamed or embarrassed about their injuries.

It is important when assessing patients for domestic violence that the screening tool used is effective for determining current and ongoing abuse and not just past abuse. Although there are many assessment tools to detect domestic violence, including the Index of Spouse Abuse and the Abuse Assessment Screen, some, such as the Ongoing Abuse Screen, address current abuse.[36] In addition, the Ongoing Abuse Screen was developed specifically for use in the ED.

Sidebar 2-1. Suicide Risk Factors in Patients

If a patient presenting to the ED seems depressed, clinicians should assess the patient for common suicide risk factors such as a profound sense of hopelessness, a history of depression or substance abuse, or a previous suicide attempt.

Consider the patient to be at risk if he or she does one or more of the following:

- Verbalizes suicidal thoughts, wishes, or a plan
- Has a history of one or more suicide attempts
- Has a family history of suicide
- Feels depressed or anxious or expresses feelings of hopelessness
- Has a chronic mental illness or history of mental illness
- Abuses alcohol or another substance
- Has a physical illness with a poor prognosis
- Has impulsive or aggressive tendencies
- Has suffered a significant loss or multiple losses (such as the death of a spouse, job loss, or financial setback)
- Has access to lethal methods, such as firearms or medications
- Feels ambivalent about treatment or does not cooperate with advice regarding treatment
- Suffers from loneliness and lacks a social network

It is okay to ask patients about any suicidal thoughts they might be having. Most patients who are suicidal are relieved to discuss their feelings and to be assured that they are not crazy for having such thoughts. Assess the patient for depression by asking if he or she is feeling depressed, sad, or discouraged. If the answer is "yes," then ask the following standard suicide assessment questions:

- How long have you felt like this?
- Do you feel that your life is no longer worth living?
- Are you thinking of acting on that feeling by hurting yourself or taking your own life?
- Do you have a suicide plan?
- Can you tell me about your plan?

Do not be afraid to ask the patient detailed information about a suicide plan. The more thought-out the plan, the more lethal it is likely to be. If the patient can discuss specific details, has made final arrangements, and has given away valued belongings, the more serious the suicidal intentions. If the patient is identified as being at risk for suicide, seek a mental health professional to provide further assessment and treatment.

Source: Captain C.: Is your patient a suicide risk? *Nursing* 36(8):43–47, 2006. Used with permission.

ED staff can start a discussion by reassuring the patient that all patients are asked routine questions about domestic abuse because so many people deal with fear and abuse in their relationships (*see* Sidebar 2-4, below, for questions to ask). Patients who are reluctant to discuss their abuse in front of others can be interviewed privately. Because the perpetrator is often unwilling to allow the victim to give a history or be alone with a clinician, the nurse might have to ask all visitors to wait in the lobby.

Domestic violence is part of the broader spectrum of family violence that includes sexual assault, as well as child and elder abuse and neglect. *Sexual assault* is defined as the sexual contact of one person with another without appropriate legal consent.[37] This includes rape, sexual abuse, and sexual misconduct. *Sexual abuse* is often used as a term for the sexual assault of children and adolescents.

Sidebar 2-4. Questions That Reveal Domestic Violence

The following questions are recommended by the American Medical Association to ask patients who might be victims of domestic violence:

- Are you in a relationship in which you have been physically hurt or threatened by your partner? Have you ever been in such a relationship?

- Are you (have you ever been) in a relationship in which you feel you are treated badly? In what ways?

- Has your partner ever destroyed things that you cared about?

- Has your partner ever threatened or abused your children?

- Has your partner ever forced you to have sex when you did not want to? Does your partner ever force you to engage in sex that makes you feel uncomfortable?

- We all fight at home. What happens when you and your partner fight or disagree?

- Do you ever feel afraid of your partner?

- Has your partner ever prevented you from leaving the house, seeing friends, getting a job, or continuing your education?

- You mentioned that your partner uses drugs/alcohol. How does he or she act when drinking or on drugs? Is he or she ever verbally or physically abusive?

- Do you have guns in your home? Has your partner ever threatened to use them when he or she was angry?

Source: American Medical Association. *Diagnostic and Treatment Guidelines on Domestic Violence.* http://www.ama-assn.org/ama1/pub/upload/mm/386/domesticviolence.pdf (accessed Dec. 3, 2006). Used with permission.

Vulnerable target populations for sexual assault include children, adolescents, elders, developmentally delayed persons, patients with physical and/or mental impairments, and persons under the influence of drugs or alcohol.

If the patient exhibits signs of domestic abuse, sexual abuse, or neglect, based on the assessment, ED staff should refer the patient to a social worker.

Additionally, ED staff should be aware of local or national resources such as the National Coalition Against Domestic Violence, the National Domestic Violence Hotline, and the Rape, Abuse, Incest National Network. Staff should pass this information along to the patient for referral.

In collaboration with a broad range of clinical, legal, forensic, judicial, and advocative organizations, ACEP has developed an approach based on consensus to assist in the care of patients with the complaint of sexual assault or sexual abuse. The handbook entitled *Evaluation and Management of the Sexually Assaulted or Sexually Abused Patient* details the clinician's responsibility for appropriately managing the sexually assaulted patient, including medical issues, emotional needs, and forensic requirements. It is available on the ACEP Web site at http://www.acep.org/NR/rdonlyres/11E6C08D-6EE7-4EE2-8E59-5E8E6E684E43/0/sxa_handbook.pdf.

Assessing Patients at Risk of Alcohol Abuse. One third of injured patients treated in the ED have an alcohol-use disorder.[38] In addition, patients who present to the ED are more likely to have alcohol-related problems than those who go to a PCP. These patients represent the spectrum of alcohol-related problems, including drinkers at risk for injury and illness, impaired drivers, and individuals who are alcohol dependent. One study found that ED patients were up to three times more likely to report heavy drinking than patients presenting to a primary care clinic.[39]

Routine screening for alcohol abuse is imperative because ED–based screenings followed by brief interventions have been shown to be effective in decreasing alcohol intake and at-risk drinking.

In one study, patients at a large public hospital ED who were screened using the Alcohol Use Disorders Identification Test (AUDIT) and identified as "drinkers" based on the screening results were provided brief, on-site counseling and referral as needed.[40] Of the 810 patients who participated, 172 were identified as "drinkers." Of the 88 patients with complete intervention data, 94% accepted the intervention, and the majority of those set goals to decrease or stop drinking. As a result, the group experienced a 68% decrease in alcohol intake, a 52% decline in alcohol-related harm, and a 61% decrease in dependence symptoms. Two thirds of the patients cited that the intervention was most helpful in their efforts to change their alcohol-related behavior.

Similarly, a computer-generated intervention was associated with a significant decrease in alcohol use and at-risk drinking in another study. This study used the AUDIT to assess 3,026 sub-critically injured patients admitted to an ED who were also assessed for motivation to reduce drinking. Patients were randomized into an intervention and control group. At 6 months, the intervention patients experienced a 36% decrease in alcohol intake compared with a 21% decrease in the control group. At 12 months, the intervention group decreased alcohol intake by 23% versus 11% for the control patients.

In addition to the AUDIT, the screening strategy recommended in the *Physician's Guide to Helping Patients with Alcohol Problems* published by the National Institute on Alcohol Abuse and Alcoholism (NIAAA) also has been proven to be a valid screening tool.[41] In a study in which 395 patients presenting to an urban ED were asked three alcohol-consumption questions, took the CAGE questionnaire (*see* Sidebar 2-5, page 45), and were questioned about past alcohol problems, the NIAAA strategy was 81% sensitive and 80% specific to the prevalence of lifetime alcohol abuse or dependence. Regarding alcohol abuse and dependence in the prior 12 months, the NIAAA strategy was 83% sensitive and 84% specific. It is well suited to the ED because of its brevity and simple interpretation.

The NIAAA strategy has become even shorter with the 2005 edition of the *Clinician's Guide to Helping Patients Who Drink Too Much.* It can now consist of a single question about heavy drinking days.

There is evidence to suggest that even asking one question from the AUDIT is sufficient to screen for patients at risk for alcohol misuse.[42] Of 149 patients admitted to the trauma service in one study, 39% had positive blood alcohol levels. The overwhelming majority of these patients had screening results consistent with harmful or dependent drinking. A cutoff of three or more drinks per day as a response to the AUDIT question "On a typical day when you are drinking, how many drinks do you have?" correlated strongly with scores on the entire AUDIT screening tool in identifying those at risk for alcohol misuse.

Based on the patient's response to the screen, ED staff might suggest further assessment by a social worker or might refer the patient for on-site counseling or a specialized treatment program. Men who drink 5 or more standard drinks in a day (or 15 or more per week) and women who drink 4 or more in a day (or 8 or more per week) are at increased risk for alcohol-related problems.[43]

In addition, staff should be aware of national resources such as Alcoholics Anonymous or the National Clearinghouse for Alcohol and Drug Information, as well as local efforts. They should pass this information on to the patient.

Case at Hand

The combination of ED–based screening for alcohol abuse and a brief intervention have been shown to decrease alcohol intake and at-risk drinking.

Strategy: Include the single-question screening method in the patient's social history. If the response is positive, consider asking the quantity-frequency and CAGE questions or the AUDIT to get a better sense of the patient's at-risk behavior.

> **Sidebar 2-5. NIAAA Recommendations**
>
> The NIAAA recommends using one of two screening methods. One method consists of a single question about heavy drinking days, and the other consists of a combination of the quantity-frequency and CAGE questions.
>
> **Option 1: How many times in the past year have you had . . .**
> - ❏ 5 or more drinks in a day? (for men)
> - ❏ 4 or more drinks in a day? (for women)
>
> **Option 2**
> **Quantity-Frequency Questions:**
> - ❏ On average, how many days per week do you drink alcohol?
> - ❏ On a typical day when you drink, how many drinks do you have?
> - ❏ What is the maximum number of drinks you have had on any given occasion during the past month?
>
> **CAGE Questionnaire: In the past 12 months . . .**
> - ❏ Have you ever felt you should <u>C</u>ut down on your drinking?
> - ❏ Have people <u>A</u>nnoyed you by criticizing your drinking?
> - ❏ Have you ever felt bad or <u>G</u>uilty about your drinking?
> - ❏ Have you ever had a drink first thing in the morning to "steady your nerves" or get rid of a hangover (<u>E</u>ye opener)?
>
> The NIAAA's *Clinician's Guide to Helping Patients Who Drink Too Much*, 2005 edition, discusses screening methods and assessment strategies for alcohol use disorders. It is available at http://pubs.niaaa.nih.gov/publications/Practitioner/CliniciansGuide2005/guide.pdf.

Desirable Outcomes Through Guideline Usage for Percutaneous Cardiac Intervention in Cardiac Patients

There is evidence to suggest that following guidelines that call for patients with ST-segment elevation myocardial infarction (STEMI) to receive primary percutaneous coronary intervention (PCI) within 90 minutes of presenting to the ED can save lives.

Studies have shown that prompt PCI for patients with STEMI significantly reduces mortality and morbidity.[44–46] One such study evaluated the effect of door-to-balloon time on in-hospital mortality using a cohort of 29,222 STEMI patients treated with PCI within six hours of presentation at 395 hospitals that participated in the National Registries of Myocardial Infarction 3 and 4 between 1999 and 2002.[47] In-hospital mortality increased for patients with door-to-balloon times greater than 90 minutes compared with those who had door-to-balloon times less than or equal to 90 minutes.

Despite the sound and growing evidence, guideline recommendations issued by the American College of Cardiology (ACC) and the AHA are being met less than 50% of the time.[48]

Case at Hand

Following guidelines that call for patients with STEMI to receive PCI within 90 minutes of presenting to the ED can significantly reduce mortality and morbidity in this patient population.

Strategy: Develop protocols that support the guidelines issued by the ACC/AHA.

Moreover, there is no substantial trend toward improvement. In 1999 35% of patients receiving PCI were treated within the recommended 90-minute door-to-balloon time, based on a retrospective observational study of the same data. By 2002 only 26% of hospitals improved their door-to-balloon time by more than 3 minutes per year.

A recent survey of Minnesota hospitals without cardiac catheterization labs reveals that one third of them are not complying with the ACC/AHA STEMI guidelines.[49] The 104 hospitals were surveyed to determine their current use of guidelines and protocols, as well as

D2B Initiative

Consider signing up as a hospital participant in the "Door to Balloon (D2B): An Alliance for Quality Campaign," an initiative aimed at reducing door-to-balloon times in U.S. hospitals performing PCI on non-transfer STEMI patients. Specifically, the goal is to increase the percentage of acute myocardial infarction patients who receive primary angioplasty within 90 minutes of hospital presentation to 75%.

To date, more than 200 hospitals have signed up for the program launched in November 2006. Strategic partners include the ACC; the AHA; the National Heart, Lung, and Blood Institute; and other health care organizations and agencies.

As a participant, hospitals are expected to attempt to implement each of the recommended evidence-based strategies. These strategies include the following:

- Have emergency physicians activate the cath lab.
- Use a single call to activate the cath lab.
- Have the cath lab team arrive and be ready within 20 to 30 minutes.
- Provide real-time data feedback in the ED and the cath lab.
- Have commitment from senior management.
- Use a team-based approach spanning multiple departments.

Participants also will be required to submit data to the alliance regarding their door-to-balloon times for analysis purposes.

To register for the D2B initiative, log on to the Web site at http://d2b.acc.org.

Table 2-2. Strategies to Reduce Door-to-Balloon Times with Mean-Time Reductions	
Strategies to Reduce Door-to-Balloon Times	**Mean Reduction in Door-to-Balloon Time (Minutes)**
Have emergency medicine physicians activate the cath lab.	8.2
Use a single call to a central page operator to activate the cath lab.	13.8
Have the ED activate the cath lab while the patient is still en route.	15.4
Expect staff to arrive in the cath lab within 20 minutes after being paged.	19.3
Keep an attending cardiologist on site at all times.	14.6
Have staff in the ED and cath lab use and receive real-time data feedback.	8.6
Source: Adapted from Bradley E.H., et al.: Strategies for reducing the door-to-balloon time in acute myocardial infarction. *N Engl J Med* 355:2308–2320, Nov. 30, 2006. Used with permission.	

their quality assessment practices regarding the management of STEMI patients. The hospitals had an average time to PCI of 192 minutes. Although 63% of respondent hospitals have guidelines or protocols and 57% use standing orders for STEMI, 33% have neither.

Overcoming Delays in Treating Cardiac Patients. Hospitals in search of ways to reduce door-to-balloon time need to look no further than a recent study that identifies six strategies significantly associated with a faster door-to-balloon time. The strategies are as follows[50]:

1. Have emergency physicians activate the cath lab.
2. Use a single call to a central page operator to activate the cath lab.
3. Have the ED activate the cath lab while the patient is en route.
4. Expect staff to arrive in the cath lab within 20 minutes after being paged.
5. Keep an attending cardiologist on site at all times.
6. Have staff in the ED and cath lab use and receive real-time data feedback.

These strategies shaved 8 to 19 minutes off door-to-balloon times; a critical amount of time

Sidebar 2-6. Reducing Delays for Transfer Patients

Smaller or rural hospitals that lack cath labs need assistance in implementing strategies to reduce door-to-balloon time. Additionally, overcrowded EDs and ambulance diversions can contribute to delays in transporting patients to the hospital for treatment (*see* Sidebar 2-7, page 49). Therefore, implementing a standardized protocol for the transfer of patients with STEMI who need PCI can also improve door-to-balloon time.

The Level 1 Heart Attack Program, a collaborative effort between the Minneapolis Heart Institute at Abbott Northwestern Hospital and 28 EDs across the state, has established a protocol that specifies what treatment is to be given before a patient is transferred. When a patient arrives at one of the participating Level 1 hospitals, clinicians rapidly assess the patient, draw essential blood studies, perform chest x-rays, and give medications, such as aspirin, nitroglycerin, heparin, and beta-blockers. The transport team, which is either helicopter or ground, is summoned simultaneously. A call to the Minneapolis Heart Institute activates a team at Abbott Northwestern to prepare for the patient in the cath lab. Clinical data are faxed while the patient is being transported. Upon arrival, the patient is taken directly to the cath lab instead of being transferred to the ED.

The program's goal is to transfer the patient within 30 minutes from community hospitals that might be as far as 170 miles away.

Implementation of the protocol and an integrated system of transfer of patients with STEMI has reduced the average door-to-balloon time from 192 minutes, which is similar to the national average, to 98 minutes.

Source: Henry T.D., et al.: Design of a standardized system for transfer of patients with ST-elevation myocardial infarction for percutaneous coronary intervention. *Am Heart J* 150:373–384, Sep. 2005.

in a group of institutions with a mean value of 100 minutes for median door-to-balloon times (*see* Table 2-2 on page 47 for exact times).

Evaluating 28 strategies in all, the researchers noted that despite the considerable time savings afforded by these measures, few hospitals used them. For example, only 14% of surveyed hospitals activated the cath lab through a single call to a central page operator. Similarly, only 23% of hospitals had an emergency physician activate the cath lab on weekdays and only 27% at night and on weekends. Although these strategies could be implemented with existing resources, study authors acknowledge that implementing some of the other strategies, such as having an attending cardiologist at the hospital 24/7, might be cost prohibitive for some organizations.

The study authors also found that false alarms were uncommon, putting to rest the fear that having ED physicians activate the cath lab would lead to staff being called in unnecessarily.

Sidebar 2-7. Does Gridlock Occur with Cardiac Patients in Your Organization?

Overcrowded EDs and ambulance diversions are associated with delays in transporting cardiac patients.

Heart attack patients treated in EDs that are experiencing significant overcrowding were 40% more likely to experience a major delay before receiving thrombolytics, according to a recent study. *Major delay* was defined as defined as a door-to-needle time of 60 minutes or more. The median door-to-needle time was 7 minutes longer for these patients than for those treated in EDs that did not experience overcrowding. Median door-to-needle time was 40, 45, and 47 minutes in EDs experiencing none, moderate, and high ED crowding, respectively. A total of 3,452 suspected acute myocardial infarction patients treated at 25 hospital EDs between 1998 and 2000 in Ontario, Canada, were evaluated in the retrospective observational study.

Similarly, ambulance diversion was associated with delays in transport of patients experiencing chest pain. However, these delays occurred only when the diversion occurred at multiple EDs at the same time, a phenomenon known as "gridlock." Gridlock occurred for slightly more than one hour a day, extending the transport interval to 17.4 minutes compared with 15.5 minutes for patients not exposed to gridlock.

In all, 11,400 patients were transported to Toronto hospitals between January 1998 and December 1999.

Sources: Schull M.J., et al.: Emergency department crowding and thrombolysis delays in acute myocardial infarction. *Ann Emerg Med* 44:577–585, Dec. 2004. Used with permission.

Schull M.J., et al.: Emergency department gridlock and out-of-hospital delays for cardiac patients. *Acad Emerg Med* 10(7):709–716, 2003. Used with permission.

Even before a heart attack patient arrives, ED staff can take some simple steps to reduce the door-to-balloon time. These steps are as follows:

- Notify the cath lab.
- Page the cardiologist.
- Prepare a critical care treatment area.

Having a fax installed near the ED will allow staff to receive electrocardiograms performed by emergency services personnel prior to the patient's arrival.

References

1. American College of Emergency Physicians (ACEP) Crowding Resources Task Force: *Responding to Emergency Department Crowding: A Guidebook for Chapters.* Washington, DC: ACEP, Aug. 2002.

2. The Lewin Group: *Emergency Department Overload: A Growing Crisis—The Results of the American Hospital Association Survey of Emergency Department (ED) and Hospital Capacity.* Falls Church, VA: American Hospital Association, 2002.

3. Burt C.W., McCaig L.F.: *Staffing, Capacity, and Ambulance Diversion in Emergency Departments: United States, 2003–2004. Advance Data from Vital and Health Statistics.* Pub. no. 376. Hyattsville, MD: National Center for Health Statistics, Sep. 27, 2006.

4. McCaig L.F., Nawar E.N.: *National Hospital Ambulatory Medical Care Survey: 2004 Emergency Department Summary. Advance Data from Vital and Health Statistics.* Pub. no. 372. Hyattsville, MD: National Center for Health Statistics, Jun. 23, 2006.

5. Center on Budget and Policy Priorities: *The Number of Uninsured Americans Is at an All-Time High.* Aug. 29, 2006. http://www.cbpp.org/8-29-06health.pdf (accessed Nov. 13, 2006).

6. Brewster L.R., Rudell L.S., Lesser C.S.: Emergency room diversions: A symptom of hospitals under stress. *Issue Brief Cent Stud Health Syst Change* 38:1–4, May 2001.

7. Schneider S.M., et al.: Emergency department crowding: A point in time. *Ann Emerg Med* 42(2):181–184, 2003.

8. Institute of Medicine: *Report Brief: The Future of Emergency Care in the United States Health System.* Jun. 2006. http://www.iom.edu/Object.File/Master/35/014/EmergencyCare.pdf (accessed Oct. 6, 2006).

9. Kennedy J., et al.: Access to emergency care: Restricted by long waiting times and cost and coverage concerns. *Ann Emerg Med* 43(5):567–573, 2004.

10. McCaig L.F., Burt C.W.: *National Hospital Ambulatory Medical Care Survey: 2001 Emergency Department Summary. Advance Data from Vital and Health Statistics.* Pub. no. 335. Hyattsville, MD: National Center for Health Statistics, Jun. 4, 2003.

11. American College of Emergency Physicians: *Emergency Department Waiting Times.* http://www.acep.org/webportal/PatientsConsumers/critissues/overcrowding/waittimes.htm (accessed Nov. 13, 2006).

12. Kuperman G.J., et al.: How promptly are inpatients treated for critical laboratory results? *J Am Med Inform Assoc* 5:112–119, Jan.–Feb. 1998.

13. U.S. General Accounting Office (GAO): *Hospital Emergency Departments: Crowded Conditions Vary Among Hospitals and Communities,* Pub. no. 03-460. Washington, DC: GAO, Mar. 2003.

14. Agency for Healthcare Research and Quality: 2005 National Healthcare Quality Report, Pub. no. 06-0018. Dec. 2005. http://www.ahrq.gov/qual/nhqr05/nhqr05.pdf (accessed Oct. 26, 2006).

15. Derlet R.W., Richards J.R.: Overcrowding in the nation's emergency departments: Complex causes and disturbing effects. *Ann Emerg Med* 35(1):63–68, 2000.

16. Fernandes C.M.B., Price A., Christenson J.M.: Does reduced length of stay decrease the number of emergency department patients who leave without seeing a physician? *J Emerg Med* 15:397–399, 1997.

17. Stock L.M., et al.: Patients who leave emergency departments without being seen by a physician: Magnitude of the problem in Los Angeles County. *Ann Emerg Med* 23(2):294–298, 1994.

18. Bindman A.B., et al.: Consequences of queuing for care at a public hospital emergency department. *JAMA* 266:1091–1096, Aug. 28, 1991.

19. Hobbs D, et al.: Hospital factors associated with emergency center patients leaving without being seen. *Am J Emerg Med* 18(7):767–772, 2000.

20. Polevoi S.K., Quinn J.V., Kramer N.R.: Factors associated with patients who leave without being seen. *Acad Emerg Med* 12(3):232–236, 2005.

21. Baker D.W., Stevens C.D., Brook R.H.: Patients who leave a public hospital emergency department without being seen by a physician, causes and consequences. *JAMA* 266(8):1085–1090, 1991.

22. Chan T.C., et al.: Impact of rapid entry and accelerated care at triage on reducing emergency department patient wait times, lengths of stay, and rate of left without being seen. *Ann Emerg Med* 46:491–497, Dec. 2005.

23. Derlet M.: *Triage.* Aug. 8, 2006. http://www.emedicine.com/emerg/topic670.htm (accessed Nov. 30, 2006).

24. Are patients with life-threatening conditions in your waiting room? *ED Nursing* Aug. 1, 2005.

25. Kuperman G.J., Boyle D., Jha A.: How promptly are inpatients treated for critical laboratory results? *J Am Med Inform Assoc* 5:112–119, Jan.–Feb. 1998.

26. Drastically cut turnaround times for lab results. *ED Nursing* 8(10):118–119, 2005.

27. Kuperman G.J., et al.: Improving response to critical laboratory results with automation: Results of a randomized controlled trial. *J Am Med Inform Assoc* 6(6):512–522, 1999.

28. Hanna D., et al.: Communicating critical test results: Safe practice recommendations. *Jt Comm J Qual Patient Saf* 31(2):68–80, 2005.

29. Hazlett S.B., et al.: Epidemiology of adult psychiatric visits to U.S. emergency departments. *Acad Emerg Med* 11(2):177–178, 2004.

30. Marshall M., et al.: Association between duration of untreated psychosis and outcome in cohorts of first-episode patients. *Arch Gen Psychiatry* 62:975–983, Sep. 2005.

31. Crandall C., et al.: Subsequent suicide mortality among emergency department patients seen for suicidal behavior. *Acad Emerg Med* 13(4):435–442, 2006.

32. Cooper J., et al.: A clinical tool for assessing risk after self-harm. *Ann Emerg Med* 48(4):459–466, 2006.

33. Horowitz L.M., et al.: Detecting suicide risk in a pediatric emergency department: Development of a brief screening tool. *Pediatrics* 107(5):1133–1137, 2001.

34. Heisel M.J., Feltt G.L.: The development and initial validation of the geriatric suicide ideation scale. *Am J Geriatr Psychiatry* 14(9):742–751, 2006.

35. Nucero P., O'Connor P.: Identification of domestic violence in the emergency department. *N J Nurse* 32(7):15, 2002.

36. Ernst A.A., et al.: Comparison of three instruments for assessing ongoing intimate partner violence. *Med Sci Monit* 8(3):CR197–CR201, 2002.

37. American College of Physicians: *Evaluation and Management of the Sexually Assaulted or Sexually Abused Patient.* http://www.acep.org/NR/rdonlyres/11E6C08D-6EE7-4EE2-8E59-5E8E6E684E43/0/sxa_handbook.pdf (accessed Nov. 30, 2006).

38. Neumann T., et al.: The effect of computerized tailored brief advice on at-risk drinking in subcritically injured trauma patients. *J Trauma* 61(4):805–814, 2006.

39. Wilk A.I., Jensen N.M., Havigurst T.C.: Meta-analysis of randomized control trials addressing brief interventions in heavy alcohol drinkers. *J Gen Intern Med* 12(5):274–283, 1997.

40. Hungerford D.W., Pollock D.A., Todd K.H.: Acceptability of emergency department-based screening and brief intervention for alcohol problems. *Acad Emerg Med* 7(12):1383–1392, 2000.

41. Friedmann P.D, et al.: Validation of the screening strategy in the NIAAA "Physician's guide to helping patients with alcohol problems." *J Stud Alcohol* 62(2):234–238, 2001.

42. Reed D.N., et al.: Use of a single question to screen trauma patients for alcohol dependence. *J Trauma* 59(3):619–622, 2005.

43. Dawson D.A., Grant B.F., Li T.K.: Quantifying the risks associated with exceeding recommended drinking limits. *Alcohol Clin Exp Res* 29(5):902–908, 2005.

44. Bradley E.H., et al.: Achieving door-to-balloon times that meet quality guidelines: How do successful hospitals do it? *J Am Coll Cardiol* 46:1236–1241, Oct. 5, 2005.

45. Cannon C.P., et al.: Relationship of symptom-onset-to-balloon time and door-to-balloon time with mortality in patients undergoing angioplasty for acute myocardial infarction. *JAMA* 283:2941–2947, Jun. 14, 2000.

46. Berger P.B., et al.: Relationship between delay in performing direct coronary angioplasty and early clinical outcome in patients with acute myocardial infarction. *Circulation* 100:14–20, 1999.

47. McNamara R.L., et al.: Effect of door-to-balloon time on mortality in patients with ST-segment elevation myocardial infarction. *J Am Coll Cardiol* 47:2180–2186, Jun. 6, 2006.

48. McNamara R.L., et al.: Hospital improvement in time to reperfusion in patients with acute myocardial infarction. *J Am Coll Cardiol* 47:45–51, Jan. 3, 2006.

49. Larson D.M., et al.: Implementation of acute myocardial infarction guidelines in community hospitals. *Acad Emerg Med* 12(6):522–527, 2005.

50. Bradley E.H., et al.: Strategies for reducing the door-to-balloon time in acute myocardial infarction. *N Engl J Med* 355:2308–2320, Nov. 30, 2006.

Chapter 3

Automation and Information Technology Strategies to Reduce Treatment Delays

"Greater reliance on electronic health records means that information needed to treat patients effectively will be a few computer clicks away, no matter where the patient is receiving care."

Source: The White House National Economic Council: *Reforming Health Care for the 21st Century: Health Information Technology.* Feb. 15, 2006. http://www.whitehouse.gov/stateoftheunion/2006/healthcare/#section11 (accessed Jan. 5, 2007).

Many health care organizations are turning to automation and technology to improve patient safety. This automation is the primary reason that health care leaders are citing for their institutions' growing investment in technology. Specifically, improving decision support for clinicians and improving patient care capabilities are the top two reasons for embracing technology cited by respondents to the 2005 *Modern Healthcare*/PricewaterhouseCoopers IT Survey. The chief executive officers and chief financial officers from 394 hospitals who responded to the survey had planned to spend 2.5% of their operating budgets on information systems, an increase from 2.2% in 2004.[1]

Organizations are using technology to enhance care by accessing patient health information, retrieving test results, ordering prescriptions, and making point-of-care decisions. The most important technologies that hospitals plan to invest in are electronic medical records (EMRs), bar-coded medication management systems, and computerized prescriber order entry (CPOE) systems, reports the 17th Annual Healthcare Information and Management Systems Society (HIMSS) Leadership Survey sponsored by ACS Healthcare Solutions.[2] *See* Figure 3-1, page 54, for a full list of technologies hospitals plan to adopt over the next couple of years.

Benefits of health information technology (HIT) include increased adherence to guideline-based care, enhanced surveillance and monitoring, and decreased medication errors.[3]

Many technologies are being implemented in hospitals and physician practices across the country. Technology is viewed as an important tool for addressing delays in treatment by streamlining processes to allow clinicians to provide patient care more quickly and efficiently. The automation of processes can dramatically reduce the time a provider spends looking for charts, tracking down laboratory results, mobilizing staff, and repeatedly recording information that someone else already recorded.

To begin, organizations instituting new technologies require implementation strategies to

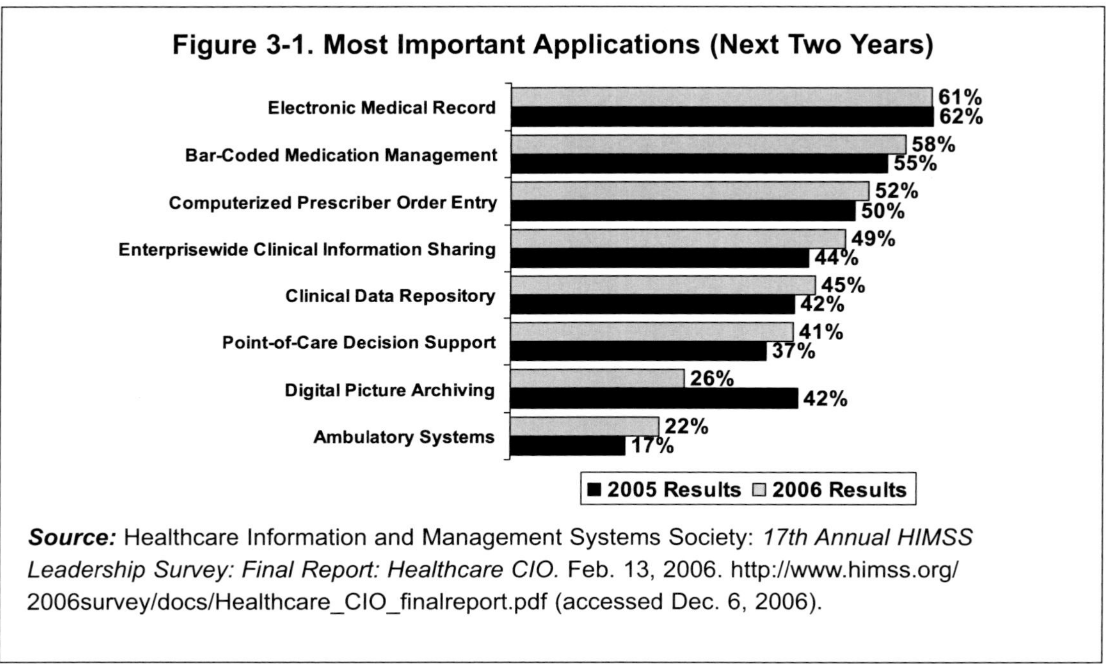

Source: Healthcare Information and Management Systems Society: *17th Annual HIMSS Leadership Survey: Final Report: Healthcare CIO.* Feb. 13, 2006. http://www.himss.org/2006survey/docs/Healthcare_CIO_finalreport.pdf (accessed Dec. 6, 2006).

ensure that the technology is used to its maximum capability by end users (for example, physicians, nurses, pharmacists).

Effectively Implementing New Technology

Health care organizations that focus on work process design and integration of new technology with existing ones can successfully implement new technologies that promote efficient treatment plans for patients.

Work Process Design

The work process design is vital to any technology implementation effort. Many technologies have been abandoned, not because of their inability to improve care, but because of problems with their design, their impact on work flow, and general dissatisfaction by end users.[4] Organizations that ignore the design principles of implementation increase the risk that end users will reject technologies that could reduce treatment delays.

Fortunately, process design principles can be followed to reduce the likelihood of end users rejecting new technology. The factors discussed in the following sections affect technology acceptance and are integral to enhancing design criteria for implementation purposes. (*See* Table 3-1, page 55, for a list of implementation design principles and the reasons why they are important.)

Organizational Factors. Individuals responsible for implementing new technology must have an understanding of the existing systems, how these systems work, and how the new technol-

Table 3-1. Implementation Design Principles: Why They Are Important

Design Principle	Reason for Importance
Top management commitment	Enables additional design principles
Responsibility/accountability	Promotes success by showing end users the importance of the change and lets them know who to go to with ideas or concerns
Structured program	Provides end users with a road map, which can reduce uncertainty and promote feelings of control. It also reduces fears associated with new technology.
Training	Targets self-efficacy, ease of use, and usefulness. It reduces uncertainty and fear while promoting control because users gain knowledge and skills.
Pilot testing	Involves users with the technology and creates a test to uncover and solve problems. It also promotes an understanding of integration needs.
Communication	Early and clear communication about the purpose of the technology reduces uncertainty and promotes perceptions of procedural justice.
Feedback	Prompt feedback to end users about concerns and ideas lets staff know they are being taken seriously.
Simulation	Simulation (for example, having the technology available to use in the intended manner without the negative consequences) promotes self-efficacy, usefulness, ease of use, and control.
End user participation	Enhances perceptions of justice, self-efficacy, and control. It also reduces fears and uncertainty.

Source: Adapted from Karsh B.T.: Beyond usability: Designing effective technology implementation systems to promote patient safety. *Qual Saf Health Care* 13:388–394, Oct. 2004.

ogy will interact with current processes and existing technologies. For example, a hospital implementing a CPOE has to consider how it will interact with the current medical records, pharmacy information systems, laboratory systems, methods of ordering and dispensing medications, and work flow. One study cited inadequate communication for the lack of understanding among staff as to why the physicians in the practice decided to adopt an EMR system and what purposes it should serve.[5] The technology's ability for monitoring patient wellness and assessment of health are key factors associated with using an EMR system.

A structured implementation program is another critical element. This could be represented by a multidisciplinary transition team, a destination where staff can go for assistance (for example, a help desk), or structured communication networks between supervisors and workers to address problems (for example, a hotline). Top hospitals have physicians and nurses dedicated to educating and training staff in order to ensure that staff have the skills to use the technologies, according to the American Hospital Association's *2004 Most Wired Survey and Benchmarking Study*.[6]

Job Factors. When a general medicine practice implemented computer-based prescribing, the new technology resulted in significant changes in the type of work being performed by hospital-based outpatient pharmacists.[7] After computer prescribing was implemented, pharmacists spent nearly 13% more time correcting prescription problems, had almost 4% less idle time, and spent roughly 2% less time in discussions with others. Pharmacists also spent 34% less time filling prescriptions, nearly 46% more time in problem-solving activities involving prescriptions, and approximately 3% less time providing advice. The new technology had a profound effect on the pharmacists' work patterns, but it did not affect the amount of time they spent with patients and physicians. The study authors did not anticipate the enormous effect the new technology would have on pharmacist work patterns and had even hypothesized that it would not have any effect.

Individual Factors. Self-efficacy refers to the end users' perception that they are confident they can use the new technology.

Integration

Integration of a new technology involves considering how well it will work with existing technologies, in the work flow processes, and within the environment. Integration must be carefully considered before a new technology is introduced.

S T R A T E G Y

Design principles that can improve the process of implementing new technologies include the following:

Designate an individual to be responsible and accountable for the success of the implementation.

Seek appropriate end user participation in all phases of the implementation.

Assess the effect of new technologies on current work flow processes and existing technologies to effectively incorporate the new technology.

Conduct pilot testing of the system in a sufficient number of departments so that the results can be applied throughout the facility.

The new and existing technologies should do the following:

- Communicate with each other
- Facilitate the integration of processes (for example, clinical and financial) across the organization
- Avoid duplicating functions
- Meet all information-related requirements for the institution (for example, comply with the Health Information Portability and Accountability Act [HIPAA] and data quality)

Implementation Strategies

Physicians attempting to implement technology in their practices should do so in tandem with redesigning the entire practice, according to Mark Leavitt, M.D., HIMSS medical director.[8] Simply implementing HIT neither eliminates duplicate work nor helps practices realize the full potential of the technology unless the practice is redesigned to conform to the new technological work processes, according to Leavitt. Using HIT in conjunction with practice redesign can improve the patient's access to information and help the physician make effective, well-informed decisions, both of which have the potential to reduce treatment delays.

The following suggested tips can help organizations implement a new technology:

- Define a structured implementation program that provides end users with a time line.
- Pilot test a new technology in one department and use the lessons learned to more efficiently implement the technology in other departments. Be sure the department chosen for pilot testing is similar enough to other departments in the organization so that the technology can be easily adapted throughout the system.
- Maintain clear and open communication channels between prospective end users, decision makers, and technical support personnel.
- Assess the organization's readiness for new technologies. Take time to slowly acclimate staff members. For example, leaders can post standardized order sets on the institution's intranet as a means to prepare for implementation of a CPOE system. The intranet site would promote safety by including legible, preprinted order forms and by directing staff members toward educational information. In this way, the facility would achieve some of the benefits of a CPOE before actually implementing one.
- Create a team of staff members to guide the implementation process of the new technology. Be sure this team is endorsed by the leadership.
- Consider cost-effective alternatives when implementing technologies.
- Make sure the balance between customization and standardization has been considered so that the new technology not only can be integrated with existing technologies within the organization and/or system, but can meet the standards of technologies that are implemented regionally and nationally.
- Flowchart current work processes of physicians, nurses, pharmacists, and other staff members. Then consider how these processes will change with the new technology. Ask several staff members from throughout the organization to contribute to this step

to ensure the flowchart's accuracy and to maintain staff buy-in.
- ■ Emphasize the need for teamwork throughout the implementation process (*see* Case Study 3-1 beginning below for more information about building a team-oriented implementation process).

The Computerized Patient Record

The adoption of EMRs—also referred to as electronic health records—has accelerated in recent years with no reason to believe that it will slow in the future.

The top HIT priority for hospitals over the next two years is implementing an EMR system, according to the 17th Annual HIMSS Leadership Survey. This was the most frequently cited

---

Case Study 3-1. Seton Healthcare Tackles Technology Implementation

Description of organization: Seton Healthcare Network is a leading provider of health care services in central Texas, serving an 11-county population of 1.4 million. The network includes five urban acute care hospitals, two rural hospitals, one mental health hospital and facilities that provide medical care for well patients.

Purpose of the project: The Network Medication Use Committee (NMUC) uses multiple teams and disciplines to tackle the myriad medication-related patient safety issues, including technology implementation.

Staff involved: 20 to 25 members attend each of the NMUC meetings.
Lessons learned: It is important to do a good job leading and managing the initial steps of any serial implementation. Be sure to set up the necessary teams and structures, make assignments, and hold people accountable.

When it comes to implementing new technologies, Seton Healthcare Network has a master plan.

The Austin, Texas–based network uses several systems and technologies designed to improve patient safety, and it is always evaluating new technologies to put in place. Among those in current use are a dispensing robot that fills medications for four of its hospitals and automated medication-dispensing cabinets at all eight of its sites.

Orchestrating all of its medication-related patient safety issues—including technology implementation—is the Network Medication Use Committee (NMUC). Between 20 and 25 members attend this interdisciplinary committee's meetings on a regular basis. Additionally, the NMUC has chartered more than 12 interdisciplinary project teams to work on a host of safety issues. The interdisciplinary structure of the teams makes getting complex issues resolved, implemented, and spread across the entire organization easier, according to Gregory R. Behrens, R.Ph., M.S.H.A., Seton's network director of pharmacy services.

(continued)

Case Study 3-1. Seton Healthcare Tackles Technology Implementation (continued)

Seton's master plan highlights the importance of integrating the technologies. According to Behrens, it is important to first link together comprehensive medication-management software, bar code technology, and a computerized prescriber order entry (CPOE) system. This should be accomplished in a sequential way, he adds. The next step is to tackle the other components, such as enhanced and updated medication cabinet automation, drug carousel technology, robotics, and smart pump technology. These should be handled separately and apart from the three initial developments. With all six systems
integrated, it is possible to drive the majority of adverse drug events out of an organization, he explains. The bar code technology alone could reduce as much as 40% of medication-related errors, says Behrens. Health care partnering at the bedside will soon become a reality at Seton.

In the meantime, Behrens offers the following strategies to implement value-added systems and technologies:

- Conduct a literature and marketplace review to determine best practices and emerging technologies, and other systems solutions to the myriad challenges facing health care organizations.
- Think out of the box—take the time to visualize one's own view of responsible and safe care combined with organizational efficiency.
- Solicit and assess the vision of other respected leaders.
- Decide on the technology and systems strategy that best fits the organization.
- Take time to think the issues through and answer questions such as "Is this organization an early, middle, or late adapter of technology?" and "What can the institution do to improve safety or effectiveness?"
- Map out the implementation strategy that makes the most sense to individuals within the organization, making sure the planned systems and technological sequencing are logical and methodical and that they flow correctly.
- Sell the vision of technology implementation as a long-term process. Reminding others about the benefits of the new technology should occur at various venues and for multiple levels of leadership. It should be part of every step in any implementation process.
- Emphasize the added value the institution will achieve from the various system improvements.
- Move through the organization's formal hierarchy to achieve the necessary approvals for the systems improvements or technologies.
- Listen to stakeholders and partners. Be dynamic, responsive, and willing to modify the plan along the way.

Source: Joint Commission Resources: *Using Technology to Improve Medication Safety.* Oakbrook Terrace, IL: The Joint Commission, 2005.

response given by 46% of respondents. In 2006, 24% of organizations had a fully operational EMR system in place, compared with 18% in 2005. An additional 36% of organizations are presently installing EMR hardware and software. Four percent have signed a contract for an EMR system, but have not yet installed it.[2]

The Rand Corporation, in its 2005 report *The State and Pattern of Health Information Technology Adoption,* suggests that the overall EMR adoption rate is between 20% and 30% for hospitals.[9]

An ambulatory care survey conducted from 2001 to 2003 by the Centers for Disease Control and Prevention (CDC) notes that EMRs were used in 31% of emergency departments (EDs) and 29% of outpatient departments.[10]

Although the CDC indicates that the technology is being used in 17% of physician's offices, researchers note that larger practices and those owned by health maintenance organizations were significantly more likely to use this technology.[11]

Benefits of EMRs

The primary benefit of an EMR is that it contains all the information the provider needs to understand a patient's treatment history. This might include the patient's health problems, medication history, laboratory and diagnostic test results, allergies, and other pertinent health information.

An EMR system can improve a provider's ability to not only access, but also to track, patient information (*see* Case Study 3-2, page 61). Given that vital clinical information is missing in nearly one in seven primary care visits, accounting for delayed care or additional services in nearly 60% of visits,[12] having a computerized patient record could potentially reduce treatment delays. This missing information included lab results, letters/dictation, radiology results, history and physical examination, and medications, all of which are typically included in an EMR. It also allows for the simultaneous review of patient records by multiple clinicians, which could improve the timeliness of their reviews, resulting in a quicker diagnosis and treatment for the patient. The same study notes that clinicians using a complete EMR system were significantly less likely to report missing clinical information.

Other benefits have been cited in several studies. Overall, the use of an EMR system can improve quality of care by improving the following:

- Access to patient clinical information
- Efficiency of documentation
- Decision support through use of reminders
- Adherence to clinical practice guidelines
- Delivery of medications, resulting in reduced medication errors
- Delivery of preventive health services
- Access to educational materials for patients

Security. As more health care organizations and providers implement the technology needed for EMRs, patient privacy protection should be considered. The possibility of violations against identifiable health information must be considered in order to protect patient information and rights.

The federal law applies to health information created or maintained by health care providers who engage in certain electronic transactions, health plans, and health care clearinghouses. Under its security regulations, health care organizations must apply reasonable and appropriate safeguards and controls to protect electronic health information. Electronic health information includes patient information stored on magnetic tapes or disks, optical discs, hard drives, servers, floppy disks, and memory cards. Protecting the integrity of health information

---

Case Study 3-2. EMR Use Reduces Treatment Delays

Name of organization: The University of Pittsburgh Medical Center (UPMC) in Pennsylvania has more than 4,000 licensed beds, with 174,000 admissions per year and 3 million outpatient visits. An academic medical center, UPMC spans the spectrum of health care delivery with its network of 19 tertiary, specialty, and community hospitals, as well as 400 outpatient sites and physician offices.

Purpose of the project: e-Record is designed to provide physicians at UPMC with EMRs to improve patient safety by reducing medication error rates and by making patient records instantly available at the point of care throughout the system.

Lessons learned: It is important to understand the culture of the organization and then identify areas of opportunity. If the area of opportunity is medication errors, the first step is to measure the medication error rate.

The University of Pittsburgh Medical Center's (UPMC) goal is to provide technological interconnectivity to all its clinicians, allowing them to securely share patient-specific data whether they are on site at one of the hospitals, in their office or clinic, at home, or anywhere in between.

To date, nearly all of its 2,500 employed physicians use the e-Record system, with more than 400 physicians using an office-based EMR system in addition to the hospital-based applications. Inpatient e-Record use has slashed UPMC's medication delivery time in half. The medical center also has launched a computerized prescribed order entry system at three of its hospitals, with another to follow in the next year. In addition, it is deploying a personal health record that will allow patients to use a secure Web site to view test results, e-mail their physicians, schedule appointments, and help manage chronic conditions such as diabetes and asthma.

EMR use also means that staff members no longer have to call the medical records office at another location to find patients' records and have them faxed over, thus eliminating potential treatment delays. The instant availability of records reduces potential test duplication, another reason for delays in treatment.

includes preventing unauthorized breaches of privacy due to theft, human errors, or natural disaster. The security rules specify a series of administrative, technical, and physical security procedures. Administrative measures could involve implementing security awareness and training programs for all staff. Technical procedures could include attaching safeguards to the EMR system to prevent tampering. Physical measures could include locking doors to rooms in which electronic health information files are kept.

STRATEGY

EMRs can be configured to restrict access to only portions of the medical record based on job function.
Many EMRs have audit trails that identify anyone who has accessed or added to the record.

The *HIPAA Compliance Journal* is devoted to news, strategies, and tips for complying with the federal law for all types of health care organizations. For the latest HIPAA information, go to the Web site at http://www.hipaacompliancejournal.com.

The privacy rule of HIPAA addresses the organization's obligation to inform the patient how his or her information will be used. It does not allow institutions to disclose health information without the patient's authorization (*see* Sidebar 3-1, page 63, for how organizations can integrate HIPAA compliance into their privacy policies).

Computerized Patient Tracking Systems

Patient tracking systems can be used to eliminate treatment delays caused by staff trying to locate patients when they begin their care. These systems are either active or passive. Active systems involve staff tracking and recording all patient movements by making entries into a computer system. Passive systems use technologies to track most movements and interactions without active input from staff. Although bar codes using infrared technology are commonly used to track patients, they are being replaced with radio frequency identification (RFID), which is considered a step up from bar coding.[13] The RFID tags, which consist of small integrated circuits with attached antennae, are worn by patients on ankle bracelets. The tags announce the patients' locations whenever they are in the proximity of a tag reader, several of which are strategically located throughout a facility. One hospital estimated that physicians and nurses spent 10% of the average shift looking for patients, equipment, or each other, a task that was eliminated with the implementation of an RFID tracking system.[14]

The use of patient tracking systems is particularly beneficial in the ED because it is such a fast-paced and chaotic environment. Beds turn over rapidly, and patients, who often start out in one location, can be moved several times between triage and treatment during a relatively short period of time. Having real-time access to patients' whereabouts allows hospital staff to accurately determine ED occupancy and capacity. Some computer-based systems update the data hourly to monitor patient flow into and out of units.[15] Knowing how long patients wait to be registered, evaluated by a physician, tested and treated, and discharged or admitted can be helpful in reducing patient wait times.

Patient tracking systems can be used to follow inpatients as well. For example, in this setting,

Sidebar 3-1. Handling Privacy Issues in the Health Care Setting

Addressing privacy and confidentiality in a health care organization involves more than being HIPAA compliant. Many health care regulatory agencies, such as The Joint Commission, have established standards calling for the development of privacy policies.

The following tips are designed to help organizations meet HIPAA requirements along with Joint Commission standards requiring a privacy policy.

Ensure that all elements of a patient's record are present. Whether patient health information is in an electronic medical record or paper records, the organization is responsible for protecting its data. Procedures should define who is authorized to request access to records and under what conditions access is allowed. In addition, methods should be in place for ensuring that appropriate patient authorizations are obtained or for tracking disclosures.

Know the difference between consent and authorization requirements. HIPAA does not require organizations to obtain patient consent to use information for care, treatment, or services. It does, however, require patient authorization if the organization is planning to disclose patient information for reasons other than treatment, such as for marketing purposes.

Handle outside requests for information consistently. Organizations should take reasonable steps to limit the use and disclosure of, and requests for, protected health information. They should know when disclosures are required or not required under HIPAA. For example, disclosures are not required for requests by a health care provider for treatment purposes. Policies and procedures should address how outside requests for information will be handled. This should include verifying the authority of the person/agency receiving the information, as well as monitoring the requests and release of information.

Know what violates privacy. White boards used to record patient-related information in hospitals do not breach a patient's right to privacy as long as no diagnostic or clinical information can be linked with the patient's name. Stickers used to identify such patient information as allergies or do-not-resuscitate orders are also permitted. The organization should implement reasonable safeguards and practices to avoid disclosure to individuals who do not have a need to know.

Source: Joint Commission Resources: Handling privacy in the health care setting. *Joint Commission: The Source* 3(1):6–7, 2005.

a tracking system eliminates the need for staff to inform other various department staff of the patient's progress as he or she moves from pre-op to post-op.[16] When involved departments are prepared and ready for the next step in the patient care process, patients are less likely to have to wait for an available bed. The system can also collect and analyze data related to operating room use, delays, and average time and volume flow, all of which impact the delivery of timely care.

An Automatic Alerting System

An automatic alerting system deployed at a large academic medical center reduced the time frame in which patients who had critical lab results were treated.[17] The computer system was designed to automatically notify the covering physician about test results involving 12 conditions in a study conducted over a two-month period. For the 94 intervention patients, the covering physician was automatically notified about the test results. For the 98 control patients, no automatic notification was made. The median time interval—the time between when the test results were available for review and when an appropriate treatment was ordered—was 38% less for patients in the intervention group, or 1 hour versus 1.6 hours for the patients in the control group. The time in which the alerting condition was resolved also was less for the intervention group: 8.4 hours versus 8.9 hours for their counterparts in the control group.

In the same study, the time differences were more significant for the 95 test results that did not meet the lab's critical reporting criteria. The median time until treatment was ordered for the 51 intervention patients was 1.2 hours compared with 2.5 hours for the 44 control patients.

The authors conclude that the alerting system was effective because it informed the patient's key provider directly, highlighting the pertinent data, which made ordering the correct treatment easier.

An Alphanumeric Page

An alphanumeric page that notifies clinicians of test results in real time was designed by researchers at Brigham and Women's Hospital in Boston.[18] Added to the hospital's clinical information system, the application allows clinicians who expect a lab result for a specific patient to request the result report via an alphanumeric pager as soon as the result is filed into the patient database. During a year-long trial, this feature was used in both inpatient and outpatient settings at a rate of roughly 2,300 times per month. Approximately 75% of the requests were made for hospitalized patients and 25% for patients seen in the ambulatory care setting. The majority of users (99%) preferred to be notified via alphanumeric pager as opposed to e-mail. Tests for electrolytes, complete blood count, and coagulation accounted for 78% of all requests.

The authors conclude that this application offers clinicians the opportunity to reduce unnecessary delays in patient care by allowing them to receive lab results in real time.

Bedside Care

Automating processes through the use of technology has made it possible for some procedures to occur at the bedside, typically reducing the time it takes to perform them.

Point-of-Care Testing

Two types of technology support point-of-care testing (POCT): small benchtop analyzers (for example, blood gas and electrolyte systems) and handheld, single-use devices (for example, urine albumin, blood glucose, and coagulation tests).[19]

Portable chemistry analyzers can read a few drops of blood from a patient's finger and provide six different laboratory test results in approximately 90 seconds.[20] Reducing the time it takes to receive test results allows patients to be diagnosed more rapidly.

Although POCT is not new, the range of tests that can be undertaken at the point of care is new. POCT is commonly used for urinalysis and to test for glucose levels and arterial blood gases. Over the last few years, this list has expanded to include the rapid analysis of cardiac biomarkers, which can help clinicians identify patients with chest pains who will benefit from early treatment and those at greatest risk of future cardiac events; POCT for D-dimer, which can help identify patients at risk of deep vein thrombosis or pulmonary embolism; and on-site screening for microbial antigens or inflammatory markers, which can help determine whether or not antibiotic therapy is appropriate even before culture test results have been returned.

The ability to make a quicker diagnosis also facilitates more rapid clinical decision making and treatment. The ability to make appropriate treatment decisions in a shorter time period can be especially helpful in the ED.

In one study, patients presenting to an ED who had POCT waited 14 minutes less to have their blood drawn than their counterparts who were allocated to have their tests performed by the hospital's central lab.[21] Moreover, treatment decisions for the POCT patients were made 74 minutes earlier for hematology tests, 86 minutes earlier for biochemical tests, and 21 minutes earlier for analyses of blood gases. Treatment decisions were considered to be critical in 7% of the 1,728 patients evaluated in the study conducted at a large teaching hospital.

Similarly, rapid testing for HIV not only results in quicker turnaround times, but in prompt administration of antiretroviral prophylaxis.[22] In a CDC–funded study at four Chicago hospitals, the feasibility of rapid HIV testing—which typically takes 20 minutes—of women with undocumented HIV status in labor and delivery units was evaluated. A total of 225 women were tested at three hospitals using POCT, and 155 were tested at a hospital using a central lab. The median turnaround time for the HIV POCT was 45 minutes compared with 3.5 hours for lab testing. The three pregnant women who tested HIV positive were provided timely therapy to reduce perinatal transmission of the virus.

Facilities that link their POCT equipment to lab services enable real-time monitoring and integration of test results into the patient's EMR.

Bedside Ultrasound

Ultrasounds can now be obtained at the bedside, which contributes to rapid diagnosis and treatment.

When bedside ultrasound was used to evaluate patients with blunt abdominal trauma, it rapidly helped distinguish patients with injuries requiring computerized tomography or surgery from those who did not experience abdominal injury.[23] Moreover, bedside ultrasound integrates easily into the resuscitation of trauma victims without causing delay in therapy. It is portable, noninvasive, and lacks any associated morbidity.

Routinely used in the ED, bedside ultrasound is especially useful for unstable patients who might not be candidates for other imaging procedures.

E-Visits

Some physicians are beginning to use e-visits to substitute for face-to-face visits. E-visits can reduce treatment delays resulting from patients not being able to schedule timely appointments. It is also a strategy that physicians can use to decrease the demand for unnecessary face-to-face visits.

Dartmouth-Hitchcock Alliance, a multispecialty group practice in northern New England comprising more than 900 primary- and specialty-care providers, recently began offering e-visits to longstanding patients.[24] Patients can choose an e-visit when seeking advice, a diagnosis, or treatment that previously would have required an office visit. The most common uses have been for follow-up care regarding chronic conditions (for example, diabetes, hypertension, anemia, depression) and acute episodes of chronic conditions (for example, back pain, sinusitis). After reviewing the patient's request, the provider determines whether an e-visit is appropriate. E-visits are not intended for emergency care, conditions with a significant visual diagnostic component, clarification of issues from previous visits, or diagnostic results reporting.

Remote ICU Care

More recently, clinicians are using medical technology to remotely monitor patients in the intensive care unit (ICU), a practice known as the use of telemedicine. In an electronic ICU, critical care physicians interact with patients and hospital staff while assessing clinical data via dedicated computer-based videoconferencing and data transmission equipment at a location physically remote from the hospital grounds. Electronic ICU members are assigned to workstations at which they receive clinical information from the hospital via remote-controlled cameras set up in each ICU patient room.

Videoconferencing equipment enables the clinicians to see patients and staff, as well as to communicate in real time with on-site caregivers. Bedside-monitoring data, such as vital signs, are transmitted in real time via a telephone access system. Critical pieces of patient information such as electrocardiograms, radiographs, consultant notes, and bedside flow sheets are scanned and transmitted digitally. Lab test results can be accessed through a telephone-based access system.

The overriding benefit of using telemedicine in the ICU is having the physician coverage necessary for the optimal care of critically ill patients who require close monitoring and frequent interventions.[25] Such coverage is especially important during off hours when care can best be characterized as crisis intervention.[26] Studies have shown that the use of an e-ICU results in improved patient outcomes.[27,28] The immediate access to key patient data plays a critical role in providing timely care to critically ill patients.

Two community hospitals that effectively deployed telemedicine to provide acute stroke consultative services concluded that its use facilitated thrombolytic therapy for acute stroke patients and that it is particularly helpful in addressing time- and spatially related emergency needs.[29] When a patient is a thrombolytic candidate, the telemedicine consultant discusses the risks and benefits of such treatment with the patient and/or family members. In addition, the consultant provides them with information on a stroke's potential disability effects, as well as the option of foregoing treatment with tPA. The patient or family can then make an informed decision regarding treatment.

Applied to emergency care, telemedicine can include real-time video and data links between EDs and ambulances, allowing remote patient assessments, automatic crash notification systems that are fully integrated with public safety dispatch systems, and hazardous material alert systems to identify harmful substances and immediately dispatch appropriate rescue and recovery resources.

Personal Digital Assistants (PDAs)

According to the HIMSS/AstraZeneca Clinician Wireless Survey conducted in 2002, 64% of physicians use PDAs.[15] The majority of respondents (70%) used them as a portable drug reference. Approximately 41% of providers used the PDA to schedule appointments, 12% used the handheld technology to interface to hospital data, and 9% used it to download lab values. All these activities are associated with treatment delays. Consequently, the use of PDAs has the potential to reduce such delays by allowing clinicians to gain immediate access to their schedules and patient health information.

When a state psychiatric hospital implemented a PDA system that included a psychopharmacology database, it reduced requests made by the medical staff for drug information by 45% during the first six months of use, reflecting better access to medication information.[30] The PDAs also allowed clinicians access to patient information, including previous psychiatric evaluations and medication profiles. Consequently, they served in a similar capacity as an EMR, which this particular hospital did not have.

Picture Archiving and Communication Systems

Picture archiving and communication system (PACS) refers to the archiving, processing, and viewing of digital radiological images, including x-rays, computed tomography, magnetic resonance imaging, and ultrasound. The use of a PACS can reduce exam-to-diagnosis time by providing rapid access to images, which is especially useful in EDs and operating rooms. Providers no longer have to wait long periods of time to view such images, as they are instantly available on the network when ready. A PACS implemented in a 20-bed ICU over a two-month period decreased the time to obtain an image from 90 to 60 minutes.[31]

Users, who included physicians, nurses, physiotherapists, and radiographers, were asked about their perceptions of the PACS. Of the 39 respondents, 99% believed the images were available more quickly than in the past, and 72% believed the use of the PACS workstation led to faster decision making with regard to patient management.

The use of a PACS also offers simultaneous access to the same images by multiple clinicians, thus facilitating the consultative process. In one study that evaluated the use of a PACS six months after implementation, users said the system offered better access to x-rays.[32] After the radiographers processed the images and checked their quality, the x-rays were readily available to authorized users at multiple locations.

Finally, the use of a PACS eliminates the need for staff to spend time searching for lost diagnostic test results. In fact, this was one of the biggest benefits noted by nurses working in the ED and ICU.[33]

Automated Drug Dispensing Systems

Automated drug dispensing systems (ADDSs) allow prescription orders to be entered into computers that automatically alert pharmacists when there are drug interaction problems or if dosages conflict with a patient's drug history.

According to the CDC's ambulatory care survey, 40% of EDs and 18% of outpatient departments use ADDSs.

This technology can be used to decrease medication turnaround times. In fact, that was one of the goals that El Camino Hospital in the heart of Silicon Valley hoped to accomplish by implementing an automated medication dispensing station.[34] Specifically, the goal was to decrease the medication turnaround time of more than 90% of medications. The system enabled the pharmacist to evaluate the appropriateness of medication orders and make alternative treatment recommendations, when appropriate. Prior to the ADDS, pharmacists manually checked and dispensed medications without having a readily retrievable medication profile. To install the ADDS, an interface with the existing CPOE and an expanded formulary to support the interface had to be created. Among the improved patient safety results achieved through the implementation of the ADDS was the verification of 94% of the medication orders in less than 15 minutes.

Continuity of Care Record

When an EMR is not an option, the Continuity of Care Record (CCR)—a proposed standard for exchanging basic patient data between providers—might be the technological answer to providing immediate access to patient information across health care settings.

The CCR contains the following patient information: diagnosis, problems and conditions, family history, social history and health risk factors, adverse reactions/alerts, current medications and relevant history, immunizations, vital signs and physiological measurements, lab results, procedures/imaging, and health status assessments.[35]

The use of the CCR could eliminate the need for providers to spend time tracking down patient data[36], as the CCR can be accessed via portable memory devices such as PDAs, secure e-mail, or Web servers, and does not require interfacing to an EMR.

References

1. Health Research Institute: 2005 *Modern Healthcare*/PricewaterhouseCoopers IT survey: Trends in IT spending among hospitals, *Health Brief,* PricewaterhouseCoopers. Apr. 2005. http://pwchealth.com/pdf/itsurvey.pdf (accessed Jan. 8, 2007).

2. Healthcare Information and Management Systems Society: *17th Annual HIMSS Leadership Survey: Final Report: Healthcare CIO.* Feb. 13, 2006. http://www.himss.org/2006survey/docs/Healthcare_CIO_finalreport.pdf (accessed Jan. 8, 2007).

3. Chaudhry B., et al.: Systematic review: Impact of health information technology on quality, efficiency, and costs of medical care. *Ann Intern Med* 144:742–752, May 16, 2006.

4. Karsh B.T.: Beyond usability: Designing effective technology implementation systems to promote patient safety. *Qual Saf Health Care* 13:388–394, Oct. 2004.

5. Crosson J.C., et al.: Implementing an electronic medical record in a family medicine practice: Communication, decision making, and conflict. *Ann Fam Med* 3(4):301–311, 2005.

6. Millard E: *CRM Buyer Special Report: Survey shows hospitals getting wired.* Jul. 21, 2004. http://www.crmbuyer.com/story/35247.html (accessed Jan. 4, 2007).

7. Murray M.D., et al.: Effects of computer-based prescribing on pharmacist work patterns. *J Am Med Inform Assoc* 5(6):546–553, 1998.

8. Broder, C.: Speaker: Practice redesign, technology should go together. *Healthcare IT News,* Apr. 4, 2005. http://www.healthcareitnews.com/NewsArticleView.aspx?ContentID=2763 (accessed Jan. 3, 2007).

9. Fonkych K., Taylor R.: *The State and Pattern of Health Information Technology Adoption.* 2005. http://www.rand.org/pubs/monographs/2005/RAND_MG409.pdf (accessed Jan. 9, 2007).

10. Burt C., Hing E.: *Use of Computerized Clinical Support Systems in Medical Settings: United States, 2001–03. Advance Data from Vital and Health Statistics.* Pub. no. 353. Hyattsville, MD: National Center for Health Statistics, Mar. 15, 2005.

11. Simon J.S., Rundall T.G., Shortell S.M.: Drivers of electronic medical record adoption among medical groups. *Jt Comm J Qual Patient Saf* 31:631–639, Nov. 5, 2005.

12. Smith P.C., et al.: Missing clinical information during primary care visits. *JAMA* 293:565–571, Feb. 2, 2005.

13. Breslow M.J., et al.: Effect of a multiple-site intensive care unit telemedicine program on clinical and economic outcomes: An alternative paradigm for intensivist staffing. *Crit Care Med* 32(1):31–38, 2004.

14. Choi J.Y., et al.: Using telemedicine to facilitate thrombolytic therapy for patients with acute stroke. *Jt Comm J Qual Patient Saf* 32(4):199–205, 2006.

15. Healthcare Information and Management Systems Society: *2002 HIMSS/AstraZeneca Clinician Survey,* Nov. 4, 2002. http://www.himss.org/content/files/surveyresults/Final%20Final%20Report.pdf (accessed Jan. 7, 2007).

16. New tracking system improves patient flow. *ED Management.* Aug. 1, 2005.

17. Franczyk A.: Surgery tracker may save millions. *Business First of Buffalo.* Sep. 1, 2006.

18. Kuperman G.J., Boyle D., Jha A.: How promptly are inpatients treated for critical laboratory results? *J Am Med Inform Assoc* 5:112–119, Jan.–Feb. 1998.

19. Kuperman G.J., et al.: Improving response to critical laboratory results with automation: Results of a randomized controlled trial. *J Am Med Inform Assoc* 6:512–522, Nov.–Dec. 1999.

20. Poon E.G., et al.: Real-time notification of laboratory data requested by users through alphanumeric pagers. *J Am Med Inform Assoc* 9:217–222, May–Jun. 2002.

21. Price C.P.: Point of care testing. *BMJ* 322:1285–1288, May 26, 2001.

22. Centers for Disease Control and Prevention: Rapid point-of-care testing for HIV-1 during labor and delivery— Chicago, Illinois, 2002. *MMWR Morb Mortal Wkly Rep* 52, Sep. 12, 2003. http://www.cdc.gov/MMWR/preview/mmwrhtml/mm5236a4.htm (accessed Jan. 16, 2007).

23. Brown M.A., et al.: Screening ultrasound in blunt abdominal trauma. *J Intensive Care Med* 18:253–260, Sep.–Oct. 2003.

24. Walters B., Barnard D., Paris S.: "Patient portals" and "e-visits." *J Ambul Care Manage* 29(3):222–224, 2006.

25. Breslow M.J.: ICU telemedicine: Organization and communication. *Crit Care Clin* 16(4):707–722, 2000.

26. Celi L.A., et al.: The eICU: It's not just telemedicine. *Crit Care Med* 29(suppl. 8):N183–N189, 2001.

27. Rosenfeld B.A., et al.: Intensive care unit telemedicine: Alternate paradigm for providing continuous intensivist care.

Crit Care Med 28(12):3925–3931, 2000.

28. Breslow M.J., et al.: Effect of a multiple-site intensive care unit telemedicine program on clinical and economic outcomes: An alternative paradigm for intensivist staffing. *Crit Care Med* 32(1):31–38, 2004.

29. Choi J.Y., et al.: Using telemedicine to facilitate thrombolytic therapy for patients with acute stroke. *Jt Comm J Qual Patient Saf* 32(4):199–205, 2006.

30. Grasso B.C., Genest R.: Use of a personal digital assistant in reducing medication error rates. *Psychiatr Serv* 52(7):883–886, 2001.

31. Cox B., Dawe N.: Evaluation of the impact of a PACS system on an intensive care unit. *J Health Organ Manag* 16(2–3):199–205, 2002.

32. Yu P., Hilton P.: Work practice changes caused by the introduction of a picture archiving and communication system. *J Telemed Telecare* 11(suppl. 2):S104–S107, 2005.

33. Bukunt S., et al.: El Camino Hospital: Using health information technology to promote patient safety. *Jt Comm J Qual Patient Saf* 31(10):561–565, 2005.

34. Healthcare Information and Management Systems Society (HIMSS): The continuity of care record standard initiative. *HIMSS Standards Insight,* Dec. 2003. http://www.himss.org/content/files/StandardsInsight/2003/12-2003.pdf (accessed Jan. 15, 2007).

35. Kibbe D.C., Phillips R.L., Green L.A.: The continuity of care record. *Am Fam Physician* 70, Oct. 1, 2004. http://www.aafp.org/afp/20041001/editorials.html (accessed Jan. 15, 2007).

Appendix
Resource Strategies Related to Reducing Delays in Treatment

Strategies to reduce treatment delays can be evaluated in several ways: They can be viewed in terms of the disease that is being treated or the type of setting in which the patient is receiving treatment.

This Appendix includes journal articles that highlight strategies for the following:

- Myocardial infarction patients
- Specialty care
- Patient access strategies
- Ventilator-associated pneumonia
- Improving primary care access

A list of journal references is included that are relevant to the following topics:

- Acute heart failure
- Stroke
- Ventilator-associated pneumonia
- Tuberculosis
- Transfer delays
- Care coordination
- Emergency departments
- Appointment delays in the physician's office

These selected resource articles represent a small portion of literature on reducing treatment delays and should not be considered as all-inclusive of available material or resources.

Articles

Boushon B., et al.: Using a virtual breakthrough series collaborative to improve access in primary care. *Jt Comm J Qual Patient Saf* 32(10):573–584, 2006.

Green L.V., Savin S., Murray M.: Providing timely access to care: What is the right patient panel size? *Jt Comm J Qual Patient Saf* 33(4):211–218, 2007.

Jacobs A.K., et al.: Recommendation to develop strategies to increase the number of ST-segment–elevation myocardial infarction patients with timely access to primary percutaneous coronary intervention. *Circulation* 113:2115–2163, 2006.

Murray, M.F.: Improving access to specialty care. *Jt Comm J Qual Patient Saf* 33(3):125–135, 2007.

Nolan K., et al.: Using a framework for spread: The case of patient access in the Veterans Health Administration. *Jt Comm J Qual Patient Saf* 31(6):339–347, 2005.

Youngquist P., et al.: Implementing a ventilator bundle in a community hospital. *Jt Comm J Qual Patient Saf* 33(4):219–225, 2007.

Joint Commission Journal **on** QUALITY **and** PATIENT SAFETY

Methods, Tools, and Strategies

Using a Virtual Breakthrough Series Collaborative to Improve Access in Primary Care

Barbara Boushon, B.S.N.
Lloyd Provost, M.S.
Janice Gagnon
Penny Carver

In January 2004, the Institute for Healthcare Improvement (IHI) launched an initiative designed to develop and test an exclusively Internet- and phone-based system of adult learning dedicated to improving access in primary care. Called the "Virtual Breakthrough Series," or VBTS, the initiative was modeled on the methodology used in IHI's Breakthrough Series (BTS) for collaborative improvement.[1] The VBTS was designed as a demonstration project, not a research project, to show that it was feasible to conduct a Breakthrough Series collaborative virtually and produce outcomes comparable to those of a traditional BTS, at substantially reduced cost. The specific outcomes to be measured were reductions in waiting time both for and at an appointment in physician office practices.

The project's ultimate aim was to improve outcomes and quality of care by using IHI's BTS collaborative model, which is designed to rapidly diffuse knowledge and spread best practices on the basis of an "all teach, all learn" philosophy—but at greatly reduced cost and to a much broader audience than can feasibly be reached through the traditional face-to-face BTS model. A traditional, face-to-face IHI collaborative is a short-term (6–15-month) learning-and-action project that brings together a large number of teams (usually 20 to 40) from hospitals or clinics to achieve rapid, significant improvement in a specific area. Each team typically consists of three members who attend three learning sessions (LSs), with an additional two or three members who work on improvements in their local organization. The total number of people participating in collaborative LSs has ranged from 40 to more than 700.

Article-at-a-Glance

Background: The Institute for Healthcare Improvement (IHI) pioneered the Breakthrough Series (BTS), a short-term improvement project that convenes, in three face-to-face meetings, hospital or clinic teams to make rapid, significant improvement. A distance-learning (virtual) version of the BTS—a VBTS—was conducted.

Methods: A model VBTS was tested with 20 organizations, using a well-established topic: improving access and efficiency in primary care. This VBTS took place by Internet and telephone, using Web-based collaboration software and audioconferencing.

Results: For the 17 organizations completing the VBTS, the average number of days to third-next-available appointment fell from 23 to 10 days (July 2004–June 2005). The Improvement Assessment Scale showed 59% of teams at level 4 or above ("significant" improvement, with most changes implemented, and evidence of sustained improvement in outcomes and plans for spread). Potential direct cost savings were about $12,000 as compared with a traditional collaborative. Six months after the VBTS's conclusion, 70% of the teams that achieved significant improvement either maintained gains or improved their results.

Discussion: Outcomes in a VBTS are potentially comparable to those in a traditional collaborative, at substantially lower cost. Prerequisites for success include senior leadership's involvement, team members' ability to participate, and information technology support.

Journal on Quality and Patient Safety

Since 1995, IHI has sponsored more than 50 BTS collaboratives, on dozens of topics, involving more than 2,000 teams from more than 1,000 health care organizations. A growing body of literature has considered the effectiveness of the BTS model, with some studies finding some significant improvements, while other studies find little or no improvement.[2-8] Although IHI has demonstrated that the BTS collaborative model can be a valuable change agent,[9,10] the model's design of face-to-face meetings carries inherent limitations. A BTS collaborative is both expensive and time-consuming, with the result that many individuals and organizations cannot participate. The virtual BTS (VBTS) was a test of a new model to determine if an entirely electronic version of the BTS collaborative, using Internet and phone, would be feasible and could produce outcomes comparable to those of a traditional, face-to-face BTS. Further, we predicted that a VBTS would significantly reduce costs to participating hospitals and clinics through conservation of staff time, elimination of travel costs, and reduction in tuition costs. We also predicted that the speed, immediacy, and convenience of synchronous and asynchronous distance communication would allow for knowledge transfer and spread of change concepts comparable to a traditional BTS.

The main outcome measure for the VBTS, as for traditional BTS collaboratives working on reduction in waiting times, was the average number of days to third-next-available appointment. The ultimate aim of the VBTS was to decrease delays both for and at appointments, by using IHI's BTS methodology, but at greatly reduced cost and involving many more organizations than can feasibly be reached through a traditional face-to-face model. This article reports the results of the demonstration project and its implications.

Developing the Collaborative
Topic
The topic chosen for the VBTS prototype was "improving access and office efficiency in primary care" (defined as a system in which patients can be seen by their primary care provider when they choose, even on the same day). Because four traditional national BTS Collaboratives had already addressed this topic, IHI had established materials already in place, as well as benchmark results for comparison.[11,12] Teams in the VBTS tested specific change ideas within the

Access and Efficiency Change Package, a collection of 11 change concepts that have been shown to improve outcomes in previous Collaboratives (Table 1, pages 575–576).

Participating Organizations
Twenty health care organizations were selected to participate in the VBTS. Organizations were selected on the basis of documented characteristics of successful improvement teams,[13] including senior leadership involvement, plans to spread the improvement, access to appropriate technology, and assurance that improving access is a primary goal of the organization. IHI's usual fees for this initial prototype were covered by a grant from the Alfred P. Sloan Foundation.

BTS Model
In the traditional BTS model, participants learn about the topic in face-to-face LSs from faculty experts, who present a vision for ideal care and specific changes necessary to achieve the ideal. A change package is designed to improve performance in the local system, and an improvement advisor guides team members through the steps needed to test, adapt, and implement the changes. Teams test these process changes using the Model for Improvement[14] during action periods between the LSs. Teams report on and share their experiences, both successes and failures, during monthly phone calls and at the second and third LSs. Each team documents, measures, and reports on its progress monthly through a shared Internet site. Faculty and staff also make monthly assessments of each team's progress. The final results of collaborative work are presented at a National Congress and at other meetings.

VBTS Model
To adapt the classic BTS model to a virtual model, we conducted a literature and expert review of e-learning. We incorporated lessons about issues such as the best way to prepare faculty, deliver content, and conduct sessions in the virtual environment[15,16] into the VBTS design.

Technology Issues
Selecting and implementing new technologies was the first step in transforming the face-to-face BTS into a virtual model (Figure 1, page 577). We evaluated

Journal on QUALITY and PATIENT SAFETY

Table 1. Improving Access to Primary Care: Change Package

Understand Supply and Demand

Understanding the patterns of both supply and demand on a weekly, monthly, or seasonal basis allows for focused efforts to shape demand to match supply, and/or increase (or decrease) supply during periods of high (or low) demand. Measure supply, measure demand, and then compare the two.

Reduce the Backlog

Backlog consists of appointments on the future schedule that have been put off due to lack of space on the schedule to do this work sooner; working down the backlog recalibrates the system to improve access. To reduce and eliminate backlog, first measure it, and then create and use a deliberate backlog reduction plan (e.g., temporarily add appointment slots; temporarily add staff and/or schedule additional overtime hours; determine if patient needs can be met without an office visit).

Reduce Appointment Types

Practices with improved access make no distinction between urgent and routine appointments because the goal is to do today's work today. When the provider is present the patient is seen, and when the provider is absent the patient is offered the choice of an appointment the next time the provider is present or today with another care team member. All other special appointment types, such as those for disease entity or physicals by age groups, can be eliminated.

Develop Contingency Plans

Even if the supply and demand in a clinic are generally in balance, there will be times when there is a surge in demand (demand outstrips supply) that is either expected (e.g., flu season) or unexpected (e.g., many walk-ins on one day). Expected and unexpected variations in supply can also occur (e.g., vacations or emergency sick leaves). To avoid disrupting the normal flow of clinic practice, clinics agree upon a standard protocol to follow for each event, including clear responsibilities for each staff member. Examples include a policy for late patients; scripts for common occurrences; plans for vacations and sudden provider absences.

Reduce Demand

One key way to improve access is to reduce unnecessary demand for various services so that those patients needing a particular service can receive it in a timely way.

Examples of reducing demand include creating alternatives to one-on-one visits; managing and decreasing no-show appointments; increasing the interval for return appointments; using "max-packing" to address as many patient needs as possible during the visit in order to reduce future work.

Optimize the Care Team to Increase Supply

The clinic has to understand the types of services it provides, and then decide who should be involved in the work and how the work should be divided among the care team. This approach begins with demand and adjusts supply to meet the demand (within the limits of clinic resources). This is different from an approach that sets an arbitrary care team mix and then tries to fit the demand into the supply. Examples include cross-training staff; reducing variation in provider styles; ensuring that clinicians and staff work to their highest level of experience and skills; establishing standard protocols to move work away from providers.

Balance Supply and Demand for Non–Appointment Work

The supply and demand for non-appointment work (messages, refills, lab review, etc.) needs to be balanced within the timeframe of a day. First, measure the non-appointment work by category for each type of staff member (provider, nurse, medical assistant, receptionist, other), and then compare it to the amount of work time that the worker can deliver. If any one worker has more work (demand) than they can do (supply) each day, that work will either not get done or it will get pushed off to the future. Next, shape the demand, match the appropriate supply to the demand, and work on improving the process.

Synchronize Patient, Provider, and Information

To eliminate delays and smooth the flow for both providers and patients during an office visit, the patient and provider should be in the exam room along with all needed equipment and information (including test results, preventive care screens, etc.) at the stated appointment time. Some specific ideas for synchronizing the appointment processes include start every appointment on time; ensure that all needed information, equipment, and supplies are available for visit; use rooming criteria check sheets to ensure the patient is prepared for the provider (e.g., "shoes off" for diabetes patients).

continued

Journal on QUALITY and PATIENT SAFETY

Table 1. Improving Access to Primary Care: Change Package *(continued)*

Predict and Anticipate Patient Needs

To ensure that patient needs are met and that patients flow smoothly through the clinic process, staff look ahead on the schedule to identify patient needs for a given day or week. This advance planning allows the clinic staff time to arrange for specific equipment or tests that may be needed either prior to or at the time of the visit, to obtain or prepare all required information for the visit, and to implement a planned care approach.

Optimize the Environment

Improving the flow of work and eliminating waste ensures that the clinical office runs as efficiently and effectively as possible. Examples include moving steps in the system closer together (e.g., staff that need to communicate regularly should be in the same physical location); standardizing room equipment and set-up; ensuring there are enough exam rooms for each provider to optimize patient flow.

Manage the Constraint

Constraints, or bottlenecks, occur when the demand for a particular resource (e.g., rooms, providers, tests) or part of the system is greater than the available supply. If changes are made to improve parts of a system without addressing the constraint, the changes may not result in reduction of delays and waiting times for the entire system. To identify the constraint, observe where the work is piling up, or where the queues are forming. Look for certain signals within the system, such as places where material or information is in short supply, or where patients or staff are waiting, to help identify constraints. Clinics usually expect that the physician is the constraint, but there may be other factors. To manage the constraint, the practice must first identify the constraint and then drive unnecessary work away from it.

---

several types of collaboration software, with the intention of supporting not only the first VBTS but also other IHI projects with Web conferencing needs. The Web communication company we selected provides integrated telephony (audio is available through the Web connection), as well as video- and audio-conferencing capabilities.

IHI's extranet, a secure section of IHI's Web site, was used as a central platform on which teams could enter data and track their measures, as well as post qualitative, narrative descriptions of their work (for example, changes tested, barriers experienced), and share presentations, team storyboards, and other documents. A collaborative listserv (e-mail distribution list) was established for both administrative communication and to facilitate content discussion. In addition, the change package, with detailed explanation, was made available on IHI.org.

Planning

The VBTS planning group consisted of three faculty members, chosen for their experience and expertise in the topic; four IHI staff members (authors); and one IHI staff member, who provided technology expertise. As is done for all collaboratives, the planning group developed a project charter that specified the goals, measures, and

expectations of participating teams and IHI; conducted informational phone calls with prospective teams; developed the collaborative time line and monthly review and assessment schedule; and designed the collaborative pre-work. Selection criteria for the organizations to be chosen were refined to ensure the greatest likelihood of success, and teams participated in an electronic application process on the basis of these criteria—which included a willingness to participate in a test of the virtual model.

IHI developed measurement strategies to evaluate the progress and results of the participating sites, as well as the measures that would evaluate the VBTS's success. Experts in distance learning worked with the faculty to adapt the traditional curriculum to a virtual one, and faculty and staff received training and coaching in online teaching and learning.

Conducting the Collaborative
Pre-Launch Activities

In the pre-launch period (the six weeks before the first virtual LS), IHI conducted several activities with the teams that were designed to build community, including training on the IHI extranet and Web communication technologies, presentation of Web-based storyboards, and clinic walkthrough summaries.

Joint Commission **Journal** on **Quality** and **Patient Safety**

In the storyboard activity, teams created graphics presentation using a template that described the organizations, the team members and their roles, information on the numbers of patients that would be affected by their improvement work, and data on current delays at appointments and days until third-next-available appointment. Teams posted their storyboards on the extranet for other teams to review and then presented them during the all-team storyboard call.

Teams also completed a clinic walk-through, in which members "became" patients with a specified clinical issue, making an appointment, driving to the clinic, finding a parking space, filling out forms, and waiting for a provider—in short, experiencing each step of the process patients go through at the local site. Team members documented their ideas for improvement, as well as their feelings about the experience. These results were posted on the extranet for access by all teams.

All these activities were aimed at helping teams get to know one another, identifying other teams with similar data and challenges, increasing comfort with the VBTS technology, introducing the models and measurement system, and setting expectations. A particular focus of the pre-launch period was building the collaborative community culture that develops at traditional, face-to-face LSs.

Learning Sessions

The first LS was presented via the Internet and telephone for five hours daily for three days, for a total of 15 content hours. The agenda included much interaction during lectures, with frequent breaks and breakout time for teams to work together with faculty assistance. Faculty and teams used the Web-based chat modality extensively during the session, giving faculty who were not formally presenting an opportunity to clarify or augment pertinent points and giving team members an opportunity to ask questions. During the first LS, teams learned about (1) the online collaborative technology and the implications of distance collaboration and (2)

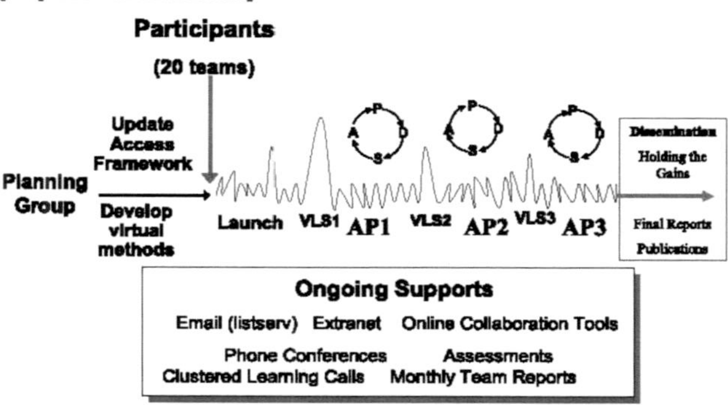

Figure 1. *Selecting and implementing new technologies was the first step in transforming the face-to-face BTS into a virtual model. AP, action period; VLS, virtual learning session.*

the change package and Model for Improvement. Each team developed an aim statement and set specific goals for reduction in delays (both for and at appointments) and determined the initial changes they would test.

The schedule for the second LS was modified based on feedback from the first session. This session was held on two consecutive six-hour days and included more interaction among teams and between teams and faculty; longer breaks; and more time built in between activities. The third LS was similar to the second but was characterized by more team input (as opposed to faculty presentation) than the second LS. As in a traditional BTS, the VBTS used an "all teach, all learn" environment, in which the faculty selected the top two performing teams to present their tests and data.

Because the LSs were offered online, requiring no travel outside of the community, many organizations set up conference rooms where additional members of the organization beyond the immediate improvement team could attend these important events. The conference room was set up with a speaker phone, computer, projector, and screen, allowing many more people to hear, see, and participate in the session. These participants included additional members of the direct care team,

Journal on QUALITY and PATIENT SAFETY

members of new teams to whom spread of the improvements was intended, and senior leadership. While some of these additional participants attended the entire session, others selected the sessions that were of particular interest to them, and simply went to the conference room at the time when the session that they were most interested in was being presented.

Action Periods

The action periods, which occur between LSs, were generally the same as those that take place in a traditional BTS. In the VBTS, they included additional synchronous work (via large all-collaborative conference calls and small-group cluster phone calls, held monthly, led by faculty, and organized by time zone). The smaller groups allowed teams to work on solving specific problems with input from others. Asynchronous work also took place (for example, listserv communication, discussion groups, team reports on changes and measures). Content information about how to improve access was available to the teams at IHI.org. Discussion groups, project management tools, and reporting tools were located on IHI's extranet, where each team maintained their own data and their own team home page.

Each month, teams submitted a report including data for each of their key measures, along with an update on changes tested and implemented, barriers encountered, and lessons learned. Faculty read and analyzed the reports, and responded with coaching via the listserv and through small-group cluster calls. Teams were encouraged to read each other's reports, looking for tips, ideas, and common experiences.

National Congress

The final event of the VBTS was a virtual National Congress, held in June 2005, at which teams shared their learning with the public. Public members received materials via e-mail and were given an electronic link to use to participate in the Congress. Registrants were encouraged to test their ability to connect days to weeks in advance by participating in an electronic session set up for that purpose. On the day of the event, the public connected via phone and Internet to the Web communication company's platform and participated in plenary and breakout sessions, as well as the chat room.

Measures

Measures designed to evaluate the success of the VBTS fell into the following two main categories:
- Access measures, which showed whether the changes the teams made on site led to reductions in delays for and at appointments (for example, number of days to third-next-available appointment, cycle time, daily supply and demand, and panel size).
- VBTS versus BTS comparison measures, which were used to evaluate the relative success of the VBTS compared with either the target for any BTS or with a traditional face-to-face BTS collaborative. A 1-to-5 Improvement Assessment Scale (IAS) was used; the scale helps collaborative directors and improvement advisors determine how well teams are doing in meeting improvement goals and implementing changes. (A detailed description of the assessment scale is provided in Table 2, page 579.) IHI, which developed the IAS in 1998, has used it to assess all teams participating in its BTS collaborative projects.

Results

Seventeen of the initial 20 organizations completed the collaborative. Three organizations elected to drop out of the collaborative, owing to a change in senior leadership, a change in day-to-day leadership, and competing priorities.

Days to Third-Next-Available Appointment

Average days to third-next-available appointment is a measure used by teams to track performance at the individual clinician level. In the VBTS collaborative, this measure fell from 23 days to 10 days during 12 months (60% reduction), as shown in Figure 2 (page 580). The Shewhart statistical process control (SPC) chart shown in this figure, with limits calculated to the end of the collaborative, indicates that this improvement trend was significant. A comparison of the same measure in a traditional BTS collaborative that IHI also conducted in 2004–2005 (Figure 3, page 581) shows a decline from 60 days at the start to just under 10 days during a 9-month period (83% reduction). Although the starting points for days to third-next-available appointment for teams in the VBTS and BTS differ considerably, more research is necessary to ascertain the reasons for this difference; it may have reflected the selection of organizations more

Journal on QUALITY and PATIENT SAFETY

Table 2. Improvement Assessment Scale for Virtual Breakthrough Series Collaborative	
Assessment/Description	Definition
1 Forming team	Team is formed; target population is identified; aim is determined; and baseline measurement begins.
1.5 Planning for the project begins	Team is meeting, discussion is occurring. Plans for the project are made.
2 Activity, but no changes	Team actively engaged in development, research, discussion but no changes are tested.
2.5 Changes tested, but no improvement	Components of the model being tested but no improvement in measures. Data on key measures are reported.
3 Modest improvement	Initial test cycles are completed and implementation begun for several components. Evidence of moderate improvement in process measures (daily demand, daily capacity, team member/patient continuity).
3.5 Improvement	Some improvement in outcome measures (third-next-available appointment and office visit cycle time); process measures of daily demand, daily capacity, and team member/patient continuity continuing to improve; Plan-Do-Study-Act test cycles on all components of the change package; changes implemented for many components of the change package.
4 Significant improvement	Most components of the change package are implemented for the population of focus. Evidence of sustained improvement in outcome measures (third-next-available appointment and office visit cycle time); halfway toward accomplishing all of the goals. Plans for spread, consistent with the team's aims, are prepared.
4.5 Sustainable improvement	Sustained improvement in most outcome measures (third-next-available appointment, future capacity, and office visit cycle time); 75% of goals achieved; plans for spread of the changes are in place.
5 Outstanding sustainable results	All components of the change package implemented, all goals of the aim are accomplished, outcome measures at national benchmark levels, and spread to a larger population begins.

experienced in improvement for the VBTS. However, teams in both the VBTS and the BTS made significant improvements, with reduction in days to third-next-available appointment to an average of about 10 days.

IAS Assessments

As shown in Figure 4 (page 582), average monthly VBTS assessments were comparable to those in the traditional BTS.

A follow-up study completed six months after the VBTS's conclusion showed that of the 10 teams that had achieved significant improvement (assessment of $\geq$ 4) by the collaborative's end, 7 had maintained their gains or improved their results six months later (Table 3, page 582). Figure 2 shows average waiting time data for the six months after the conclusion of the VBTS (July through December 2005).

Discussion

This demonstration project shows that the VBTS collaborative achieved results that are comparable to those of a traditional collaborative on the same topic and at significantly reduced costs for both the participating and host organizations. However, further testing and refinement of the VBTS model, as well as ongoing comparison with traditional face-to-face collaboratives should help establish over time the conditions under which the VBTS can continue to achieve similar results to the traditional method. For example, in this first test of the VBTS, the number of teams was limited to 20, and faculty and staff with proven track records were selected to lead this work. In addition, the topic and measures selected were mature and robust. We recommend that future tests of the VBTS add more wide-ranging conditions such as a greater number of teams, less-experienced faculty, and use of a

Joint Commission™ Journal on QUALITY and PATIENT SAFETY

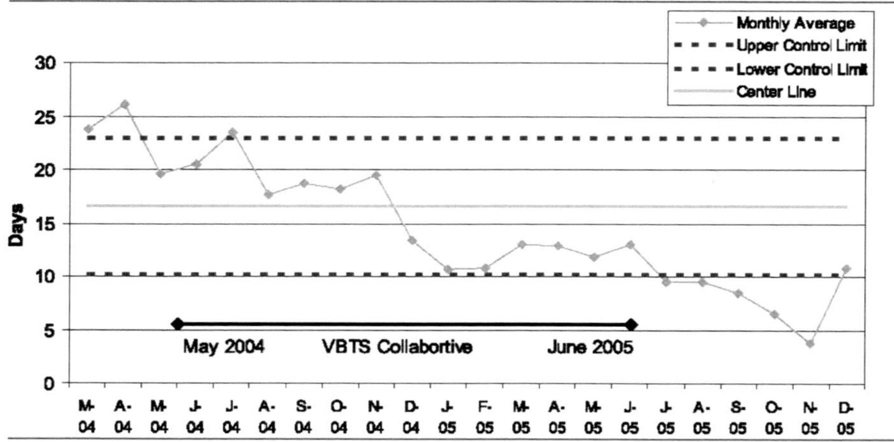

Figure 2. *In the Virtual Breakthrough Series (VBTS) collaborative, the average number of days to third-next-available appointment fell from 23 days to 10 days during 12 months (60% reduction).*

less-developed topic. By testing the VBTS under broader conditions, an even more robust model should emerge.

Because the results from this first VBTS are comparable to those of the traditional BTS model on the same topic, the business impact is based on potential cost savings not benefits. For a participating organization, the expected savings in direct costs that can be realized from participation in a VBTS and not having to travel to sessions is $11,979 (Table 4, page 582). These potential differences in cost are associated with the three LSs (since the action periods and other work do not differ between the models). Reductions in costs are achieved by not using staff time to travel to LSs and by not incurring travel costs. Newly incurred costs, however, are those associated with hosting the LSs at the participant's home site and with long-distance phone charges for the LSs.

On the basis of the results from this initial demonstration, future VBTS collaboratives will require some modifications to maximize the likelihood of success and sustained improvement. Although the Web communication technology was well received by most of the participants, support is needed at local sites, both from information technology (IT) and from senior leadership. IT support must be available, especially before and at the

first LS, to ensure access and connectivity. For example, some participants were unable to get online or did not know that they could not dial long distance from their conference room. For Web-based sessions, IHI now implements connection testing, in which participants can test their audio and Web connection within a certain time interval before the actual session. Streamlining of the electronic platforms for reporting is also needed (for both VBTS and traditional BTS) to eliminate potential confusion and thus to increase reporting and participation. For example, participants were required to enter data on the extranet as well as complete a monthly progress report spreadsheet and upload this document to the extranet, which some participants felt was a bit extraneous.

Changes at the participating organizations, which are needed to help ensure success, are the same as those identified in traditional collaboratives, such as a greater involvement by senior leadership, stable staffing and balanced supply (clinician availability) and demand (for services), and a committed core group and an organized team. Even though the participants do not travel to the collaborative, time must be built in to the providers' schedules to ensure their availability when the sessions take place; clinic and personnel schedules and team members'

Journal on QUALITY and PATIENT SAFETY

workloads must be modified to accommodate these sessions and to prevent team members from being distracted to attend to local "urgent matters." Participation in distance learning may be more "invisible" and thus seem less important than traveling to meetings. The time and effort commitment for the participants are the same, except for actual travel time, but this may not be readily apparent to those outside the team.

The key success factors for teams in the VBTS, which are similar to those identified for teams in a traditional BTS, include the following:

■ Senior leader oversight, commitment, and involvement

■ High degree of physician involvement and championship of the improvements

■ Vigilance and attention to detail from the day-to-day manager of this work

■ Diligent testing and implementation of a high percentage of the change concepts

■ The ability to modify supply to balance demand during the collaborative's time frame

■ Deliberate collection and analysis of data

On the basis of these results, IHI is considering VBTS collaboratives for future projects. Larger groups will be enrolled to assess scalability, and additional topic areas will be tested to ensure generalizability. Although IHI has more to learn from further testing, we hope that other health care organizations will test the virtual approach to conduct their own collaboratives to provide more insights into the virtual model's performance.

Two VBTS Teams

Sidebar 1 (pages 583–584) highlights the work of two of the more successful teams in the VBTS. The biggest factor separating the best teams from others was the ability to balance supply and demand—that is, to make the changes necessary to bring the demand for their services in line

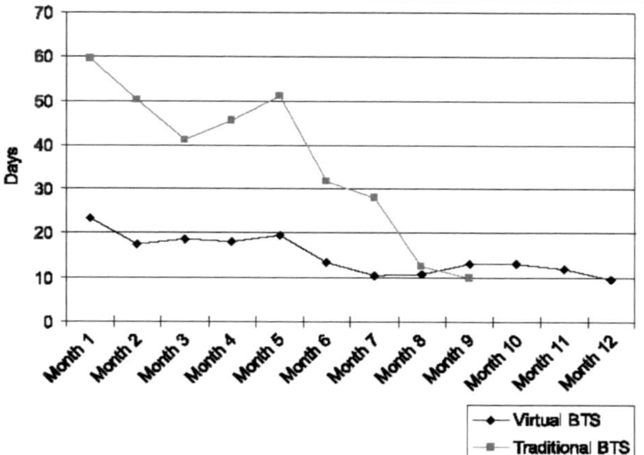

Figure 3. *The averages of this metric across participating clinicians, taken monthly, are shown. For clinicians taking multiple measurements per month, those values were aggregated (averaged) within that month before the general aggregation was made. Some clinicians did not have data for some months in the measurement period, but those clinicians' data were still included in the aggregate for periods in which they had data. Data are drawn from IHI's Improving Access and Efficiency in Primary Care BTS, October 2004–June 2005. BTS, Breakthrough Series.*

with the supply (mostly clinicians) available. Some teams were not able to make this happen completely within the collaborative's time period. Without this, it is impossible to greatly reduce or maintain the core outcome measure of days to third-next-available appointment. ∎

The work reported in this article was supported in part by a grant from the Alfred P. Sloan Foundation. The authors express their thanks to Faith McLellan, Ph.D.; Jane Roessner, Ph.D.; Val Weber, Frank Davidoff, M.D.; and Andrew Hackbarth for their assistance in the preparation and revision of this manuscript. The Institute for Healthcare Improvement is grateful to its faculty, including Mark Murray M.D., M.P.A.; Michael Davies, M.D.; and L. Gordon Moore, M.D.; Erik Bailey, technical director; and the pioneering organizations that participated in the Virtual Breakthrough Series for their support and contributions to this work.

Barbara Boushon, B.S.N., is Director, Institute for Healthcare Improvement (IHI), Cambridge, Massachusetts. **Lloyd Provost, M.S.,** is Statistician, Associates in Process Improvement, Cambridge. **Janice Gagnon** is Manager, New Product Development, and **Penny Carver** is Senior Vice President, IHI. Please address correspondence to Penny Carver, pcarver@ihi.org.

JOINT COMMISSION™ Journal on QUALITY AND PATIENT SAFETY

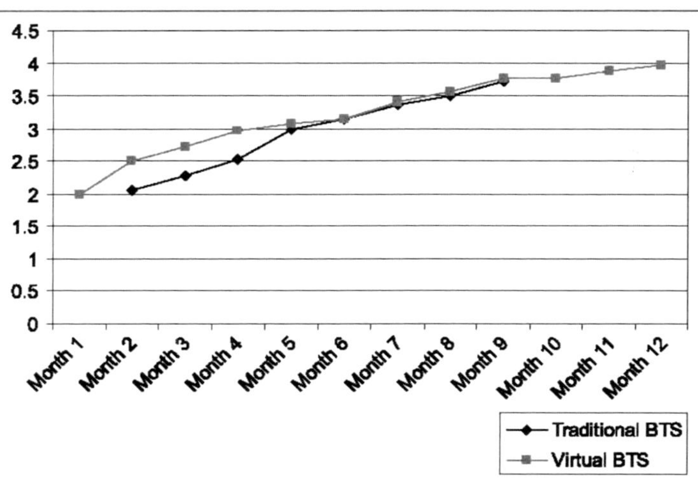

Figure 4. *Average monthly assessments were comparable between the Virtual Breakthrough Series (VBTS) and the traditional BTS. IAS, Improvement Assessment Scale.*

Table 3. Improvement Assessment Scale (IAS) Results for Virtual Breakthrough Series Teams After Six Months*

	< 4 IAS assessment at end of Collaborative	≥ 4 IAS assessment at end of Collaborative
< 4 IAS assessment six months later	3 (43%) *Still no breakthrough, but continued to improve*	2 (20%) *Did not hold gains*
≥ 4 IAS assessment six months later	0 (0%) *Breakthrough after end*	7 (70%) *Held gains*
Did not report six months later	4 (57%)	1 (10%)
Total teams	7	10

* "4" refers to the assessment in Table 3.

Table 4. Direct Cost Savings in a Virtual Breakthrough Series (VBTS) and a Traditional BTS

Cost Impact	Changes in Participant Costs	Participant	Assumptions
–	Travel costs to learning session (LS)	–$9,000	3 LSs x 3 people x $1000 = $9000
–	Time saved from not traveling to LS	–$3,600	3 LSs x 3 people x 1 day x $400 = $3,600
+	Supplies and printing costs for participants at site	+$405	($17 per person x 5 +$50 labor) x 3 LS = $405
+	Long-distance phone charges for LS ($.08–$.05/min, < $200)	+$216	3 LSs x 10 hours = $216
	Net change in participant costs	–$11,979	

JOINT COMMISSION™
Journal ON QUALITY AND PATIENT SAFETY

Sidebar 1. Two of the Virtual Breakthrough Series Collaborative Teams

**Marshfield Clinic, Indianhead Center,
Rice Lake, Wisconsin**

The pilot began with an initial group of five family practice physicians. Marshfield Clinic tested and eventually implemented the following changes, among others:

- **Synchronize patient, provider, and information:** Start every appointment on time by asking patients to arrive 15 minutes before a scheduled appointment.

- **Understand supply and demand:** The fact that Monday had much more demand than supply resulted in a change to a provider's usual day off.

- **Obtain physician and staff buy-in:** Set expectations, trained staff on the concepts of advanced access, and shared data to display positive changes for patients.

- **Assign physician champion:** Instrumental in coaching and communicating with providers the need for change and how it would benefit them.

- **Reduce the backlog:** Physicians created backlog reduction plans.

- **Used future capacity chart** to determine when several providers would be out of the office on a given day and created contingency plan.

- **Created and implemented service agreements** between primary care and specialty care offices, including urology, ENT, nephrology, and orthopedics.

After achieving same-day access, Marshfield Clinic spread the changes to all 12 family practice physicians in the clinic, plus the pediatrician. The initiative was adopted systemwide, with spread to other departments in the clinic (internal medicine, ophthalmology, urology, and surgery).

Results

Days to third-next-available appointment decreased in all departments (data not shown). In family practice and pediatrics, waiting times fell from a high of 24 days to 1 day (Figure, below).

PracticePartners, Greater Portland Medical Group, Westbrook, Maine

PracticePartners was a five-provider practice, including four physicians and one physician assistant. The physician assistant left the practice and was not replaced, which caused many access issues with appointment scheduling, telephones, and so on. PracticePartners tested and eventually implemented the following changes, among others:

- **Understand and balance supply and demand:** Provider schedules are reviewed during morning huddles and are used to anticipate needs and prevent constraints. Trends are identified and schedules are altered to satisfy demand. For example, high-demand days have fewer physicals to accommodate acute visits. Physicals are scheduled on days with lower call volume.

- **Reduce the backlog:** Providers created backlog reduction plans.

- **Reduce appointment types:** Appointment types were reduced to three types: OV15 (sick visits, follow-up visits); OV30 (male physical exams, new patients); and OV45 (female physical exams with Pap tests).

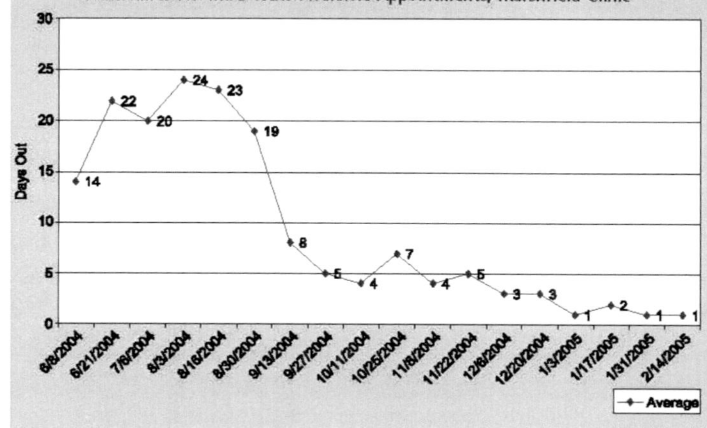

continued

Journal on Quality and Patient Safety

Sidebar 1. Two of the Virtual Breakthrough Series Collaborative Teams, *continued*

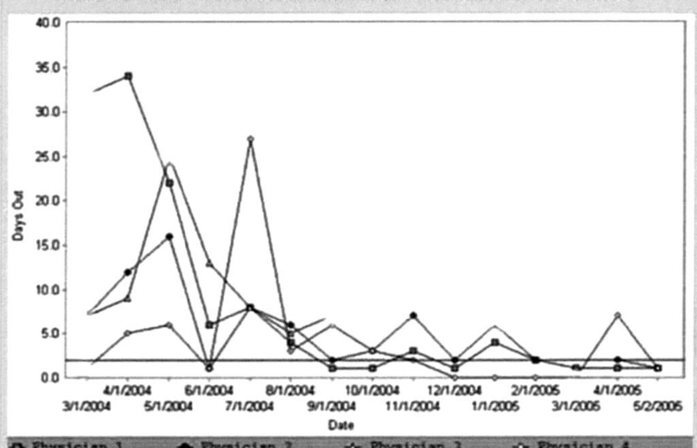

■ Develop contingency plans: Freeze providers' schedules for two weeks after doctors are on service at the hospital or on vacation. Open up first week during the last week that the provider is on service, filling in prebook slots as patients call. Open up second week the first week that the provider is back. Office also freezes some prebook slots in remaining providers' schedules to accommodate patients of the provider who is away.

Results

The practice's goal was to reduce days to third-next-available appointment to less than 1 day (when the project started, average time was 30–35 days). By the end of the VBTS, the number of days to the third-next-available appointment for all providers was less than two days (Figure, left; each line represents one physician).

The practice found that the key to success was buy-in from all physicians and staff.

References

1. Institute for Healthcare Improvement: *The Breakthrough Series: IHI's Collaborative Model for Achieving Breakthrough Improvement,* 2003. http://www.ihi.org/IHI/Results/WhitePapers/TheBreakthroughSeries IHIsCollaborativeModelforAchieving+BreakthroughImprovement.htm (last accessed Aug. 4, 2006).

2. Øvretveit J., et al.: Quality collaboratives: Lessons from research. *Qual Saf Health Care* 11:345–351, Dec. 2002.

3. Mittman B.S.: Creating the evidence base for quality improvement collaboratives. *Ann Intern Med* 140:897–901, Jun. 2004.

4. Landon E., et al.: Effects of a quality improvement collaborative on the outcome of care of patients with HIV infection: The EQHIV Study. *Ann Intern Med* 140:887–896, Jun. 1, 2004.

5. Schonlau M., et al.: Evaluation of a quality improvement collaborative in asthma care: Does it improve processes and outcomes of care? *Ann Fam Med* 3:200–208, May–Jun. 2005.

6. Horbar J.D., et al.: Collaborative quality improvement to promote evidence based surfactant for preterm infants: A cluster randomised trial. *BMJ* 329:1004, Oct. 30, 2004.

7. Cretin S., Shortell S.M., Keeler E.B.: An evaluation of collaborative interventions to improve chronic illness care: Framework and study design. *Eval Rev* 28:28–51, Feb. 2004.

8. Weeks W.B., et al.: Using an improvement model to reduce adverse drug events in VA facilities. *Jt Comm J Qual Improv* 27:243–254, May 2001.

9. Horbar J.D., et al.: Collaborative quality improvement for neonatal intensive care. NIC/Q Project Investigators of the Vermont Oxford Network. *Pediatrics* 107:14–22, Jan. 2001.

10. Flamm B.L., Berwick D.M., Kabcenell A.: Reducing cesarean section rates safely: Lessons from a "breakthrough series" collaborative. *Birth* 25:117–124, Jun. 1998.

11. Nolan T.W., et al.: *Reducing Delays and Waiting Times Throughout the Healthcare System.* Boston: Institute for Healthcare Improvement, 1996.

12. Murray M., Berwick D.M.: Advanced access: Reducing waiting and delays in primary care. *JAMA* 289:1035–1040, Feb. 26, 2003.

13. Mills P.D., Weeks W.B.: Characteristics of successful quality improvement teams: Lessons from five collaborative projects in the VHA. *Jt Comm J Qual Saf* 30:152–162, 2004.

14. Institute for Healthcare Improvement: *How to Improve.* http://www.ihi.org/IHI/Topics/Improvement/ImprovementMethods/HowToImprove/ (last accessed Aug. 4, 2006).

15. Palloff R., Pratt K.: *Building Learning Communities in Cyberspace.* San Francisco: Jossey-Bass Publishers, 1999.

16. Aragon S.R. (ed): Facilitating Learning in Online Environments. *New Directions for Adults and Continuing Education,* no. 100, Winter 2003.

The Joint Commission Journal on Quality and Patient Safety

Timeliness and Efficiency

Providing Timely Access to Care:
What is the Right Patient Panel Size?

Linda V. Green, Ph.D.
Sergei Savin, Ph.D.
Mark Murray, M.D., M.P.A.

Difficulty in obtaining a timely appointment to see a physician is a common problem. In one study, 33% of patients cited "inability to get an appointment soon" as a significant obstacle to care,[1] and the Institute of Medicine has identified "timeliness" as one of the six key "aims for improvement" in its major report on quality of health care.[2]

Primary Care and Advanced Access

For most patients, their primary care physician is their major access point into the health care system. Yet primary care practices often have long waits for appointments and may have difficulty in accommodating patients who have potentially urgent problems. As a result, patients experience delays in treatment and may be seen by someone other than their own physician, potentially leading to adverse clinical consequences, patient dissatisfaction, and loss of revenue for the practice. Large backlogs may require additional staff and resources to deal with patients trying to get appointments for the same day and are often correlated with a high rate of cancellations or "no-shows," which can result in lost income and wasted capacity.[3]

To remedy this problem, some primary care practices have adopted a patient scheduling approach known as *advanced access*. As opposed to a "traditional" system where each physician's daily schedule is fully booked in advance or a "carve-out" model in which a fixed number of appointment slots are held open for urgent cases, the goal of the advanced access approach is to reduce delays by offering every patient a same-day appointment, regardless of the urgency of the problem. The fundamental idea behind advanced access is to "do all of today's work today"

Article-at-a-Glance

Background: Delays for appointments are prevalent, resulting in patient dissatisfaction, higher costs, and possible adverse clinical consequences. A "just-in-time" approach to patient scheduling, called advanced access, has been effective in reducing delays in multiple clinical settings. Offering most patients appointments on the same day requires achieving an appropriate balance between supply of and demand for appointments, but no methods have been previously proposed to determine what this balance should be.

Methods: A measure of balance is termed the *overflow frequency level*—the fraction of days when demand exceeds the average number of appointment slots available. A probability model was developed to estimate this measure for any practice. The model can be used in identifying an appropriate panel size or, conversely, the physician capacity needed to provide timely access.

Results: Delays for appointments will be excessive unless the ratio of the average daily demand for appointments to the average daily capacity is less than one. This ratio's appropriate value is dependent on the desired *overflow frequency level*, which indicates the fraction of days for which physician overtime would be necessary to offer most patients same-day appointments. A table provides suggested panel sizes for a range of practice types, and a spreadsheet file is available on request to help determine panel size or physician capacity in any specific situation.

Conclusion: The simple probability model can be used to improve the timeliness of care while considering the constraints on physicians' working hours.

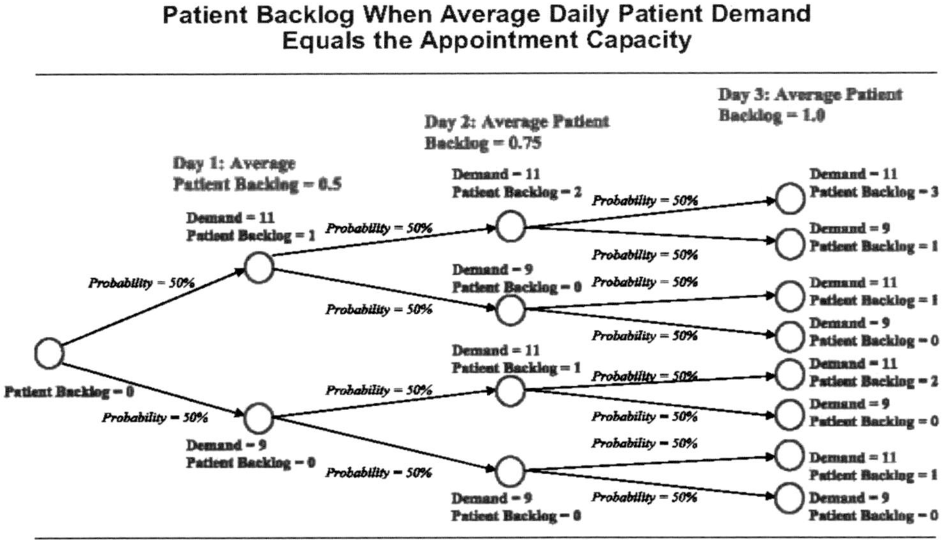

The Joint Commission Journal on Quality and Patient Safety

Patient Backlog When Average Daily Patient Demand Equals the Appointment Capacity

Figure 1. *The example illustrates the growing patient backlog in the case when average daily patient demand equals the appointment capacity.*

so that patients don't have to wait for appointments, practices don't waste capacity holding appointments in anticipation of same-day needs, and patients have a greater likelihood of seeing their own physician. Several success stories have documented the benefits of this approach in both managed care and fee-for-service environments, including dramatically shorter waits, higher levels of continuity of care, less wasted capacity for the practice, and increased patient, staff, and physician satisfaction.[3]

Advanced access can only work if patient demand for visits and physician capacity to see patients are "in balance." Advocates of advanced access have identified several ways in which the number of visits can be reduced, physician time can be better leveraged, and scheduling practices can be streamlined so as to achieve a better balance between supply and demand.[3,4] However, in discussions with practitioners, we have found that questions remain about what constitutes an appropriate balance and, more specifically, what is a "manageable" panel size. The answers to these questions are not obvious and require a quantitative approach.

The Need for "Safety" Capacity

A fundamental feature of patient demand for primary care is its random nature: the actual number of patients requesting care on any particular day will vary around the average daily value, sometimes substantially. It is this inherent randomness that makes it difficult to determine the answers to questions such as: "How large a panel size can be served by a given physician practice?" If not for this variability in demand, the answer would be obvious—the panel size would be the one that made the daily demand for care equal to the daily number of physician appointment slots available. However, with this variability, making supply and demand equal on average would create chronic backlogs for care and waits for appointments that would likely get longer and longer.[5] Although this characteristic of service systems has been known to operations professionals for decades, it may seem counterintuitive. A simple example, illustrated in Figure 1 (above), may help explain this critically important concept.

Consider a primary care practice that has a daily patient demand for appointments that takes on only two

The Joint Commission Journal on Quality and Patient Safety

possible values—11 and 9, each with 50% probability. Suppose the maximum number of patients that can be seen each day is exactly equal to 10, so that any "excess" demand must be pushed to the next day that has available appointment slots. Figure 1 illustrates all possible realizations of patient backlog values for a period of three days, assuming we start with no backlog. As shown, the average backlog grows from 0.5 patients at the end of the first day to 0.75 at the end of the second day to 1.0 at the end of the third day. If this exercise is carried out further, the average patient backlog will continue to grow from day to day. This may be surprising because it seems logical to assume that "bad" days, that is, days with a demand of 11, will be balanced out by "good" days, those with only 9 new patient demands.

So why doesn't this balancing out happen? As our simple example shows, when patient demand is less than the appointment capacity, *the extra service capacity cannot be transferred to the next day* to serve future patient demand and is therefore lost. On the other hand, on the "bad" days, when patient demand exceeds service capacity, the unserved demand does not disappear and has to be satisfied in the future. So "good" days cannot clear the backlog created by the equal number of "bad" days. Furthermore, if the demand variability is increased, for example, by adding possible demands of 8 and 12 patients, the average backlog will grow faster.

Thus, if the goal is to provide immediate access to care with a high probability, then the average daily demand for appointments must be *strictly less* than the maximum capacity to see patients. Another way of saying this is that there must be some *safety capacity* relative to demand. Safety capacity, the amount of capacity in excess of average demand, serves as a hedge against demand variability. Without it, a practice will be unable to offer timely care to its patients.

Finding the Right Balance Between Supply and Demand

How much safety capacity does any specific practice need? This depends primarily on the desired *overflow frequency level*—the percentage of days when demand exceeds the number of appointment slots for that day. In the example illustrated in Figure 1, the overflow frequency is 50%. The lower the overflow frequency level, the easier it will be to

offer same-day appointments by occasional use of physician overtime. Decreasing the overflow frequency level can only be accomplished by increasing the safety capacity. However, more safety capacity also means more days and hours when physicians are not seeing patients. So the "right" level of safety capacity for any given office must be a subjective determination that will likely be based on the trade-off between the revenue associated with seeing more patients and the amount of overtime the practice is willing to undertake to keep patient delays minimal. To evaluate the possible trade-offs, it is necessary to understand the relationship between safety capacity, patient panel size, and overflow frequency.

A Modeling Approach

Safety capacity can be created by either increasing physician capacity or decreasing demand. Physician capacity may be increased by adding appointment slots to the day, and demand might be reduced by using tactics such as greater use of telephone and e-mail and the use of group visits. However, panel size is the major determinant of demand and the prime lever for achieving the right balance between supply and demand.

We have developed a simple quantitative model to help evaluate the trade-offs associated with a given panel size. Since the only objective of the model is to help identify a good balance of overall supply and demand for a given practice, it is not necessary for the model to distinguish between "external" demands, that is, those that are generated by patients' actions, and "internal" demands, that is, those that are the result of the physician's decision to see a patient for follow-up work or chronic care. No matter the source of the demand, all demands must be satisfied in a timely fashion, and doing so requires a panel size that allows for sufficient safety capacity.

The model does not address the "micro-management" issues such as daily scheduling of follow-up visits, dealing with cancellations, or scheduling of physicians' office hours and vacations. Although these are all important factors for the efficient functioning of the practice, they do not significantly affect the best choice of panel size and so are not needed in our "macro" model. We will revisit these issues later in the article.

Although about $^2/_3$ of all primary care physicians work in group practices,[6] a number of studies[7-10] have

The Joint Commission Journal on Quality and Patient Safety

documented the benefits of continuity of care. These observations support the view that a patient should be seen, whenever possible, by his or her physician, and therefore, that a panel should be associated with an individual physician. However, as described later, our approach can easily be extended to allow for determining a panel size for multiple physicians working as a team.

Finding the Right Panel Size

Establishing an appropriate panel size for an existing practice consists of the following six steps:
1. Identifying the current panel size
2. Estimating the daily visit rate per patient
3. Fixing the number of daily appointment slots
4. Calculating the current overflow frequency
5. Setting the target overflow frequency
6. Computing the panel size based on the target flow frequency

Steps 5 and 6 can be done iteratively to identify a desirable trade-off between panel size and overflow frequency.*

1. IDENTIFYING THE CURRENT PANEL SIZE

In many managed care practices, the patient panel size N_{cur} is simply the number of patients enrolled with a physician. However, in fee-for-service or mixed practices, the number of patients "on file" may be misleading because it is not uncommon to preserve files for patients who may no longer be using the practice's services. In these situations, it has been found that the panel size will be most accurately estimated by calculating the total number of distinct patients seen by a physician in the last 18 months. (Use of a year may underestimate the effective panel size, whereas the two-year count typically produces an overestimated value[4]).

In a multiphysician practice, estimating the current panel size for each physician may be more complicated because a given physician's patient may see another physician if his or her preferred provider is unavailable. Therefore, in these practices, it is important to track for each physician the number of requests for appointments rather than the number of actual visits.

*A spreadsheet file that provides all necessary computations for these six steps is available from the authors by e-mail request.

2. ESTIMATING THE DAILY VISIT RATE PER PATIENT

The most accurate assessment of daily demand requires prospective measurement of the specific appointment dates that patients actually ask for, including walk-ins (external demand), as well as the follow-up visit dates that physicians actually request (internal demand). If prospective data are not available, an estimate can be obtained by examining appointment logs for a recent period of time, for example, 18 months, and counting the number of appointments over that period of time.

Let T be the number of working days for the period of time being examined and let A be the number of patient appointments (or, if available, requests for appointments) for those T days. Then, as shown in Figure 2 (page 215), the daily visit rate per patient p is calculated by dividing A by the product of the number of patients on the current panel, N_{cur} and T: $p = \dfrac{A}{N_{cur} \times T}$

For example, consider a general/family practitioner with a current panel of $N_{cur} = 2500$ patients who had $A = 6500$ office visits during the last 18 months ($T = 315$ days). For this practice, $p = \dfrac{A}{N_{cur} \times T} = \dfrac{6500}{2500 \times 315} = 0.008$ visits/day per patient.

3. ESTABLISHING THE NUMBER OF DAILY APPOINTMENT SLOTS

The average daily supply of appointment slots, C, is determined by the average length of an appointment slot and the average daily number of hours devoted to direct patient care. So if a physician spends an average of 7 hours per day in patient care and appointments are scheduled 20 minutes apart, the daily appointment capacity is $C = 7$ hours $\times$ 3 appointments/hour = 21 appointments. If a practice has a varying number of appointment slots per day during the week, C should be the *average* number of slots per day.

4. CALCULATING THE OVERFLOW FREQUENCY

Consider a practice with panel size N and with daily demand rate p. If each patient request for care is generated independently of any other patient's request, the total daily demand for primary care services on any given day can be modeled as a *binomial* random variable with expectation equal to Np and variance equal to $Np(1-p)$. The binomial random variable with parameters N and $0 < p < 1$ describes the random number of "successes" in N independent trials when the probability of success in any single trial is p. In

The Joint Commission Journal on Quality and Patient Safety

the primary care environment, this binomial random variable corresponds to the number of appointment requests that a patient panel of size N generates on a given day. (A more detailed description of the properties of the binomial random variable can be found, for example, in Bertsekas and Tsitsiklis.[11])

Using this model and the number of appointment slots each day C, we can estimate the effect of *any* panel size on the overflow frequency by calculating the probability that the demand for appointments exceeds the supply of slots on any given day, as illustrated by the formula in Figure 3 (page 216). Using this formula with $N = 2700$, $p = 0.008$, and $C = 21$, results in an estimated overflow frequency of 49.4%.

6. Computing the Appropriate Panel Size

For a practice that operates five days a week, an overflow frequency of 49.4% implies that to avoid patient delays, the physician will need to see patients during "overtime" more than twice a week on average. It is important to note that the higher the overflow frequency, the greater the average backlog and so the longer the overtime needed to "do today's work today." For the parameters used in the previous example, the average duration of overtime when it occurs can be shown to be more than an hour. It is also important to understand that because overtime frequency is a long-term average, in any given week it could be considerably higher, leading not only to substantial overtime but long backlogs for appointments as well.

So, in our example, the current panel size would need to be reduced to be able to comfortably and consistently offer same-day appointments. This does not mean that the panel size would need to be small enough to lead to a near-zero likelihood of overflow frequency. Infrequent overflows, for example, 5%, 10%, or even 20%, are likely to be small enough that they can usually be handled with occasional and modest levels of overtime and therefore not jeopardize future appointment capacity. On the other hand, the smaller the overflow frequency, the lower will be the average daily utilization of the practice, pN/C. In selecting a target panel size and therefore a target level of overflow frequency, a physician should take into account

Calculation of the Daily Demand Rate for a Panel of Current Size N_{cur}

Calculating the daily demand rate for a panel of current size N_{cur}

1. Choose an observation period (for example, 18 months) and calculate the number of working days T within this period.

2. Count the number of patient visits, A, over those T days.

3. The daily demand rate for appointments (per day per patient) is

$$p = \frac{A}{N_{cur} \times T}, \text{ where } N_{cur} \text{ is the current panel size.}$$

Figure 2. *The calculation of the daily demand rate for a panel of current size N_{cur} is shown.*

his or her own tolerance for overtime work—5% (approximately once a month), 10% (once in two weeks), or 20% (once a week).

If the current panel size results in an overflow frequency that is too high, as in our example, a more appropriate panel size can be found by decreasing it and recalculating the overflow frequency using the formula in Figure 3. On the other hand, if the computed overflow frequency is lower than desired, the panel size should be adjusted upward. This process of adjustment and recalculation should be repeated until the overflow frequency computed for the trial value of the panel size is close enough to the desired overflow frequency.

Consider our previous example with initial panel size of 2,700 and assume that the desired overflow frequency level is 20%. Because the computed current value of the overflow frequency (49.4%) is much higher than the target, we might try a panel size of $N = 2000$. Using the Figure 3 calculation for this value of N, we obtain an overflow frequency of 8.8%, which is lower than our target. So on the next iteration, we can try a somewhat larger panel, $N = 2300$, which produces an overflow frequency of 22.8%. Because this is an estimate, this is probably sufficiently close to the target to be considered a good choice. Alternately, continuing iterations, one discovers that for the panel size of $N = 2250$ the overflow frequency comes very close to 20%.

Examples Based on Other Data

Table 1 (page 217) shows the patient panel sizes (and attained utilizations) for a "typical" general and family

The Joint Commission Journal on Quality and Patient Safety

Calculation of the Overflow Frequency

Calculating the overflow frequency

If the daily patient demand is modeled as a binomial random variable with parameters N (panel size) and p (demand rate), the probability that the number of patients will exceed the number of available slots C (overflow frequency) can be calculated as :

$$\text{Overflow frequency} = 1 - (1-p)^N - \sum_{k=1}^{C} \frac{(N-k+1)(N-k+2)\times...\times N}{1\times 2\times...\times k} p^k (1-p)^{N-k}$$

where k is the index of summation.

This expression can also be rewritten as

$$\text{Overflow frequency} = 1 - (1-p)^N - \frac{N}{1} p(1-p)^{N-1} - \frac{N(N-1)}{1\times 2} p^2 (1-p)^{N-2}$$

$$- \frac{N(N-1)(N-2)}{1\times 2\times 3} p^3 (1-p)^{N-3} - ... - \frac{N(N-1)(N-2)...(N-C+1)}{1\times 2\times 3\times...\times C} p^C (1-p)^{N-C}$$

Figure 3. *The calculation of the overflow frequency—the fraction of days when demand exceeds the average number of appointment slots available—is shown.*

practitioner (on average, 1.575 annual visits per patient,* according to Murray and Berwick[4]) and a "typical" pediatrician (on average, 1.98 annual visits per child according to the 2002 NAMCS[5]), which would result in an overflow frequency of 5% (approximately, once a month), 10% (twice a month), or 20% (once a week). The 2002 NAMCS reported that the average duration of the "face-to-face" part of the office visit is 16.1 minutes for general/family and pediatrics practices, 18.1 minutes for obstetrics/gynecology (OB/GYN) practices, and 20.0 minutes for internal medicine practices. In our calculations we considered appointment intervals of 20 minutes. Under the assumption of an 8-hour workday (for a 5-day work week this roughly corresponds to the 40.2 hours spent by a family physician on direct patient care or patient-related service during a complete week of practice[12]), this results in 24 daily appointment slots. Because the actual daily appointment capacity is likely to be somewhat lower, we also consider a daily capacity of 20 appointment slots. The calculations were performed using the formula in Figure 3 under the assumption of 210 work days per year. This value, in our estimate, is a good representation of the annual number of work days for a large number of primary care practices.

Adjusting Supply for a Fixed Panel Size

Although the above analyses addressed the issue of determining panel size, the same approach can be used to determine appropriate physician capacity for a given panel size. For the case where continuity of care is considered important, capacity will be the number of daily appointment slots needed by a single physician to handle the proportion of the panel that represents his or her patients. This can be done by using the binomial formula in Figure 3 to assess the overflow that would result from each possible alternative and choosing the minimum number of slots that keeps the overflow within a "tolerable" limit. In a multiphysician setting where continuity is not considered critical, the daily capacity would be the number of slots per day for each physician multiplied by the number of physicians, and the analysis would be done using the possible alternatives as before. It is important to note that the total panel size that can be handled by a group practice in which continuity of care is not considered paramount will likely be significantly larger than the sum of the individual panel

* Although the National Ambulatory Medical Care Survey Series (NAMCS) 2002 survey reports the total number of annual visits to general and family practitioners in the United States (215,466,000), the annual visit rate per patient is not easy to estimate because we could not find reliable statistics on the number of people who actually use (or even have) a primary care physician. The rate of 0.761 annual office visits per person, reported in NAMCS 2002 survey, was obtained by dividing the total number of visits to general and family practitioners by the entire size of the United States population (283,135,000), taken from 2000 U.S. Census data. Clearly, using this value would result in a gross underestimation of actual patient visit rates. The rate we use (1.575 annual visits per patient) is calculated on the basis of the assumption of 210 annual in-office days and on the assumption (used in Murray and Berwick[4]) that in an average patient panel not overly weighted with elderly and chronically ill patients, 0.07%-0.08% of patients will request a visit on an average day. We note that this estimate is somewhat higher than the 0.05% figure used by Smoller (Smoller M.: Telephone calls and appointment requests: Predictability in an unpredictable world. *HMO Practice* 6:25–29, Jun. 1992.)

The Joint Commission Journal on Quality and Patient Safety

Table 1. Panel Sizes (Capacity Utilizations) for Different Parameter Values, Primary Care Type: General and Family Practice and Pediatrics*				
	General and Family Practice		**Pediatrics**	
	Daily Appt. Slots = 24	Daily Appt. Slots = 20	Daily Appt. Slots = 24	Daily Appt. Slots = 20
Overflow frequency = 5%	2321 (73%)	1879 (70%)	1848 (73%)	1496 (70%)
Overflow frequency = 10%	2515 (79%)	2053 (77%)	2002 (79%)	1635 (77%)
Overflow frequency = 20%	2765 (86%)	2279 (85%)	2200 (86%)	1813 (85%)

* Appt., appointment

sizes of the individual physicians in the practice if the goal is that patients see their preferred physician with high probability.

Achieving the Right Balance

The analyses provided can be easily modified for any particular physician practice. This requires that data be collected to accurately assess both supply and demand. As Murray and Berwick point out,[4] historical visit data may be misleading because they measure activity that may be less than actual demand if a practice has experienced lost and deferred demands. Therefore, it is important that demand be measured prospectively. In doing so, both weekly and seasonal patterns should be considered to identify times of particularly high (and low) levels of demand.

For example, there may be several months each year with particularly high demand because of flu season. In this case, accurate records of demand are important to estimate a seasonally adjusted patient visit rate per day, which can then be used in the binomial model to help identify capacity needs during these times. Physician supply can then be adjusted accordingly if part-time physicians are available. Vacation times and other activities should be scheduled during lower-demand seasons and days if possible to ensure sufficient capacity during higher-demand times. In addition, it is important to identify the fraction of the demand that can be managed to offset the variability in the unscheduled demand.[3] Patients who need follow-up appointments should be scheduled early in the day on

lower demand days and/or during lower demand times of the year. Of course, in any given practice, there will be constraints on both physician and patient scheduling and the above guidelines are just that—goals to work toward. To the extent that they can be followed, daily delays for appointments will be reduced.

Conclusion

Ensuring timely access to medical care is an important goal for any physician practice and advanced access requires some specific guidance in achieving it. However, the variability inherent in the demand and delivery of health care makes it impossible to determine specific answers to questions about panel size or, conversely, physician practice size by using guesswork or intuition. In this article, we have described a simple probability model that can be used to supplement the qualitative approach of advanced access to make major improvements in the timeliness of care while considering the constraints on physicians' working hours. ∎

Linda V. Green, Ph.D., is Armand G. Erpf Professor and **Sergei Savin, Ph.D.,** is Associate Professor, Columbia Business School, Columbia University, New York City. **Mark Murray, M.D., M.P.A.,** is Principal, Mark Murray & Associates, Sacramento, California. Please address correspondence to Linda V. Green, lvg1@columbia.edu.

93

The Joint Commission Journal on Quality and Patient Safety

References

1. Strunk B.C., Cunningham, P.J.: Treading Water: Americans' Access to Needed Medical Care, 1997-2001. Washington, D.C.: Center for Studying Health System Change, Mar. 2002. http://www.hschange.com/CONTENT/421/?words (last accessed Feb. 6, 2007).

2. Institute of Medicine: Crossing the Quality Chasm: A New Health System for the 21st Century. Washington, D.C.: National Academy Press, 2001.

3. Murray M., Tantau C.: Same-day appointments: Exploding the access paradigm. Fam Pract Manag 7:45-50, Sep. 2000.

4. Murray M., Berwick D.M.: Advance access: Reducing waiting and delays in primary care. JAMA 289:1035-1040, Feb. 26, 2003.

5. Hall R.: Queueing Methods for Services and Manufacturing. Englewood Cliffs, N.J.: Prentice Hall, 1991.

6. Hing E., Cherry D.K., Woodwell D.A.: National Ambulatory Medical Care Survey: 2002 Summary. Advance Data from Vital and Health Statistics; No. 346. Hyattsville, MD: National Center for Health Statistics, 2004.

7. Christakis D.A., et al.: The association between greater continuity of care and timely measles-mumps-rubella vaccination. Am J Public Health 90:962-965, Jun. 2000.

8. Becker M.H., Drachman R.H., Kirscht J.P.: Continuity of pediatrician: New support for an old shibboleth. J Pediatr 84:599-605, Apr. 1974.

9. Gill J.M., Mainous A.G.: The role of provider continuity in preventing hospitalizations. Arch Fam Med 7:352-357, Jul.–Aug. 1998.

10. Gill J.M., Mainous A.G. III, Nsereko M.: The effect of continuity of care on emergency department use. Arch Fam Med 9:333-338, Apr. 2000.

11. Bertsekas D.P., Tsitsiklis J.N.: Introduction to Probability. Boston: Athena Scientific Publishing, 2002.

12. American Academy of Family Physicians: About Us: Table 14. Average number of patient contact hours per week by family physicians, May 2005. http://www.aafp.org/online/en/home/aboutus/specialty/facts/14.html (last accessed Feb. 6, 2007).

AHA Consensus Statement

Recommendation to Develop Strategies to Increase the Number of ST-Segment–Elevation Myocardial Infarction Patients With Timely Access to Primary Percutaneous Coronary Intervention

The American Heart Association's Acute Myocardial Infarction (AMI) Advisory Working Group

Alice K. Jacobs, MD, FAHA, Chair; Elliott M. Antman, MD, FAHA; Gray Ellrodt, MD; David P. Faxon, MD, FAHA; Tammy Gregory; George A. Mensah, MD, FAHA*; Peter Moyer, MD; Joseph Ornato, MD, FAHA; Eric D. Peterson, MD, FAHA; Larry Sadwin; Sidney C. Smith, MD, FAHA

Abstract—Although evidence suggests that primary percutaneous coronary intervention (PCI) is the preferred reperfusion strategy in the majority of patients with ST-segment–elevation myocardial infarction (STEMI), only a minority of patients with STEMI are treated with primary PCI, and of those, only a minority receive the treatment within the recommended 90 minutes after entry into the medical system. Market research conducted by the American Heart Association revealed that those involved in the care of patients with STEMI recognize the multiple barriers that prevent the prompt delivery of primary PCI and agree that it is necessary to develop systems or centers of care that will allow STEMI patients to benefit from primary PCI. The American Heart Association will convene a group of stakeholders (representing the interests of patients, physicians, emergency medical systems, community hospitals, tertiary hospitals, and payers) and quality-of-care and outcomes experts to identify the gaps between the existing and ideal delivery of care for STEMI patients, as well as the requisite policy implications. Working within a framework of guiding principles, the group will recommend strategies to increase the number of STEMI patients with timely access to primary PCI. (***Circulation.*** 2006;113:2152-2163.)

Key Words: AHA Consensus Statements ■ myocardial infarction ■ revascularization ■ quality of health care ■ triage

Mounting evidence from randomized trials suggests that for patients with ST-segment–elevation myocardial infarction (STEMI), primary percutaneous coronary intervention (PCI) is superior to fibrinolytic therapy alone in reducing the composite end points of death, reinfarction, intracranial bleeding, reocclusion of the infarct artery, and recurrent ischemia. The benefits of primary PCI are greatest if it is performed in an expeditious manner after the onset of symptoms. This requires a highly coordinated effort, especially when interhospital transport is needed to provide PCI.[1,2] In the United States, however, only a minority of patients with STEMI receive primary PCI, and in those who

do, fewer than 40% are treated within 90 minutes after arrival at the initial hospital as recommended (as a goal) by the American College of Cardiology (ACC)/American Heart Association (AHA) guidelines.[3] Given that the majority of hospitals do not have PCI capability, physicians, hospitals, and the Department of Public Health in several states have been faced with the challenge of providing primary PCI to STEMI patients in a timely fashion. In fact, several regions have established both triage and transfer protocols for PCI in patients with STEMI.[4,5]

The AHA, which is dedicated to reducing disability and death due to cardiovascular diseases and stroke, has recog-

*The opinions expressed in this manuscript are those of the authors and should not be construed as necessarily representing an official position of the Centers for Disease Control and Prevention, the United States Department of Health and Human Services, or the United States Government.

The American Heart Association makes every effort to avoid any actual or potential conflicts of interest that may arise as a result of an outside relationship or a personal, professional, or business interest of a member of the writing panel. Specifically, all members of the writing group are required to complete and submit a Disclosure Questionnaire showing all such relationships that might be perceived as real or potential conflicts of interest.

This statement was approved by the American Heart Association Science Advisory and Coordinating Committee on February 28, 2006. A single reprint is available by calling 800-242-8721 (US only) or writing the American Heart Association, Public Information, 7272 Greenville Ave, Dallas, TX 75231-4596. Ask for reprint No. 71-0360. To purchase additional reprints: up to 999 copies, call 800-611-6083 (US only) or fax 413-665-2671; 1000 or more copies, call 410-528-4121, fax 410-528-4264, or e-mail kramsay@lww.com. To make photocopies for personal or educational use, call the Copyright Clearance Center, 978-750-8400.

Expert peer review of AHA Scientific Statements is conducted at the AHA National Center. For more on AHA statements and guidelines development, visit http://www.americanheart.org/presenter.jhtml?identifier=3023366.

Circulation is available at http://www.circulationaha.org   DOI: 10.1161/CIRCULATIONAHA.106.174477

nized the unmet need in the care of many of the nearly 400 000 patients per year with STEMI in the United States and the potential benefits of regionalized care.[6,7] Therefore, the AHA convened a multidisciplinary group of experts, the Acute Myocardial Infarction (AMI) Advisory Working Group (AWG), to develop recommendations for a strategy to increase the number of STEMI patients with timely access to primary PCI and to explore the role the AHA should play in this endeavor. After review of the state of the science and the current status of reperfusion therapy in the United States (below), the AWG recommended that the AHA commit to exploring both systems and centers of care that would allow more rapid access to primary PCI for a greater number of patients. In this context, *systems* are defined as integrated, regionalized groups of separate entities that provide specific services for the system, which could include tertiary centers, community hospitals, emergency medical services (EMS) providers, and others. *Centers* are defined as entities that provide patient care services for a specific specialty or service, such as a community or tertiary hospital. The attainment of this goal will likely require cross-system regional collaboration that may or may not be in the interest of a single provider. Accordingly, this initiative could benefit from the attention, motivation, and expertise of the AHA. PricewaterhouseCoopers (PwC) was selected to prepare a report on the desirability, feasibility, and potential effectiveness of establishing (regional) systems and/or centers of care for STEMI patients with a focus on whether and how this might improve patient access to quality care and outcomes. The primary goal of the report was to assist the AHA in developing its position and role in defining the optimal care for patients treated with primary PCI.

After analysis of PwC's findings, the AWG recommended that the AHA convene all the stakeholders involved in the care of patients with STEMI to begin to discuss the issues involved in expanding access to timely primary PCI. This will be accomplished at a 3-day conference in Boston, Mass, beginning on March 30, 2006. The AWG then developed a list of principles (below) to guide the AHA in leading this initiative.

The purpose of this report is to briefly summarize the evidence supporting primary PCI as the preferred reperfusion strategy for patients with STEMI, share the market research supporting the development of systems and centers of care, define the guiding principles that will serve as the basis and framework for all subsequent discussions and recommendations, and issue a "call to action" to convene all constituents involved in the care of STEMI patients at the AHA conference, "Development of Systems of Care for STEMI Patients."

State of the Science

Reperfusion with either fibrinolytic therapy or PCI early after the onset of coronary occlusion in patients with STEMI has been shown unequivocally to improve short- and long-term patient outcomes.[8] Despite that evidence, several large-scale registries have reported that strategies for reperfusion therapy are not well implemented in many countries.[9,10] In the United States, approximately one third of patients with STEMI do not receive any reperfusion therapy despite its availability

and the absence of any contraindication.[11] Furthermore, disparities exist with regard to delivery of reperfusion therapy, with lower rates reported for women and for black patients.[12,13]

The ability to achieve timely reperfusion for patients with STEMI is limited by the patient's ability to recognize their symptoms and to promptly contact the medical system, the time necessary to transport the patient to the hospital, the decision process on arrival, and the requisite time to implement the reperfusion strategy (Figure). Multimedia public education campaigns and community intervention programs aimed at reducing patient delay between symptom onset and hospital presentation and at increasing activation of EMS have not yet proven sufficiently effective.[14,15] Rapid transport of patients with STEMI to the most appropriate facility is hampered by several factors: A minority (10%) of EMS systems have 12-lead ECG capabilities[16]; a minority (4% to 5%) of EMS patients with chest pain have STEMI[17]; a mandate exists to deliver the patient to the nearest facility even when fibrinolysis may be contraindicated and the facility does not provide primary PCI; and transport times may be long in rural areas. If a patient is brought to a non–PCI-capable facility and primary PCI is necessary, it is not unusual for the patient to wait for the next available ambulance to gain access to PCI. Furthermore, critically ill patients often require stabilization before transport.

The decision about the appropriate reperfusion modality is most often made at the receiving facility. Even at institutions that frequently use both strategies, the decision process can be delayed, particularly if primary PCI is not routinely available at all times.[18] In addition, primary PCI has been underutilized in patients with cardiogenic shock and in those with contraindications to fibrinolytic therapy. Finally, relatively late presentation after symptom onset, comorbid conditions, the absence of chest pain, and presentation during off-hours have been reported to increase the time to reperfusion.[19]

Fibrinolytic Therapy Versus Primary PCI

The AWG reviewed the status of both pharmacological and catheter-based reperfusion therapy to identify the gaps between the current system and the ideal system(s) of care that will be developed, to recognize a subset of patients (ie, in rural areas) that may not be able to obtain timely PCI despite implementation of ideal systems, and to attempt to decrease the number of patients who do not receive any reperfusion therapy. This group also thoroughly reviewed the ACC/AHA Guidelines for the Management of Patients With STEMI and noted that the guidelines writing committee concluded that it was not possible to produce a simple algorithm for a reperfusion strategy given the heterogeneity of patient profiles and availability of resources in various clinical settings at various times of day.[20] The overarching recommendation from the ACC/AHA STEMI guidelines writing committee was for healthcare providers to aggressively attempt to minimize the time from entry into the medical system to implementation of the reperfusion strategy. This is best accomplished using the concept of medical system goals (Figure).

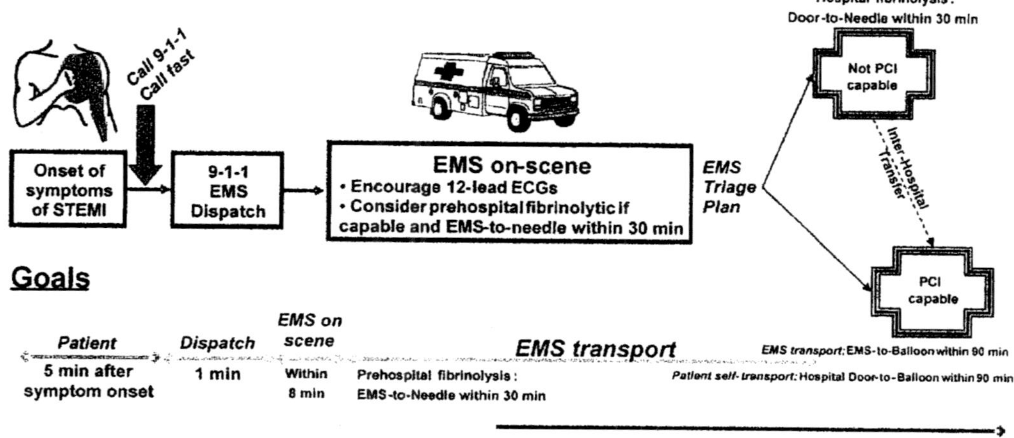

***Golden Hour = First 60 minutes**

Options for transportation of patients with STEMI and initial reperfusion treatment (reproduced with permission from Antman et al[20]).

To facilitate rapid initiation of reperfusion therapy, the medical system goal for patients receiving fibrinolysis is a door-to-needle (or medical contact–to-needle) time of within 30 minutes; for those undergoing PCI, a door-to-balloon (or medical contact–to-balloon) time of <90 minutes is recommended.[20] No evidence exists that there is a threshold effect for the benefit of shorter times to reperfusion, which underscores the fact that the goals delineated in the STEMI guidelines are not "ideal" times but rather the longest times that should be considered acceptable by the medical system. Another important physiological principle is that the goal of reperfusion is to restore flow in the infarct artery not only as quickly as possible but also as completely as possible, which includes attaining enhanced myocardial perfusion in the infarct zone.[21] A variety of treatments are used for both pharmacological and catheter-based methods of reperfusion to optimize epicardial and myocardial reperfusion.

Comparisons of pharmacological and PCI strategies in the literature are confounded by a number of methodological difficulties. For example, an overview of 23 trials that compared fibrinolysis with PCI had a total sample size of only 7739 patients and spanned a 10- to 15-year period that concluded before the advent of substantial improvements in both pharmacological and PCI strategies. These limitations notwithstanding, the rate of the composite end point of death/myocardial infarction/cerebrovascular accident was 13% in the fibrinolysis trials and 8% in the PCI trials, which represents a 5% absolute risk difference and a 38% relative risk difference (*P*<0.0001). Much of the difference in this composite end point was driven by the rate of recurrent myocardial infarction, although there was a significant difference in both short- and long-term mortality.[1]

When selecting the type of reperfusion strategy, clinicians have to consider 4 critical questions[20]:

1. *The time from onset of symptoms.* Data exist that indicate that there is a time-dependent decrease in the efficacy of fibrinolytic therapy after the onset of symptoms.[22] In contrast, the ability to produce a patent infarct artery is much less dependent on symptom duration in patients undergoing primary PCI, although mortality is time dependent even with PCI.[20] However, the delay to PCI should be considered even in patients who present relatively late (>2 to 3 hours) after the onset of symptoms.

2. *The risk of STEMI.* The benefit of primary PCI rises with increasing risk of STEMI. When the estimated mortality in patients treated with fibrinolysis is extremely high, as in the setting of cardiogenic shock, compelling evidence exists that favors the PCI strategy. As the estimated mortality rate with fibrinolysis declines, the relative mortality advantage of PCI also declines, with equipoise being attained at approximately a 3% estimated mortality rate with fibrinolysis.[23]

3. *Risk of fibrinolytic therapy.* When both fibrinolysis and PCI are available, the higher the patient's risk of bleeding with fibrinolytic therapy, the more strongly the decision should favor PCI.[20] However, it is important to consider relative versus absolute contraindications to fibrinolytic therapy, particularly in patients in whom timely access to primary PCI is not currently feasible. In addition, in the setting of cardiogenic shock, fibrinolytic therapy is less effective.[20]

4. *Time required for transport to a skilled PCI laboratory.* Critical to the success of the PCI-based strategy are the experience and location of the PCI laboratory, as well as the experience of the operator. Trials that support an advantage of PCI over fibrinolysis were performed in centers with highly experienced teams committed to a rapid delivery of reperfusion therapy. For example, in the DANAMI-2 (DANish trial in Acute Myocardial Infarction-2) and PRAGUE-2 (PRimary Angioplasty after

transport of patients from General community hospitals to catheterization Units with/without Emergency thrombolytic infusion-2) studies, patients who were transferred from community hospitals to an invasive center underwent PCI with a door-to-balloon time that averaged 26 minutes once they arrived at the invasive center.[24,25] The time for transportation from the community hospital to the invasive center averaged 32 minutes in DANAMI-2 and 48 minutes in PRAGUE-2. By contrast, reports from the National Registry of Myocardial Infarction in the United States for patients with STEMI who undergo transfer for PCI show an unacceptably long time between initial presentation at the first hospital to balloon inflation at an invasive center, at a median of 180 minutes.[19] This is composed of a median of 120 minutes for decision making in the first hospital plus transportation and arrival in the PCI hospital, and 53 minutes between PCI hospital arrival and balloon inflation. An additional report from the National Registry of Myocardial Infarction that evaluated the times to implementation of reperfusion strategies during regular work hours versus off-hours and for weekday (Monday through Friday) versus weekend (Saturday or Sunday) presentations showed important differences between fibrinolytic therapy and PCI.[26] The door-to-needle time during regular hours was 33.2 minutes and increased slightly to 34.3 minutes during off-hours. In contrast, door-to-balloon times during regular hours were 94.8 minutes but increased by 21.3 minutes to 116.1 minutes during off-hours. Longer off-hours door-to-balloon times were primarily due to a longer interval between obtaining the ECG and patient arrival at the catheterization laboratory.

A relationship between the onset of symptoms and the time to initiation of reperfusion has been established previously for fibrinolytic-treated patients. Although the data remain somewhat controversial, the bulk of the evidence also suggests that prolonged times from symptom onset to balloon inflation are associated with an increased risk of mortality.[20] The Zwolle Group reported, after adjustment for baseline characteristics, that each 30-minute delay between the onset of symptoms and balloon inflation was associated with a relative risk of 1-year mortality of 1.08 ($P=0.04$).[27] Furthermore, it has been reported that in patients undergoing primary PCI at a single center between 1984 and 2003, door-to-balloon times ≥ 2 hours versus <2 hours were associated with a higher mortality at 7 years in high-risk but not in low-risk patients and in patients who presented early (≤ 3 hours) but not in those who presented late (>3 hours) after symptom onset.[28]

Healthcare systems in many communities have adopted a variety of approaches for more timely delivery of reperfusion therapy for STEMI. Those communities that are supported predominantly by single, close-knit EMS and ambulance systems have generally adopted the practice of obtaining a prehospital 12-lead ECG and then initiating prehospital fibrinolysis, except for patients for whom PCI would clearly be preferable (eg, those with cardiogenic shock).[29] Other communities, typically urban in location, have adopted a strategy of direct transportation for all STEMI patients to a dedicated primary PCI center that is available 24 hours a day, 7 days per week.[4]

No large-scale randomized trials comparing such reperfusion strategies have been reported to date; however, it is recognized by the writing committee for the ACC/AHA Guidelines for the Management of Patients With STEMI and the AWG that the critical considerations in the delivery of primary PCI are the interrelated issues of timeliness and access. If timely access to primary PCI is available, the evidence suggests that PCI is the preferred reperfusion strategy, especially in those presenting late after symptom onset, those who are considered high risk, and those in whom fibrinolysis is contraindicated. Thus, primary PCI is the focus of this AHA initiative. Facilitated PCI, which involves prompt performance of PCI after an initial preparatory pharmacological regimen, has not been proven to be an effective or safe alternative to primary PCI.[30] In fact, in the Assessment of the Safety and Efficacy of a New Treatment Strategy with Percutaneous Coronary Intervention trial (ASSENT-4 PCI), a randomized trial of tenecteplase before PCI versus primary PCI alone that tested the strategy of facilitated PCI in patients with STEMI, the primary end point of death, heart failure, and shock at 90 days was significantly higher in patients treated with combination therapy.[31] A hybrid approach, referred to as a pharmacoinvasive reperfusion strategy, that involves initial treatment with fibrinolytic therapy followed routinely by cardiac catheterization and PCI as indicated on a nonurgent basis has also been proposed as an approach to reperfusion for STEMI,[8] but at the present time, the evidence supporting such a strategy is not robust.

Market Research Findings

Given the evidence that timely performance of primary PCI is superior to fibrinolytic therapy in the majority of patients with STEMI, the future design for the provision of cardiac services will play a critical role in providing prompt access to this therapy. However, it is anticipated that multiple barriers and problems will be encountered if the current environment is disrupted by the establishment of systems and centers of care, particularly to the degree that those systems exclude certain providers. Spending and utilization growth have made cardiac services a multibillion dollar business and a critical component of the operations of acute care providers. In many urban hospitals, cardiac-related diagnosis and treatment account for roughly 40% of net revenues. These financial trends have fueled cardiac competition among hospitals and have resulted in an outgrowth of physician-owned cardiac specialty hospitals in several markets.

PwC was directed by the AHA to carefully explore all strategies that could potentially increase the number of STEMI patients with access to timely primary PCI with a minimum negative impact on existing care in a particular local area. Specifically, the analysis was to include an assessment of the market and financial impact for hospitals that provide these services.

Research Methods

The research approach was both qualitative and quantitative. Phone interviews and Web-based surveys were conducted to gauge support and solicit input from key stakeholders. The interview and survey instruments were designed in a collab-

TABLE 1. STEMI-Related State Statutes[36]

State	Reference	Statute
Arizona	Ariz Rev Stat §36-2205 (1998)	The Department of Health Services, in consultation with the medical director of EMS, can establish protocols relating to the transportation of patients based on the patient's condition.
Delaware	Del Code Ann tit 16, §97 (1996)	A voluntary and inclusive statewide trauma care system has been established and provides for the creation of a statewide trauma plan specifically addressing prehospital care.
Florida	Fla Stat §212.055 (2003)	Certain counties are authorized to levy surtax to fund trauma care. Florida law also sets boundaries for state trauma system plans.
Illinois	Ill Rev Stat ch 730 §5/5-9, ch 705 §105/27.6, ch 20 §3960/6.01 (1996)	The Department of Public Health will investigate a hospital in an EMS system that goes on "bypass status" to determine whether the action was reasonable. Hospitals improperly diverting will receive a fine.
Nebraska	Neb Rev Stat §71-2017 and 71-2029 (1997)	The statewide trauma system allows facilities to be designated for care based on the patient's intensity of injury.
Oklahoma	Okla Stat tit 63 §1-2530 (2003)	The Trauma Systems Improvement and Development Act requires facilities to meet standards set by the state Board of Health to designate themselves as trauma centers.

orative effort, with input from AWG members. Each instrument was pilot tested with appropriate audiences before survey launch. Additional information about the research methods and the financial modeling is included in the Appendix.

Key Findings

Policy

Certification of primary PCI centers could impact payers, especially Medicare, which is the single largest payer of cardiac services and influences how, when, and where cardiac care services are delivered. For hospitals, Medicare often represents more than half of the payer mix. The Centers for Medicare and Medicaid Services (CMS), which administers the Medicare program, has put into place pay-for-performance programs intended to align financial incentives with desired improvements in patient care. As the agency that ensures access to care for more than 40 million elderly Americans, it must consider how a diversion or certification policy might affect access to care, not only for patients with STEMI but also for those with other disorders who are currently cared for at hospitals without primary PCI capability.

The new outpatient drug benefit is expected to spike growth in Medicare spending unmatched by growth in the federal budget. Owing to this, Medicare could face budgetary pressures that may negatively impact payment for hospitals and physicians. Attempts to correct the current discrepancy in payment for procedural versus evaluation and management services that fueled the wave of new specialty hospitals may also impact cardiac services. This wave has created a debate in the industry about the quality and cost-effectiveness of specialty hospitals and their effect on community hospitals. In response to concerns raised by the American Hospital Association, Congress put an 18-month moratorium on new physician-owned specialty hospitals in place. As part of that moratorium, the Medicare Payment Advisory Commission (MedPAC),[32] the commission that advises Congress on Medicare issues, is reviewing how cardiac care should be delivered and paid for. Depending on how a system is structured,

regionalization of care for STEMI patients could put financial stress on hospitals that depend on cardiac care to subsidize unprofitable services.

Simultaneously, Congress and MedPAC[33] are interested in improving quality and moving ahead with a pay-for-performance strategy that focuses, in part, on cardiac care. For example, 5 of Medicare's 10 quality indicators focus on AMI care. MedPAC is currently reviewing the types of data collected on AMI to determine how to extend pay-for-performance metrics. Movement to a system of care for STEMI patients could be complementary to Medicare's move toward pay-for-performance if it increases quality for Medicare beneficiaries and reduces costs from unnecessary readmissions without unreasonably restricting access.

Commercial payers are also quickly moving toward pay-for-performance metrics. In fact, the Leapfrog Group has collected summaries of more than 100 pay-for-performance programs.[34] As healthcare costs increase, all payers want to see more evidence that their patients are receiving timely and appropriate care. In some cases, payers are contracting only with "centers of excellence" in an attempt to divert their patients to hospitals that provide higher quality of care. These factors will influence how a system of care for STEMI patients could be developed.

In addition to the impact of federal programs and legislation, the differing state regulatory frameworks and the landscape of "certificate of need" (CON) programs must be taken into account when one considers a primary PCI certification program. Intended to manage healthcare costs by controlling supply, CON laws provide an avenue for state health planning agencies to review access to and quality and costs of healthcare services before the development of any additional services. Approximately half the states have cardiac-specific CON requirements. CON laws regulate the number of hospitals that deliver cardiac catheterization and cardiac surgery procedures. In a state where CON is mandated for cardiac care, hospital programs must justify their community needs (eg, volume projections, use rates, and access to care), capital expenditures, staffing requirements, and impact on providers to the state health planning agency for consideration. Once

TABLE 2. Response to Interview/Survey Question: Would You/Your Organization Support the Establishment of a Certification/Designation Program for the Treatment of Myocardial Infarction Through Primary Angioplasty?

Interview/Survey Cohort	Yes, %	No, %	Don't Know, %
Physicians (n=100)	75	14	11
Urban hospitals (n=14)	72	7	21
Rural hospitals (n=5)	60	20	20
EMS (n=2)	50	0	50

TABLE 3. Operating Margin and Case-Mix Index 2002

	Overall	PCI Procedures	Cardiac Surgical Procedures
Operating margin			
Community hospitals	4.3%	3.6%	8.7%
System-affiliated hospitals		9.5%	14.1%
Case-mix index	1.3	2.7	5.9

the formal CON application is submitted, the state agency evaluates these criteria before granting an approval determination.

However, the evolution of technology in health care has resulted in a recent shift in decision making about where cardiac services can be delivered. Since 1994, 6 states have repealed their CON requirements for cardiac surgery, and in a program originally developed by the Cardiovascular Patient Outcomes Research Team (C-PORT) at Johns Hopkins Hospital and Health System, 50 hospitals from Queens, NY, to rural Massachusetts are piloting programs that allow them to perform angioplasty procedures without an on-site cardiac surgery program.[35]

A review of state EMS laws showed that 6 states have statutes relevant to primary PCI centers (mainly with regard to trauma care; Table 1).[36] These statutes will have to be considered in the approach to certification, specifically when incorporating the EMS component.

EMS regions are governed separately by state and create their own protocols. There are 329 different regions in the United States, with >993 hospital-based EMS systems.[37] Hospital-based EMS systems only make up 6.51% of the total number of EMS systems (48.6% are private, third-party systems and 44.89% are fire station based). This variation among states will add to the complexity of incorporating the prehospital component of any proposed certification program.

Stakeholder Interviews/Surveys
The majority of physicians, hospitals, and EMS officials interviewed support a primary PCI certification program. As Table 2 indicates, there was strong support among providers; however, many expressed concerns. For example, some rural hospitals, operating with fewer resources than their larger urban counterparts, are concerned about their ability to achieve certification and maintain cardiac revenue streams, an important subsidy for other service lines. Some physicians and urban hospitals questioned the need for such certification and redundancy with existing programs. Other unintended consequences discussed included a negative halo effect caused by the diversion of EMS such that hospitals without the primary PCI certification might find themselves bypassed for other services as well.

Federal policymakers interviewed shared concerns that some hospitals may see this effort as a threat that ultimately eliminates their cardiac business. Furthermore, the additional cost of another certification may not be perceived as a good investment by certain hospitals. Federal policymakers were also concerned about the potential to increase the number of

uninsured patients who are transferred to accredited centers. Specifically, certification may create "patient dumping" issues if providers use their noncertification as an excuse to transfer uninsured patients to certified centers. Such transfers under a reorganized system might allow them to avoid penalties under the Emergency Medical Treatment and Active Labor Act (EMTALA).[38]

Respondents were also questioned about the design of the potential program and specifically about a systems-versus-centers approach (ie, certification of a PCI-capable hospital). Overall, respondents did not believe access and quality were mutually exclusive and did not provide a consensus of opinions as to whether a systems or centers approach would be optimal.

The majority of respondents believed that a systems approach would increase coordination of care, reduce redundancies, and provide a consistent level of emergency care to all communities; however, they also believed that a systems approach would be difficult to implement and could lead to conflicting policies among the various providers. As noted earlier, rural respondents believed that a systems approach might exclude them in spite of the high quality of their programs.

The centers approach also received mixed reviews. Although some respondents believed that the focus of a centers approach would improve outcomes, others believed associated access issues would delay treatment and negatively impact outcomes. Others were concerned that a centers approach might shift focus from community interest to return on investment.

Respondents did agree on the impact a primary PCI certification program would have on individual healthcare stakeholders. All interview/survey cohorts agreed that the hospitals and health systems would be affected most intensely, ahead of both consumers and physicians. It was predicted that payers, both public and private, would be the least impacted. This point was validated in conversations with health plan officials who indicated that they already certify and designate centers along these lines when negotiating rates for nonacute conditions. However, it was acknowledged that payers, both public and private, would need to play a role in ensuring the viability of non-PCI/STEMI hospitals if regionalization were to be implemented.

The impact on hospitals and health systems will primarily involve a need for collaboration with their physicians to meet established certification guidelines and performance standards. When physician respondents were asked which performance standards would be most relevant for a primary PCI certification program, the most often cited responses were quality outcomes, treatment times, and volume, and the majority of hospital leaders interviewed indicated they were

TABLE 4. STEMI Certification Program Impact Study: Market Descriptions

	Small Market	Middle Market	Large Market
Market	City No. 1	City No. 2	City No. 3
Population	195 000	823 000	1 100 000
No. of hospitals	8	14	10
No. of hospitals with cardiac surgery capabilities	2	7	4
2004 Inpatient PCI volume	153	614	883

already tracking and reporting most AMI-specific outcome measures in view of the Joint Commission on Accreditation of Healthcare Organizations and CMS performance standards for AMI.

US Market Impact

Although a certification program would likely increase quality of care, it also could financially benefit hospitals that qualify for the certification and subsequently experience increased patient volume. However, it also could financially disrupt some hospitals. As previously discussed, cardiac services supplement low margins in other services for many hospitals (Table 3). The operating margin for PCI procedures was 3.6% and 9.5% for community hospitals and system-affiliated hospitals, respectively, in 2002. For comparative purposes, cardiac surgery procedures yielded an operating margin of 8.7% and 14.1%, respectively. This range compares favorably to the overall operating margin for all hospitals in the United States during 2002 (4.3%). For system-affiliated hospitals, which constitute the majority of hospitals, margins on cardiac surgical procedures are more than 3 times higher than overall margins. As such, any shift in cardiac services will have a profound financial impact. When national averages are applied to a community of system-affiliated hospitals, the loss of 100 inpatient PCI cases would create a $350 000 to $450 000 loss in contribution margin (the margin a hospital uses to offset fixed costs). A similar-volume loss of cardiac surgery procedures would result in a contribution margin loss of $1 million to $1.25 million. Under these circumstances, a hospital would be forced to absorb fixed costs in other typically less profitable service lines.

A loss of PCI or cardiac surgical volumes would lower a hospital's case-mix index, which would lower its overall Medicare reimbursement. A reduced case-mix index could also affect commercial insurance reimbursement. In all markets, reactions from the public, changes in managed care contracting practices, and the ability to reallocate or eliminate direct operating expenses will exacerbate the financial impact of program participation and volume shifts.

To better illustrate the potential outcome associated with a primary PCI certification, PwC modeled the impact on 3 distinct markets in actual cities in the United States selected on the basis of population, level of cardiac services, and number of hospitals (Table 4). The model accounted for the capacity of a system-wide approach and the various indirect financial outcomes discussed in this report. It was projected that the certification program would create a 25% shift in cardiac volumes. The 25% volume shift was used consistently

in all 3 of the market examples to demonstrate the effect of cardiac cases moving from institutions within a service area.

The small-market example currently has 8 hospitals, 2 of which are capable of performing cardiac surgery. Conservatively speaking, the total market for cardiac surgery and PCI procedures is worth approximately $2.6 million in contribution margin. If a primary PCI certification program were developed, it is likely that both of the cardiac surgery–capable institutions would be eligible for and would seek the certification. Under this set of assumptions, should just 1 facility be selected as a program participant, 25%, or $640 000, of the potential contribution margin directly attributable to cardiac and PCI procedures could change hands. Furthermore, it is highly probable that the certification would indirectly impact other cardiac services in the market. If we assume that 25% of other cardiac service volumes (cardiac catheterization procedures, other PCI procedures, cardiac medicine) would move from the other providers in the market to the selected facility, each nonselected facility would stand to lose, on average, approximately $160 000 in contribution margin.

In the middle-market example, there are 14 hospitals, 7 of which are capable of performing cardiac surgery. Conservatively speaking, the total market for cardiac surgery and PCI procedures is worth approximately $14 million in contribution margin. Again, it is likely that each of the cardiac surgery–capable institutions would be eligible for and would seek the certification. Should 3 of these facilities be selected for program participation, each of the 2 nonselected hospitals would stand to lose $700 000 in contribution margin. With the forecasted shift of 25% of other cardiac service volumes from other providers in the market to the selected facilities, each nonselected facility would stand to lose, on average, approximately $450 000 in contribution margin.

In the large-market example, there are 10 hospitals, 4 of which are capable of performing cardiac surgery. The total market for cardiac surgery and PCI procedures is worth approximately $17.6 million in contribution margin. Again, it is likely that each of these 4 institutions would be eligible for and would seek the certification. Should 2 of these facilities be selected for program participation, each of the 2 nonselected hospitals would stand to lose $1.1 million in contribution margin. If we assume that 25% of other cardiac service volumes would move from the other providers in the market to the selected facilities, each nonselected facility would stand to lose, on average, approximately $840 000 in contribution margin.

Losses of PCI and cardiac surgery volumes could have a substantial direct financial impact on community and system-affiliated hospitals. These losses would be multiplied by changes in the overall case-mix index and other indirect, or halo, effects. These changes could ultimately impact a hospital's financial viability and limit access to healthcare services in general.

Losses to individual hospitals would need to be weighed against the benefits, in terms of reduced mortality and morbidity, to the nearly 400 000 patients who experience STEMI each year in the United States, against the cost savings to the global healthcare system, and against the economic value added to the population. However, modeling lives and costs saved if more patients had access to primary

PCI will require extensive additional study and will have to be based on the ideal system(s) and centers of care recommended after stakeholder consensus has been achieved. Therefore, PwC did not perform these analyses. The AWG reviewed a report on the estimated economic gains from declining mortality in the United States in which the authors estimated that a single percent reduction in mortality from cancer or heart disease would be worth nearly $500 billion to current and future Americans.[39] If one assumes that even half of the 33% of STEMI patients who do not receive any reperfusion therapy would be able to undergo primary PCI, with an absolute risk reduction of 4% (compared with no reperfusion), then 2640 lives per year would be saved. In addition, when performed at experienced centers in a timely fashion, primary PCI, compared with fibrinolytic therapy, saves 20 lives for every 1000 patients treated.[2] If one assumes that even half of the 31% of STEMI patients who receive fibrinolytic therapy would undergo primary PCI, with an absolute risk reduction of 2%, another 1240 lives would be saved. Therefore, implementation of strategies to increase the number of patients with access to primary PCI in a timely fashion could save nearly 4000 (or more) lives per year. In fact, in a study evaluating the projected cost-effectiveness of primary PCI, it was noted that the strategy was cost-effective at hospitals with existing catheterization laboratories under a wide range of assumptions and was cost-ineffective at low-volume or redundant laboratories, which supports the regionalization of cardiac services in urban areas.[40]

Role of the AHA

The majority of respondents believed that a coordinated effort between the AHA and an independent accreditation or medical specialty society would be the optimal structure for designing the program. The groups believed that the primary focus of the AHA should be on leveraging its relationships to ensure that the appropriate people are involved. Respondents in general said that because of the local nature of health care, the program should be developed as a broad framework that could be adapted to local processes and regulations. The experience of the American Stroke Association (a division of the AHA) with stroke certification,[41] which was developed in a similar fashion, would benefit that process. Although respondents believed the AHA should be at the forefront of organizing the program, there was a consensus that it should not regulate it. Proponents believe the AHA should remain the driving force for medical science and advocacy in cardiac care and should work with a separate entity for accreditation oversight. A certification program would ultimately benefit from the AHA's ability to bring together all interested constituents and its proficiency in disseminating information through local affiliates.

Conclusions

With a recognized need to improve the care of STEMI patients from its current state, key stakeholders would support a primary PCI certification program, with the understanding that some community hospitals might experience a negative financial impact. Each of the interview cohorts had common themes that resonated throughout the facilitated discussions. Rural hospitals, which depend heavily on cardiac service revenues, are con-

cerned with their ability to maintain cardiac services under a new designation. They will likely advocate for longer ranges in transport time standards because of the greater distances between centers in rural settings. Urban hospitals believe that a certification program will assist with increasing patient volume and increased marketing efforts for their facilities. EMS providers recognize certification as an opportunity for additional training and education, both for their staff and for the hospitals. Health plans are already supporting similar programs for non-acute care providers and could use the certification program as a means to negotiate reimbursement rates.

Guiding Principles

In view of the evidence-based treatment recommendations for patients with STEMI and the demographic, political, and financial implications inherent in the establishment of systems of care to increase the number of patients with timely access to primary PCI, the AWG developed principles (below) to guide this initiative. A system of care for STEMI patients must have the following components:

1. Patient-centered care as the No. 1 priority
2. High-quality care that is safe, effective, and timely
3. Stakeholder consensus on systems infrastructure
4. Increased operational efficiencies
5. Appropriate incentives for quality, such as "pay for performance," "pay for value," or "pay for quality"
6. Measurable patient outcomes
7. An evaluation mechanism to ensure quality-of-care measures reflect changes in evidence-based research, including consensus-based treatment guidelines
8. A role for local community hospitals so as to avoid a negative impact that could eliminate critical access to local health care
9. A reduction in disparities of healthcare delivery, such as those across economic, education, racial/ethnic, or geographic lines

Next Steps: Role of AHA and Call to Action

The AWG agreed that the next step in the process after the development of this initial consensus statement was to convene a conference for all stakeholders to begin to develop an implementation plan (which may include a call for pilot studies or targeted research) for the establishment of systems (and centers) of care to increase the number of patients with timely access to primary PCI. The conference, "Development of Systems of Care for STEMI Patients," will be held in Boston, Mass, from March 30 to April 1, 2006. The goals of the conference are as follows:

1. To convene representatives from major stakeholders in the care of STEMI patients
2. To achieve consensus on the guiding principles for the establishment of a system (urban/suburban and rural) of care for STEMI patients
3. To develop the ideal implementation system from the perspective of each stakeholder (ie, patient, physician, EMS, emergency department, local hospital, tertiary center, payer) and in terms of outcomes and quality of care
4. To understand the barriers, gaps, and policy implications
5. To develop recommendations

Below is a partial list of participating key stakeholder organizations:

- *Patient:* Centers for Disease Control and Prevention; National Heart, Lung, and Blood Institute
- *Physicians:* AHA Councils on Cardiopulmonary, Perioperative, and Critical Care; Cardiovascular Nursing; Cardiovascular Surgery and Anesthesia; Clinical Cardiology; ACC; American College of Emergency Physicians; American College of Physicians; Society for Cardiovascular Angiography and Interventions; The Society of Thoracic Surgeons
- *Nurses:* AHA Council on Cardiovascular Nursing; American Association of Critical-Care Nurses; Emergency Nurses Association
- *EMS:* American Ambulance Association; Association of Air Medical Services; National Association of State EMS (NAEMS) Directors; NAEMS Physicians; National EMS Information Systems; National EMS Management Association
- *Community hospital/regional center:* National Rural Health Association; Society for Chest Pain Centers; state hospital associations
- *Payers:* Aetna; CMS; Blue Cross Blue Shield Association; United Health Care
- *Evaluation/outcomes:* AHA Quality of Care and Outcomes Research Interdisciplinary Working Group; Agency for Healthcare Research and Quality; Food and Drug Administration; Joint Commission on Accreditation of Healthcare Organizations

The AHA is issuing a call to action to improve both the implementation and the timeliness of reperfusion with primary PCI for STEMI patients in the United States. It is clear there is a need for improvement along the continuum of the treatment pathway beginning with patient education, through EMS systems, to hospital-based strategies. This initiative is fueled by the concern about the number of patients who do not receive evidence-based therapy for STEMI and by the results of market research that indicate that those involved in the care of STEMI patients support the concept of developing ideal systems of care. The AHA is committed to mobilizing healthcare providers, policy makers, and payers to explore relative advantages, costs, and implications for the global healthcare system in pursuit of improved outcomes and quality of care delivered to patients with STEMI.

Appendix

PwC's Research Methods and Sources

Hospitals interviewed included a geographically diverse population of rural and urban hospitals, including some academic medical centers. This sample included hospitals both with and without cardiac surgery capabilities. Health plan interviews were conducted to capture opinions from the largest private payers. In all, 30 interviews were conducted.

A Web-based survey was performed with a random sample of members of the AHA Council on Clinical Cardiology to gain a thorough understanding of current clinical treatment patterns for STEMI patients in markets across the United States. E-mail surveys were received from 101 respondents.

Multiple databases were used to analyze the policy landscape for STEMI care. The MediRegs database was used to conduct stored searches that examined specific key words (eg, cardiac, centers of excellence, primary angioplasty, acute myocardial infarction, heart attack, diversion protocol, bypass, cardiac systems, and certificate of need) on a weekly basis. The search spanned the entire reimbursement library, with access to more than 40 000 documents. MediRegs's reimbursement library contains Federal legislation (US Code and public laws, Code of Federal Regulations, Federal Register); CMS, Office of Inspector General (OIG), Department of Health and Human Services, Public Health Service, Occupational Safety and Health Administration (OSHA), Food and Drug Administration (FDA), CDC, Drug Enforcement Agency, Social Security Administration (SSA), Department of Defense (DOD), and state administrative codes; CMS manuals, program memos, forms, and rulings; CMS Medicaid and managed care policy; CMS contractor local medical review policies and bulletins; OIG reports, advisory opinions, fraud alerts, and corporate integrity agreements; FDA guidelines and product approvals; OSHA directives, standard interpretations, and fact sheets; SSA manuals and rulings; DOD TRICARE and CHAMPVA (Civilian Health and Medical Program of the Department of Veterans Affairs) manuals; court and administrative decisions, including all Provider Reimbursement Review Board, CMS administrator, and Departmental Appeals Board decisions and court cases back to 1991; General Accounting Office reports; and comprehensive collections of individual state legislation, HIPAA (Health Insurance Portability and Accountability Act of 1996), Prospective Payment System, EMTALA, and Stark information. In addition to the databases, the 2004 National Directory of Health Planning, Policy and Regulatory Agencies, the 15th edition published by the American Health Planning Association, was used for the CON research.

PwC's financial model analyzed a shift in cardiac volume at 25% of business by diagnosis-related groups in the following services for cardiac care: open heart (104 to 109), cardiac catheterization (124 to 125), PCI (516, 526), PTCA (517, 518, 527), and cardiac medicine (110, 111, 115 to 117, 121 to 123, 126, 127, 130 to 145). Data sources for this modeling included the following:

- 2001, 2002, and 2003: all payer state discharge data from 25 states, 2003 Medicare hospital market area file, CMS 2003
- MEDPAR (Medicare Provider Analysis and Review) data, CMS June 2002
- TEFRA (Tax Equity and Fiscal Responsibility Act of 1982) Medicare enrollment file
- 2004 and 2009 demographic projections, Solucient Market Planner Plus; Claritas Inc

Acknowledgment

The AWG, on behalf of the AHA, thanks the AHA Council on Clinical Cardiology for its strong support of this initiative and of the market research.

Jacobs et al   Strategies to Increase Access to Primary PCI in STEMI   *2161*

Disclosures

Writing Group Disclosures

Writing Group Member	Employment	Research Grant	Other Research Support	Speakers Bureau	Honoraria	Ownership Interest	Consultant/Advisory Board	Other
Alice K. Jacobs	Boston Medical Center	None	None	None	None	None	None	Wyeth
Elliott M. Antman	Brigham and Women's Hospital	Sanofi-Aventis, Merck, Eli Lilly, Genentech, Centocor, Bristol-Myers Squibb	None	None	None	None	Sanofi-Aventis, Eli Lilly	None
Gray Ellrodt	Berkshire Medical Center	None	None	None	None	None	None	None
David P. Faxon	University of Chicago	None	None	None	None	None	Sanofi, Johnson & Johnson	None
Tammy Gregory	AHA	None	None	None	None	None	None	None
George Mensah	CDC	None	None	None	None	None	None	None
Peter Moyer	Boston University School of Medicine, Boston EMS	None	None	None	None	None	None	None
Joseph Ornato	Richmond Ambulance Authority, Hanover County EMS	None	Chairman, Data/Safety Monitor Board overseeing European TROICA study (study funded by Boehringer Ingelheim)	STRIVE lecture series (sponsored by Squibb-Sanofi)	None	None	"Heartscape," Baltimore, Md; Revivant (now owned by Zoll Medical), Sunnyvale, Calif; National Registry of Myocardial Infarction (NRMI), sponsored by Genentech but run independently	None
Eric D. Peterson	Duke University Medical Center	Schering Plough, BMS/Sanofi, BMS/Merck	None	None	None	None	None	None
Larry Sadwin	Landmark Healthcare Foundation, Torbot Group	None	None	None	None	None	JCAHO: member, Public Advisory Board; National Health Council-Putting Patients First	None
Sidney C. Smith	None	None	None	None	Sanofi-Aventis, Eli Lilly, Astra Zeneca, Pfizer	None	Sanofi-Aventis, Eli Lilly, Astra Zeneca, Pfizer	None

This table represents the relationships of writing group members that may be perceived as actual or reasonably perceived conflicts of interest as reported on the Disclosure Questionnaire, which all members of the writing group are required to complete and submit.

Reviewer Disclosures

Reviewer	Employment	Research Grant	Other Research Support	Speakers Bureau/Honoraria	Ownership Interest	Consultant/Advisory Board	Other
Harlan Krumholz	Yale University School of Medicine	None	None	None	None	None	None
Raymond Gibbons	Mayo Clinic Foundation-Gonda	Radiant Medical; Boston Scientific; Boehringer Ingelheim; Spectranetics; KAI Pharmaceuticals; TargeGen; TherOx; King Pharmaceuticals	None	None	None	Hawaii Biotech; Cardiovascular Clinical Studies (WOMEN study); Consumers Union; TIMI 37A	None
Eric Bates	University of Michigan	None	None	Genentech, Boehringer Ingelheim, Roche, PDL BioPharma	None	None	None

This table represents the relationships of reviewers that may be perceived as actual or reasonably perceived conflicts of interest as reported on the Disclosure Questionnaire, which all reviewers are required to complete and submit.

2162   Circulation   May 2, 2006

References

1. Keeley EC, Boura JA, Grines CL. Primary angioplasty versus intravenous thrombolytic therapy for acute myocardial infarction: a quantitative review of 23 randomised trials. *Lancet.* 2003;361:13–20.

2. Zijlstra F. Angioplasty vs thrombolysis for acute myocardial infarction: a quantitative overview of the effects of interhospital transportation. *Eur Heart J.* 2003;24:21–23.

3. McNamara RL, Herrin J, Bradley EH, Portnay EL, Curtis JP, Wang Y, Magid DJ, Blaney M, Krumholz HM; NRMI Investigators. Hospital improvement in time to reperfusion in patients with acute myocardial infarction, 1999 to 2002. *J Am Coll Cardiol.* 2006;47:45–51.

4. Moyer P, Feldman J, Levine J, Beshansky J, Selker HP, Barnewolt B, Brown DFM, Cardoza JP Jr, Grossman SA, Jacobs A, Kerman B, Kimmelstiel C, Larson R, Losordo D, Pearlmutter M, Pozner C, Ramirez A, Rosenfield K, Ryan TJ, Zane RD, Cannon CP. Implications of the mechanical (PCI) vs thrombolytic controversy for ST segment elevation myocardial infarction on the organization of emergency medical services: the Boston EMS experience. *Crit Path Cardiol.* 2004;3:53–61.

5. Henry TD, Unger BT, Sharkey SW, Lips DL, Pedersen WR, Madison JD, Mooney MR, Flygenring BP, Larson DM. Design of a standardized system for transfer of patients with ST-elevation myocardial infarction for percutaneous coronary intervention. *Am Heart J.* 2005;150:373–384.

6. Topol EJ, Kereiakes DJ. Regionalization of care for acute ischemic heart disease: a call for specialized centers. *Circulation.* 2003;107:1463–1466.

7. Jacobs AK. Primary angioplasty for acute myocardial infarction: is it worth the wait? *N Engl J Med.* 2003;349:798–800.

8. Antman EM, Van de Werf F. Pharmacoinvasive therapy: the future of treatment for ST-elevation myocardial infarction. *Circulation.* 2004;109:2480–2486.

9. Eagle KA, Goodman SG, Avezum A, Budaj A, Sullivan CM, Lopez-Sendon J; GRACE Investigators. Practice variation and missed opportunities for reperfusion in ST-segment–elevation myocardial infarction: findings from the Global Registry of Acute Coronary Events (GRACE). *Lancet.* 2002;359:373–377.

10. French WJ. Trends in acute myocardial infarction management: use of the National Registry of Myocardial Infarction in quality improvement. *Am J Cardiol.* 2000;85:5B–9B.

11. Fox KA. An international perspective on acute coronary syndrome care: insights from the Global Registry of Acute Coronary Events. *Am Heart J.* 2004;148:S40–S45.

12. *National Healthcare Quality Report, 2005.* Rockville, Md: Agency for Healthcare Research and Quality; 2005. Available at: http://www.ahrq.gov/qual/nhqr05/nhqr05.htm. Accessed January 25, 2006.

13. Vaccarino V, Rathore SS, Wenger NK, Frederick PD, Abramson JL, Barron HV, Manhapra A, Mallik S, Krumholz HM; National Registry of Myocardial Infarction Investigators. Sex and racial differences in the management of acute myocardial infarction, 1994 through 2002. *N Engl J Med.* 2005;353:671–682.

14. McGinn AP, Rosamond WD, Goff DC Jr, Taylor HA, Miles JS, Chambless L. Trends in prehospital delay time and use of emergency medical services for acute myocardial infarction: experience in 4 US communities from 1987–2000. *Am Heart J.* 2005;150:392–400.

15. Luepker RV, Raczynski JM, Osganian S, Goldberg RJ, Finnegan JR Jr, Hedges JR, Goff DC Jr, Eisenberg MS, Zapka JG, Feldman HA, LaBarthe DR, McGovern PG, Cornell CE, Proschan MA, Simons-Morton DG; for the REACT Study Group. Effect of a community intervention on patient delay and emergency medical service use in acute coronary heart disease: the Rapid Early Action for Coronary Treatment (REACT) Trial. *JAMA.* 2000;284:60–67.

16. Canto JG, Rogers WJ, Bowlby LJ, French WJ, Pearce DJ, Weaver WD. The prehospital electrocardiogram in acute myocardial infarction: is its full potential being realized? National Registry of Myocardial Infarction 2 Investigators. *J Am Coll Cardiol.* 1997;29:498–505.

17. Weaver WD, Eisenberg MS, Martin JS, Litwin PE, Shaeffer SM, Ho MT, Kudenchuk P, Hallstrom AP, Cerqueira MD, Copass MK, Kennedy JW, Cobb LA, Ritchie JL. Myocardial Infarction Triage and Intervention Project–phase I: patient characteristics and feasibility of prehospital initiation of thrombolytic therapy. *J Am Coll Cardiol.* 1990;15:925–931.

18. Nallamothu BK, Wang Y, Magid DJ, McNamara RL, Herrin J, Bradley EH, Bates ER, Pollack CV Jr, Krumholz HM; National Registry of Myocardial Infarction Investigators. Relation between hospital specialization with primary percutaneous coronary intervention and clinical outcomes in ST-segment elevation myocardial infarction: National Registry of Myocardial Infarction-4 analysis. *Circulation.* 2006;113:222–229.

19. Nallamothu BK, Bates ER, Herrin J, Wang Y, Bradley EH, Krumholz HM; NRMI Investigators. Times to treatment in transfer patients undergoing primary percutaneous coronary intervention in the United States: National Registry of Myocardial Infarction (NRMI)-3/4 analysis. *Circulation.* 2005;111:761–767.

20. Antman EM, Anbe DT, Armstrong PW, Bates ER, Green LA, Hand M, Hochman JS, Krumholz HM, Kushner FG, Lamas GA, Mullany CJ, Ornato JP, Pearle DL, Sloan MA, Smith SC Jr. ACC/AHA guidelines for the management of patients with ST-elevation myocardial infarction: a report of the American College of Cardiology/American Heart Association Task Force on Practice Guidelines (Committee to Revise the 1999 Guidelines for the Management of Patients With Acute Myocardial Infarction). 2004. Available at: http://www.acc.org/clinical/guidelines/stemi/index.pdf. Accessed August 24, 2005.

21. Gibson CM. Has my patient achieved adequate myocardial reperfusion? *Circulation.* 2003;108:504–507.

22. Boersma E, Maas AC, Deckers JW, Simoons ML. Early thrombolytic treatment in acute myocardial infarction: reappraisal of the golden hour. *Lancet.* 1996;348:771–775.

23. Kent DM, Schmid CH, Lau J, Selker HP. Is primary angioplasty for some as good as primary angioplasty for all? *J Gen Intern Med.* 2002;17:887–894.

24. Andersen HR, Nielsen TT, Rasmussen K, Thuesen L, Kelbaek H, Thayssen P, Abildgaard U, Pedersen F, Madsen JK, Grande P, Villadsen AB, Krusell LR, Haghfelt T, Lomholt P, Husted SE, Vigholt E, Kjaergard HK, Mortensen LS; DANAMI-2 Investigators. A comparison of coronary angioplasty with fibrinolytic therapy in acute myocardial infarction. *N Engl J Med.* 2003;349:733–742.

25. Widimsky P, Budesinsky T, Vorac D, Groch L, Zelizko M, Aschermann M, Branny M, St'asek J, Formanek P; PRAGUE Study Group Investigators. Long distance transport for primary angioplasty vs immediate thrombolysis in acute myocardial infarction: final results of the randomized national multicentre trial–PRAGUE-2. *Eur Heart J.* 2003;24:94–104.

26. Magid DJ, Wang Y, Herrin J, McNamara RL, Bradley EH, Curtis JP, Pollack CV Jr, French WJ, Blaney ME, Krumholz HM. Relationship between time of day, day of week, timeliness of reperfusion, and in-hospital mortality for patients with acute ST-segment elevation myocardial infarction. *JAMA.* 2005;294:803–812.

27. De Luca G, Suryapranata H, Ottervanger JP, Antman EM. Time delay to treatment and mortality in primary angioplasty for acute myocardial infarction: every minute of delay counts. *Circulation.* 2004;109:1223–1225.

28. Brodie BR, Hansen C, Stuckey TD, Richter S, Versteeg DS, Gupta N, Downey WE, Pulsipher M. Door-to-balloon time with primary percutaneous coronary intervention for acute myocardial infarction impacts late cardiac mortality in high-risk patients and patients presenting early after the onset of symptoms. *J Am Coll Cardiol.* 2006;47:289–295.

29. Danchin N, Blanchard D, Steg PG, Sauval P, Hanania G, Goldstein P, Cambou JP, Gueret P, Vaur L, Boutalbi Y, Genes N, LaBlanche JM; USIC 2000 Investigators. Impact of prehospital thrombolysis for acute myocardial infarction on 1-year outcome: results from the French Nationwide USIC 2000 Registry. *Circulation.* 2004;110:1909–1915.

30. Keeley EC, Boura JA, Grines CL. Comparison of primary and facilitated percutaneous coronary interventions for ST-elevation myocardial infarction: quantitative review of randomised trials. *Lancet.* 2006;367:579–588.

31. Assessment of the Safety and Efficacy of a New Treatment Strategy with Percutaneous Coronary Intervention (ASSENT-4 PCI) Investigators. Primary versus tenecteplase-facilitated percutaneous coronary intervention in patients with ST-segment elevation acute myocardial infarction (ASSENT-4 PCI): randomised trial. *Lancet.* 2006;367:569–578.

32. MedPAC. March 2005: Report to the Congress: Physician-Owned Specialty Hospitals. Washington, DC: Medicare Payment Advisory Commission; 2005.

33. MedPAC. March 2005: Report to the Congress: Medicare Payment Policy. Washington. DC: Medicare Payment Advisory Commission; 2005.
34. The Leapfrog Group. Incentives and reward compendium guide and glossary. Available at: www.leapfrog.org/compendium. Accessed May 24, 2005.
35. Aversano T, Aversano LT, Passamani E, Knatterud GL. Terrin ML, Williams DO. Forman SA; Atlantic Cardiovascular Patient Outcomes Research Team (C-PORT). Thrombolytic therapy vs primary percutaneous coronary intervention for myocardial infarction in patients presenting to hospitals without on-site cardiac surgery: a randomized controlled trial. *JAMA*. 2002;287:1943–1951.
36. National Conference of State Legislatures, 2005. Available at: http://www.ncsl.org. Accessed June 27, 2005.
37. National Association of State EMS Directors, 2004. Available at: www.jems.com/resources. Accessed July 13, 2005.
38. Emergency Medical Treatment and Active Labor Act (EMTALA). A resource for current information about the Federal Emergency Medical Treatment and Active Labor Act, also known as COBRA or the Patient Anti-Dumping Law. Maintained by Garan Lucow Miller, P.C.. a Michigan law firm. Available at: http://www.EMTALA.com. Accessed July 11, 2005.
39. Picker L. The value of health and longevity. National Bureau of Economic Research Web site. Available at: http://www.nber.org/digest/dec05/w11405.html. Accessed June 29, 2005.
40. Lieu TA, Gurley RJ, Lundstrom RJ. Ray GT. Fireman BH. Weinstein MC, Parmley WW. Projected cost-effectiveness of primary angioplasty for acute myocardial infarction. *J Am Coll Cardiol*. 1997;30: 1741–1750.
41. Schwamm LH, Pancioli A. Acker JE III. Goldstein LB, Zorowitz RD, Shephard TJ, Moyer P, Gorman M. Johnston SC, Duncan PW, Gorelick P, Frank J, Stranne SK, Smith R, Federspiel W. Horton KB, Magnis E, Adams RJ; American Stroke Association's Task Force on the Development of Stroke Systems. Recommendations for the establishment of stroke systems of care: recommendations from the American Stroke Association's Task Force on the Development of Stroke Systems. *Circulation*. 2005;111:1078–1091.

The Joint Commission Journal on Quality and Patient Safety

Timeliness and Efficiency

Improving Access to Specialty Care

Mark F. Murray, M.D., M.P.A.

Waits and delays plague health care systems worldwide. Surveys have demonstrated that wait times for most specialists exceed those for primary care practices, and, dependent on the location and the specific specialty, average five weeks for nonurgent appointments.[1] These delays lead to widespread dissatisfaction and mistrust on the part of patients, demoralization of staff and providers; adverse clinical outcomes, increased cost because of rework and redundancy, the overuse of precious resources to triage patients, high fail-to-keep appointment rates, and suboptimum revenue.[2-15] Typically, patients are seen, screened, and referred from other more primary venues of care, such as primary care, emergency department (ED), or an urgent care center, which determine that more specialized care is needed for diagnosis or treatment, yet an extended wait is a major barrier to care.[16-18]

In addition, with increased delay into any component of the specialty care practice, systemwide workload increases. The delay increases phone calls to primary care and to specialty care, increases the requirement for use of resource as "triage," and increases cancellations and no-shows as well as unnecessary visits. Although the most perceptible delay in specialty care is the delay for an initial appointment, specialists inhabit systems of care that are fraught with other patient delay: at the ED, from the ED to the hospital bed or intensive care unit (ICU), from the ICU to hospital bed, as well as delays at testing, procedure, and surgical venues.[19-21]

Delays occur as a result of a mismatch of demand for service and supply of service or as a result of flow variation on the demand or supply sides. Specialty care providers live in a world of "supply competition," with numerous activities and duties competing for limited provider supply. This

Article-at-a-Glance

Background: Waits and delays plague health care systems worldwide, and wait times for most specialists exceed those for primary care practices. In office-based practices, the provider office presence is not diluted by competing indispensable activities, and the demand for service is most often for a single type, or stream, of office-based appointment demand. In the more complex specialty practices, however, the demand streams for office visits and other services compete for provider time and dilute the supply of office visits.

Seven Flow Strategies, with a Focus on the Initial Appointment: Seven strategies for reduction of delay can be applied, not only at all steps in patient flow and for all demand streams but also at all steps (for example, office visit, diagnostic procedure, surgery, follow-up) and within all specialty care types and ranges of practice. Each specialty care practice will need to discover how to use the basic principles and implement customized solutions within its own unique environment. Although it is ultimately critical to eliminate the delays in all streams of service, the focus is on the application of change strategies at the initial step between primary care and all specialty care practice types. The strategies are (1) balance supply and demand at each step in the chain, (2) work down the backlog, (3) reduce appointment types, (4) independent contingency planning for all variation, (5) reduce the demand for visits, (6) increase the supply, and (7) improve the efficiency of the office work flow.

Summary: Specialists support various, distinct demand streams that require demand/supply balance to achieve optimal system performance. If demand/supply balance exists within any stream, waits can be minimized, and the practice can choose time frames within which to balance workload.

125

107

The Joint Commission Journal on Quality and Patient Safety

Table 1. Glossary of Terms	
System	A series of processes ordered in such a way as to achieve an aim.
Closed System	A system that has a closed, fixed enrollment, where there is a mandatory care relationship.
Open System	A system where patients, primarily due to their insurance or coverage plans, have a choice, and may or may not choose to seek a care relationship with these particular doctors.
Process	A series of tasks ordered in such a way as to achieve a specific aim; a set of processes makes up a system.
Smooth	No delays and maximum value.
Demand Streams	Distinct types of demand that require a distinctly different supply to resolve; the distinctly different supply could be a different room, a different provider, a provider doing a different kind of work, a different amount of time, a different venue, or different equipment.
External Demand	Demand generated outside the practice from referring doctors or referring venues, or directly from that population. This is demand that the practice does not directly control.
Internally Generated Demand	Return visits. Demand generated from inside the practice.
Packaging	Appropriate work-up.
Balance Box	Time frame within which the practice chooses to achieve balance of demand and supply.
Common-cause Variation	Random variation that occurs randomly in a system; cannot be controlled.
Special-cause Variation	Variation that is not inherent to the system; can be anticipated and controlled.
Backlog	Reservoir of waiting patients. Work in progress.
Provider Office Supply	The amounts of time providers spend in the office. The resource (supply) left over after all other indispensable duties is accounted for.

article explores this competition and the deeper system effects of delay to show how the initial delay "into the specialty practice"—that is, associated with the patient's access to specialty care—can be reduced.

Delays in Specialty Care

Multiple interventions, primarily focusing on "scheduling systems," have been attempted, resulting in the proliferation of multiple appointment types and guidelines, rules for demand management, increased triage and gatekeeping, and the use of mid-level providers as intermediaries. None of these interventions have succeeded in significantly altering the patient experience of delay.[22–38]

Recently, Schall et al., using principles previously developed to address delays in primary care practices, demonstrated improvements in waits and delays in both primary and specialty care settings in Veterans' Administration (VA) practices.[16] Because of the specific nature of the VA environment—primarily salaried physicians and a "closed" system (Table 1, above), this work has not been considered universally applicable.

By using the same principles with modification for each specific environment, "open" systems—generally, health care organizations with nonsalaried clinicians and a wider range of patient choice about specialists—have attained even more impressive achievements in their efforts to reduce delays. These organizations, by focusing on the various duties competing for provider (supply) time, have developed a deeper understanding that the wait time between primary care and specialty care represents one wait in a series of system steps. Isolated optimization of this step could have an adverse effect on overall system performance by "solving" the wait at the initial step while pushing the wait time deeper into the system.

Access to care in the specialty arena requires looking at patients' initial passage into specialty care, as well as analyzing their entire journey across specialty care services. Although patients, referring providers, and specialty care staff are frequently frustrated by long waits at the initial care step, specialists themselves are often inundated with another set of competing tasks: procedures, testing, surgery—both operating room (OR) or ambulatory surgery center, and ED and "on-call" coverage. Performance of these duties often takes precedence over office-based appointments. Because delays for much of this work is deemed intolerable, specialists focus their attention on these deeper system responsibilities, relegating office visits to a lower priority. Thus, office visit appointments are the point in the system

The Joint Commission Journal on Quality and Patient Safety

Table 2. Why Do Queues Form?	
Demand > Supply	When demand for service is greater than supply of service, a waiting time will ensue. Example: if daily demand is 10 units of service and daily supply is 10 units of service, there will be no waiting time. If daily demand is 11 and daily supply is 10, each day one more patient will wait.
Variation in Either Demand or Supply	If the average demand is 10 and the average supply is 10, but supply or demand is variable, a waiting time will ensue. If daily demand ranges between 5 and 15 and supply is fixed at 10, 5 units of supply go unused on days when demand is 5. On days when demand is 15 and supply is fixed at 10, 5 demand units wait. Because unused supply cannot be passed forward, variation creates an inevitable waiting time. Supply variation (e.g., the specialist cancels appointments due to emergency surgery) is more common than demand variation and creates most specialty care office delays.
Paradigm	In health care, an accepted paradigm goes: if the patient is really sick and can prove it, that patient is prioritized into a line with a short wait. Patients who cannot prove they are really sick are placed in a line with a longer wait. This prioritization inevitably lengthens delays for less acute patients.
Use of a buffer	In many specialty care environments, queues are used as a buffer for assurance of revenue or to guard against the risk of unused supply. While the attempt to get "100% utilization" seems efficient, this buffering strategy is often costly and wasteful, creating rework and redundancy, adding to fail to keep rates, and diverting resources to "triage" patients into urgent and nonurgent queues.

where the queues inevitably form. Reasons for the formation of queues are shown in Table 2 (above).

Demand Streams in Primary and Specialty Care

The single term *specialty care* obscures the wide range of dynamics at work in these practices. In office-based practices, the provider office presence is not diluted by competing indispensable activities, and the demand for service is most often for a single type of office-based appointment demand (single demand stream). Within that demand stream there is competition, of course, between new patient visits and return visits. In the more complex specialty practices, however, the demand streams for office visits and other services compete for provider time and dilute the supply of office visits.

The fundamental dynamic in primary care and the entire range of specialty care practices is the same: demand for services, whether these services are multiple or single, has to be balanced by a corresponding supply or resource for optimal system performance. The range of complexity is determined by the number of distinct types of work or demand streams addressed by the practice. Thus, some specialty care practices with a minimal number of distinct types of work (for example, dermatology with a primary focus on office workload and office procedure) act more like primary care than the more complex specialty care practices with more distinct streams of demand (for example, obstetrics/gynecology with streams of office work, "on-call" function, deliveries, OR, ambulatory surgery center, hospital, and other procedures.)

The provider office supply in specialty care, then, is the total provider supply minus the supply or resource required to support the nonoffice activities deeper inside the flow system. The competition between the various demand streams and even within the demand streams (new versus return, for example) compounded by demand variation, contributes to turbulence, unpredictability of flow, and delays. For long-term viability, any system requires a balance of the sum of the demand stream work with a sum of the supply available to support that demand. All the competing streams need an aggregate balance. Without that overall balance, and even if one stream is permanently imbalanced, an increasing wait time will be inevitable. At the same time, most specialty care practices do have an overall balance, as manifested by relatively stable but persistent wait times that fluctuate between the various and competing demand streams. For example, the delay for an appointment may be shortened but, at the same time, the delay for a surgical procedure will be lengthened, and then this situation reverses itself. The overall delay, however, remains lengthy, but persistent and stable, implying that overall demand is balanced by supply but the delivery of the service is delayed.

Practice complexity is directly related to the number and variety of competing demand streams. The strategies

The Joint Commission Journal on Quality and Patient Safety

for improvement in each stream are the same, although the specific applications of those principles often differ.

Seven Flow Strategies, with a Focus on the Initial Appointment

The seven strategies for reduction of delay, developed and derived from observation of such leading businesses as Toyota, Starbucks, and Amazon.com, and that match demand for service to supply of service, can be applied not only at all steps in patient flow and for all demand streams but also at all steps (for example, office visit, diagnostic procedure, surgery, follow-up) and within all specialty care types and ranges of practice. Each specialty care practice will need to discover how to use the basic principles and implement customized solutions within its own unique environment. Although it is ultimately critical to eliminate the delays in all streams of service, this article focuses on how the change strategies are applied at the initial step between primary care and all specialty care practice types. The specialty care delay problem cannot be definitively resolved by looking at only one step at a time, but the initial step from primary care to specialty care is often a good starting point because (a) delay is most easily viewed and measured at the initial step; (b) the greatest number of patients are delayed at that step; and (c) delays amplify as the work flows further inside the system, making it crucial to reduce the delay at the initial step.[39-42] For specialty care groups with provider supply devoted primarily to outpatient work, for example, dermatology and rheumatology, improving the flow of work at this step should solve the entire flow problem.

It is possible to solve the initial delay by temporarily pulling resources from other duties. For example, waits can be reduced for new and return orthopedic patients by adding more office hours and subtracting OR hours; the result is fewer delays in the office because of the favorable demand-supply balance but greater delay at the surgical step. Thus, improving the wait time at any step requires an understanding of the entire system flow dynamic. To improve the flow and reduce the waits across the system, each link in the chain needs to be evaluated, measured, optimized, and kept in constant balance. To achieve optimal system performance, it is critical to determine the linkages between the steps, understand and discover the system bottleneck, link all the steps, and smooth the entire

flow. This process of delay improvement is thus iterative: back and forth between the initial step and the other steps. The seven change strategies that follow can be applied at each step in the patient's journey to improve flow.

1. BALANCE SUPPLY AND DEMAND AT EACH STEP IN THE CHAIN

The first step in access improvement is to understand, measure, and achieve a balance between demand and supply at each step. Demand is commonly measured by looking at past activity, which represents a retrospective view of how much work was completed within a time frame. This may be different than the amount of work generated within the same time frame. Thus, demand must be measured prospectively, as it is generated.[2,3]

Demand at the initial step into specialty care has two components: externally generated demand (workload generated from outside the practice, either from patients or referring entities) and internally generated demand (work generated from within the practice as requests for return visits). Each of these demand streams must be measured, evaluated, and compared to the available supply of appointments.

To understand and influence external demand, it is important to stratify this demand into the following components:

a. *What is the work?* There are various categories of work sent to specialty providers, based on diagnosis, symptom, or condition.

b. *Who sends the work?* There will be variation between one primary care provider and another in terms of the amount of type of work sent.

c. *Where does the work come from?* The packaging of the work often differs significantly depending on the venue (for example, from the primary care provider versus the ED).

For specialty care practices with stable and consistent daily provider presence, it is possible to match the appointment demand with the appropriate appointment supply each day. This single-day balance box is achievable if providers are present > 60% of the time and are reasonably distributed over that time frame. For most specialty practices, however, the office supply is diluted to ≤ 50% of the total potential office time and is spread unevenly across the week. In addition, other factors are present: (a) the geographical distance of the referring venue from the specialty care practice; and (b) the need for more information, tests,

The Joint Commission Journal on Quality and Patient Safety

or procedures before the visit, which create delay for the initial specialty care visit. These factors create tension for an extended time frame; thus, most practices will widen the supply-demand balance box to five days. The system dynamics—steps required to achieve balance and deal with variation—remain the same, but instead of the primary care mantra of doing "today's work today," the goal is to do "this week's work this week." If there is a balance between demand and supply, this stability can be achieved within any chosen time frame. If there is an imbalance in any of the demand streams, however, waits will inevitably get worse, and nothing can solve the problem.

The distinct types of demand that come into specialty care practices include demand for office appointments (which can be subdivided into new patients and return patients), surgery in the OR, surgery in an ambulatory surgery center, procedure or test, hospital consultation, and the catch-all miscellaneous demand captured by the "on-call" function. These demand streams are managed by an allocation of resource or supply. Most practices use intuition, experience, and some data, as well as a concern about clinical issues to ensure that the supply is sufficient to meet these various different types of demand. The priority in the competition between demand streams is based on acuity. A demand/supply balance has to be achieved within each demand stream and across demand streams. Total demand (all demand types, converted to time and added) must equal all supply time. If one demand stream is mismatched, either permanently or temporarily, a delay will ensue. Eventually the wait gets intolerable. Practices can, however, tolerate variation as long as in the long run the demand equals the supply. This temporary mismatch is managed by tolerating a wait and then catching up. The more acute demand streams (on-call function and hospital) are always balanced without fail, and the least acute (office, primarily the return appointment demand stream) are the most tolerable and absorb the variation. For example, if half the specialty providers are not working in any venue within the practice, some demand streams are prioritized and supported at 100% (the on-call function and hospital) while the office, with low priority, is supported at far less than 50%. Hence, the longest and most variable waits are seen in the office. If this wait is temporary because of a temporary demand/supply mismatch, a practice can "get away with it," but if it is caused by a permanent mismatch, then the wait will just get worse, leading to practice system breakdown. Even though this article focuses on the office work alone, it should be noted that it is critical to measure the demand and supply in all the competing demand streams. In the office, if the total appointment demand generated during a five-day period is equal to appointment supply for the same period of time but there is an appointment delay, then the next strategies employed include the strategy to work down the backlog of work and strategies to reduce the variation in demand or supply to achieve a smoother flow and less fluctuation with these temporary delays. Palo Alto Urology and Camino Medical Group Otolaryngology (Sidebar 1, page 130, and Sidebar 2, page 131) are particularly strong examples of measurement and review of the allocation of supply for the correct ratio of supply to balance the measured demand for that service.

2. Work Down the Backlog

Backlog reduction is a necessary strategy to recalibrate a delayed system of care. In specialty care, backlogs of patients often exist at every system step. Wherever a demand/supply mismatch is present, either permanent or temporary, a delay ensues. These delays need to be measured, evaluated for stability, and then stabilized. If wait times are worsening, demand reduction and supply enhancement strategies (as described below) need to be employed first to achieve stability. Once stabilized, the backlog can be eliminated and the system recalibrated.

To eliminate backlog, a period of time must be spent completing more work than is generated. The requisite extra supply can be added within the daily schedule or as a bolus of supply somewhere within the week. Some specialty practices face a larger backlog for new patients, whereas others have a larger and expanding backlog for return patients. Both streams need to be measured and evaluated for delay and demand/supply balance. To achieve optimal system function, the new patient demand stream, in which delay and dissatisfaction occur most frequently, needs to be balanced first.

In addition to adding supply, the following enhancement strategies will indirectly help reduce backlog:
a. Getting the referred patient on the right route for care and ensuring that the appropriate specialist is consulted to reduce secondary referrals for care and ensuring that patients see the same provider of care for subsequent visits[43,44]

The Joint Commission Journal on Quality and Patient Safety

Sidebar 1. Palo Alto Urology

Palo Alto Medical Group, a division of Palo Alto Medical Foundation, is a multi-specialty medical practice staffed with 410 physicians within 34 departments. The urology group has been working on access improvement for 2 years.

Synopsis of results: Achieved aim of reducing wait time to 5 days or less. Improved referral provider satisfaction. CON, consult.

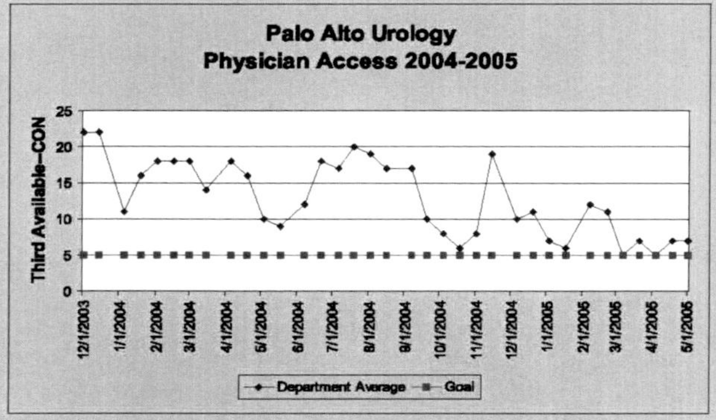

Key Changes (selected as specific changes from the high-leverage change ideas):

- Measured wait time, appointment demand, and relative supply
- Reviewed how specialists allocate time
- Reduced backlog
- Measured office lead time
- Synchronized appointment times
- Developed service agreements with primary care
- Improved "graduation" of patients back to primary care

Backlog reduction requires the support of leadership, which must aid in the development of measurement guidelines, set dates for the start and completion of backlog reduction, add support staff to aid in the work, and align the incentives so that providers who reduce their backlog early do not receive overflow from other providers. The Camino Medical Group Otolaryngology (Sidebar 2) practice had a strong backlog reduction plan.

3. Reduce Appointment Types

Reducing the appointment types in specialty care to a minimum number is one of the most powerful delay reduction strategies. An appointment type is a specific visit type that has both inclusion and exclusion criteria. A "new patient" appointment is often distinctly different than a "return follow-up patient" appointment. Pushing any work to the future, through use of multiple appointment types and their resulting queues, creates inflexibility in the future schedule, rigidity inside the scheduling system, and the necessity for triage, which uses up resources. It also increases rework, redundancy, and the likelihood of no-shows, and inevitably leads to longer waiting times.[2-3,18] Reducing appointment types allows any patient to be seen in any appointment slot, thereby reducing variation and delay.[52]

Although the goal is to minimize appointment types to achieve less patient waits, some distinct appointment types are necessary to maintain smooth flow. Any specialty care practice with a balance box larger than 24 hours, a low new-to-return patient ratio, or provider office presence of < 50% will need distinct new and return appointment slots. For example, in a strictly obstetrics practice, the ratio of new patients to returning patients is low, and the providers are often in the office < 50% of the office time.

b. Maximizing the efficiency of each visit and doing more within each visit

c. Altering return visit rates[45,46]

d. Developing appropriate care delivery models, wherein patients not appropriate for referral back to primary care can be seen by nonphysician resources within the boundaries of the specialty care practice[47-51]

e. Streamlining and improving the flow of work across the office so that, with the same intensity of effort, more patients can be seen and evaluated

f. Reviewing all venues of work (procedure, hospital, surgery) for inefficiencies—if the flow at other venues can be improved, supply can be gained to add support to office practice.

The Joint Commission Journal on Quality and Patient Safety

In this setting, a distinction between new and return appointments is necessary because without that distinction, the return patients would crowd out the new patients. In addition, distinct appointment types must be created when there is a clear need for a specific specialist, a specific room, specific support staff, a specific time frame, or specific equipment.

Although the new and return appointment types will compete within the office demand stream, from the patient and referring provider customer viewpoint, the most critical wait time is that for new patients. In specialty care practices where there is > 50% provider absence from the office because of support of numerous other demand streams, then "pooling of new patient referrals," that is, sending the work nonspecifically to the department, allows appointments to be made with the first-available new-patient appointment slot. If work is sent to specific specialty care providers in a predetermined way (nonpooled), then if a provider is absent from the office for extended periods, longer waits will inevitably result.

4. Implement Contingency Planning for All Variation

If a specialty care practice is committed to reducing the waits to within a specific time frame, it will need to plan for all demand and supply variation. In most practices, demand for new appointments is relatively stable and merely needs to be measured. Internally generated demand (return work) shows more variation because of specific provider practice styles.[45] Contingency planning requires an understanding of this variation, and, while averages of demand and supply are useful metrics, fine-tuning is necessary. Statistical process control graphs can be used to view the variation in the demand for service and the supply of resource and can help identify causes of this variation. Special cause variation (artificially created variation) must be addressed and eliminated, and common cause variation (normal expected variation) must be understood and stabilized. Improvement strategies include measurement and

> ### Sidebar 2. Camino Medical Group Otolaryngology
>
> Camino Medical Group is a multi-specialty medical practice located in San Jose, California, staffed with 223 physicians within 46 departments. The otolaryngology group has been working on access improvement for 18 months.
>
> **Synopsis of results:** Achieved aim of reducing wait time to 5 days or less. Improved referral provider satisfaction.
>
> **Key Changes** (selected as specific changes from the high-leverage change ideas):
> - Explicit backlog reduction plan
> - Service agreements with primary care
> - Standardized rooms
> - Use of physician's assistant for follow-up and minor procedures
> - Prepare in advance for visits

planning for any seasonal demand variation, bringing return discretionary visits back in times where there is less need for new visit time as a buffer to smooth demand, development of time-off policies to smooth the supply resource, and planning for providers returning from practice absences.

Equitable distribution of new patient workload among providers is another way to smooth demand. Making each provider responsible for a panel or caseload of patients helps create this equity. Panels or caseloads need not be equal but must be large enough to keep the provider busy and small enough that the provider can complete the work each day or within each week. To keep the wait time stable, providers must absorb demand variation on a daily or weekly basis; some days or weeks may be heavier than others.[2–3,16–17,42]

Specialists create unique value by seeing new patients; dividing new patients equitably among providers creates the tension to graduate patients (that is, refer them back to primary care) to open up space for the other new patients.[16–18]

Office waiting times in specialty care practices with multiple demand streams competing for allocation of supply often fluctuate widely because of prioritization based on acuity of the allocated supply. Because the work done in many practices (general surgery, for example) is done linearly and in sequence, that is, patients are initially seen, then evaluated and then sent deeper into the system for another service; if there is overallocation in one step and

The Joint Commission Journal on Quality and Patient Safety

Sidebar 3. Santa Clara Eye Care

Santa Clara Valley Medical Center, a public hospital owned and operated by Santa Clara County, is staffed by a 370-physician multispecialty medical group and supports an academic teaching program. The Eye Care service department recently completed its second year of implementation.

Synopsis of results: Achieved aim of reducing wait time to 5 days or less. Improved referral provider satisfaction. Reduced staffing cost.

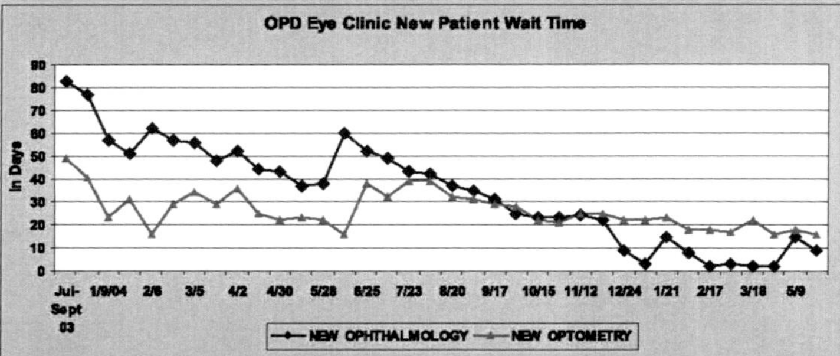

Key Changes (selected as specific changes from the high-leverage change ideas):

- Measured wait time, appointment demand, and relative supply
- Reduced backlog
- Measured office lead time
- Synchronized appointment times
- Increased number of clinics by identifying additional space
- Expanded diabetes mellitus screening clinic because patients with diabetes were seen less efficiently in the general eye clinic
- Opened one clinic just for new patients

This in turns creates an extending wait for the OR. This wide fluctuation in under- or overallocation creates temporary mismatches in each of the various demand streams, and the back-and-forth movement creates boluses, batches, delays, system turbulence, and variation—all of which can be addressed by planning for these contingencies. For example, if the office provider supply is low, the wait time goal for new patients can be maintained by a higher ratio of new patients on each office provider's schedule. Alternatively, if office provider supply is high, then the new-patient ratio per provider can be lowered, allowing more return visits on the schedule. Measurement and a conscious plan to avoid wide swings in allocation are key.

underallocation in another, temporary demand/supply mismatches result. This, in turn, creates boluses of work and work waiting. For example, if a surgeon planning an absence spends a disproportionate amount of time in the OR to reduce surgical backlog before that absence, backlog will still increase into the office—not only during but before the absence. On the surgeon's return, the first priority is often to "make up" on-call time, which in turn generates more OR cases and keeps the surgeon away from the office. The office backlog continues to build. Eventually, there are not enough surgery cases to fill the "block time," so the surgeon then withdraws from the OR and moves back to the office, where "hidden" surgical demand is uncovered within the backlog into the office.

5. Reduce the Demand for Visits

Because most work comes to specialists through a filter of primary care, the most effective demand reduction strategy is the development of service agreements.[16–19] A service agreement is an agreement between any two entities in a flow system, one of which sends work to the other.[19] It defines the proper work and outlines the correct packaging of that work, which directs the right work to the right person and ensures that it is prepared in such a way that it can be efficiently dealt with once it reaches the specialist. Service agreements also afford the opportunity to streamline the referral process itself, reducing or eliminating steps to reduce or eliminate patient delay. Service agreements between primary care and urologists, for

The Joint Commission Journal on Quality and Patient Safety

example, can define what work in the urology arena is done by primary care providers (monitoring of stable pro-static-specific antigen levels), what work is done by urologists (scrotal mass), and what is the proper packaging prior to referral (a set of defined tests for patients with microscopic hematuria). When providers recognize the commitment to stabilize patient wait times within a specific time frame, they then recognize the tension in the new-to-return-patient ratio. Because there is a limit to the potential provider supply, providers gain the incentive to optimize that ratio by graduating patients back to primary care or managing patients within the specialty practice with less direct physician contact. Other demand reduction strategies focus on continuity, individual provider return visit rates, and the use of technology.[44–46] These strategies work best in environments based on continuity, relationship, and trust, in which the patient realizes that they can see their own doctor at any time, for any problem. The Palo Alto Urology practice (Sidebar 1) developed a strong service agreement.

6. INCREASE THE SUPPLY

Practices can increase supply by adding more hours or more providers or by subtracting unnecessary work from the provider. Any flow process has a rate-limiting step, which in health care is the provider. The entire journey can move only as fast as the slowest step, that is, the greatest mismatch of demand and supply.[52] When patients traverse the specialty care network, the slowest step is commonly found in the office setting. Thus, increasing supply means driving all unnecessary appointment work away from providers for the provider to be freed to perform work for

which she or he is uniquely qualified. Hematology-oncology practices have used this strategy for years by having much of the follow-up chemotherapy work done by specialized practice nurses and not physicians. This in turn requires a care team task and workflow analysis to ensure that the right person is doing the right work.[47–51] By using a retinal camera, the Santa Clara Eye practice

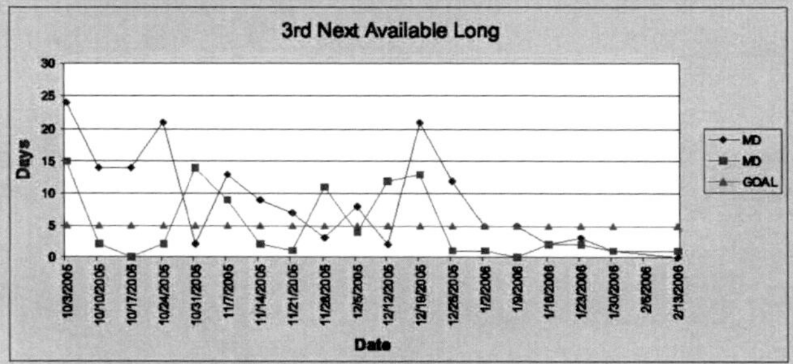

Sidebar 4. Marshfield Clinic Pain Management

Marshfield Clinic is the largest private group medical practice in Wisconsin, with more than 725 physicians representing 86 different medical specialties and serving over 360,000 unique patients. During a three-year period, Marshfield Clinic has been involved in an organization-wide effort to improve access to care for all patients to all specialties. The pain management practice has been involved in access improvement for 18 months.

Synopsis of results: Achieved access aim of offering 100% of patients an appointment within 5 days. Achieved office efficiency aim of 35% reduction of follow-up appointment cycle time. Eliminated costly overtime. Improved staff satisfaction with job.

Key Changes (selected as specific changes from the high-leverage change ideas):

- Measured wait time, appointment demand, and relative supply
- Commitment to complete all work that can arrive prior to 3:30 P.M. each day
- Reduced backlog by adding more appointments temporarily
- Standardized appointment slots
- Review future schedule on a daily basis
- Measured office lead time
- Synchronized appointment times
- Improved continuity
- Revised referral process
- Post-vacation contingency plans with "held" slots
- Revised provider schedule by adding slots when necessary and eliminating hidden time
- Standardized examination rooms and process

The Joint Commission Journal on Quality and Patient Safety

(Sidebar 3, page 132) was able to leverage the physicians' time and functionally increase the supply devoted to direct patient care.

7. IMPROVE THE EFFICIENCY OF THE OFFICE WORK FLOW

Improving the workflow within the office setting itself requires an explicit plan to address patient delays during the appointment. The plan includes flow-mapping the patient's journey, identifying the value-added steps, and eliminating non-value-added steps and waits between steps. Streamlining the patient's journey by reducing delays for the patient-provider interaction frees more time for that valuable interaction. With the same effort, specialty providers can see more patients within the same time frame. This does not mean working faster; it means that distractions and interruptions are eliminated. Streamlining the flow of work also requires synchronizing the work: consistently getting the patient, provider, information, equipment and staff to an open room on time.[53,54] The Marshfield Clinic Pain Management practice (Sidebar 4, page 133) focused attention on synchronizing the daily appointment workflow and preparing in advance for that work.

Summary

Specialists support various, distinct demand streams, all of which require a demand/supply balance to achieve optimal system performance. Each stream is linked operationally and can be linked with measurement. Movement of resource from one stream to another disrupts the delicate balance. Thus, measurement and balance of all streams is necessary. If there is a demand/supply balance within any stream, waits can be minimized, and the practice can choose the time frame within which to balance the workload. Although a complex choreography is at play, the seven flow strategies will ensure that waits and delays are reduced or eliminated. ∎

The author would like to acknowledge the work, dedication, and effort of the following individuals in improving access to specialty care at their own sites and in contributing to the article: Marshfield Clinic Pain Management, Edna Devries, M.D., Linda Pelton, Heidi Reigel; Camino Medical Group: Phil Brosterhouse, M.D., Nina Quintal; Palo Alto Medical Group, Jenny Buchanan, Susan Smith, M.D.; Santa Clara Eye Care, Kent Imai, M.D., Chris Snow, M.D., Donna Decarlo, Joe Eliason, M.D.

Mark F. Murray, M.D., M.P.A., is Principal, Mark Murray & Associates, Sacramento, California. Please address correspondence to murraytant@msn.com.

References

1. Merritt, Hawkins & Associates: *2004 Survey of Physician Appointment Wait Times.* Irving, Texas: Merritt, Hawkins & Associates, Summary Report: 1-12, 2004.
2. Murray M., Berwick D.M.: Advanced access: Reducing waiting and delays in primary care. *JAMA* 289:1035–1040, Feb. 26, 2003.
3. Murray M., et al.: Improving timely access to primary care: case studies in the advanced access model. *JAMA* 289:1042–1046, Feb. 26, 2003.
4. Kennedy J.G., Hsu J.T.: Implementation of an open access scheduling system in a residency training program. *Fam Med* 35:666–670, Oct. 2003.
5. Boelke C., Boushon B., Isensee S.: Achieving open access: The road to improved service and satisfaction. *MGM Journal* 47:58–68, Sep.–Oct. 2000.
6. Valenti W.M., Bookhardt-Murray J.: Advanced-access scheduling boosts quality, productivity and revenue. *Drug Benefit Trends.* 16:510,513–514, May 2004.
7. Lacy N.L., et al.: Why we don't come: Patient perceptions on no-shows. *Ann Fam Med* 2:541–545, Nov.–Dec. 2004.
8. Moore C.G., Wilson-Witherspoon P., Probst J.C.: Time and money: Effects of no-shows at a family practice residency clinic. *Fam Med* 33:522–527, Jul.–Aug. 2001.
9. Barron W.M.: Failed appointments: Who misses them, why they are missed, and what can be done. *Prim Care* 7:563–574, Dec. 1980.
10. Hixon A.L., Chapman R.W., Nuovo J.: Failure to keep clinic appointments: implications for residency education and productivity. *Fam Med* 31:627–630, Oct. 1999.
11. Belardi F.G., Weir S., Craig F.W.: A controlled trial of an advanced access appointment system in a residency family medicine center. *Fam Med* 36:341–345, May 2004.
12. O'Hare C.D., Corlett J.: The outcomes of open-access scheduling. *Fam Pract Manag* 11:35–38, Feb. 2004.
13. Carlson B.: Same-day appointments promise increased productivity. *Managed Care* 11:43–44, Dec. 2002.
14. Giannone J.: Open access as an alternative to patient combat. *Fam Pract Manag* 10:65, Jan. 2003.
15. Herriot S.: Reducing delays and waiting times with open-access scheduling. *Fam Pract Manag* 6:38–43, Apr. 1999.
16. Schall M., et al.: Improving patient access to the Veterans Health Administration's primary care and specialty clinics. *Joint Comm J Qual Saf* 30:415–423, 2004.
17. Duffy T.E.: Urology advanced clinic access concepts. Paper presented at the 4th Annual International Summit on Redesigning the Clinical Office Practice, St. Louis, Apr. 14, 2003.
18. Parenti C., Pierpont G., Murray M.: Reducing wait times for cardiac consultation. *Federal Practitioner* 22: pp. 24–28, 31, Feb. 2005.
19. Murray M.: Reducing waits and delays in the referral process. *Fam Pract Manag* 9:39–42, Mar. 2002.

The Joint Commission Journal on Quality and Patient Safety

References, *continued*

20. Asplin B.R., et al.: A conceptual model of emergency department crowding. *Ann Emerg Med* 42:173–180, Aug. 2003.
21. Forster A.J., et al.: The effect of hospital occupancy on emergency department length of stay and patient disposition. *Acad Emerg Med* 10:127–133, Feb. 2003.
22. Berry L.L., Seiders K., Wilder S.S.: Innovations in access to care: A patient-centered approach. *Ann Intern Med* 139:568–574, Oct. 7, 2003.
23. Bodenheimer T.: Innovations in primary care in the United States. *BMJ* 326:796–798, Apr. 12, 2003.
24. Dewitt P.: Finding the time: Clinics pursue new strategies to reduce wait time for appointments. *HealthLeaders* 11:72–73, Sep. 2004.
25. Kilo C.M., et al.: Improving access to clinical offices. *J Med Pract Manag* 16:126–132, Nov.–Dec. 2000.
26. Kofoed L., Ramirez M.E.: Improving access: A model for mental health care. *Federal Practitioner* 21:11–12,17-20,23,26, Sep. 2004.
27. Murray M.: Modernizing the NHS. Patient Care: Access. *BMJ* 320:1594–1596, Jun. 10, 2000.
28. Murray M., Tantau C.: Must patients wait? *Jt Comm J Qual Improv* 24:423–425, Aug. 1998.
29. Murray M., Tantau C.: Same-day appointments: Exploding the access paradigm. *Fam Pract Manag* 7:45–50, Sep. 2000. http://www.aafp.org/fpm/20000900/45same.html (last accessed Jan. 4, 2007).
30. Berwick D.: As good as it should get: Making health care better in the new millennium. Paper presented at the National Coalition on HealthCare, Institute for Health Care Improvement, Boston, Sep. 1998.
31. Kilo C., Endsley S.: As good as it could get: remaking the medical practice. *Fam Pract Manag* 7:48–58, 2000.
32. Singer I.: Advanced access: A new paradigm in the delivery of ambulatory care services. Paper presented at the National Association of Public Hospitals and Health Systems, Washington, D.C., Oct. 1, 2001.
33. White B.: Starting a revolution in office-based care. *Fam Pract Manag* 8:29–35, Oct. 2001.
34. Randolph G., et al.: Behind schedule: Improving access to care for children one practice at a time. *Pediatrics* 113(3 pt 1):e230–e237, Mar. 2004.
35. Murray M., Tantau C.: Redefining open access to primary care. *Managed Care Quarterly* 7:45–55, Summer 1999.
36. Smith J.: Redesigning health care. *BMJ* 322:1257–1258, May 26, 2001.
37. Murray M.: Waiting for Healthcare: Physician offices can dramatically reduce how long patients wait for appointments [editorial]. *Postgrad Med* 113:13–14, Feb. 2003.
38. Kolata G.: Harried doctors try to ease big delays and rushed visits. *The New York Times:* Jan. 4, 2001. http://www.nytimes.com/2001/01/04/science/04DOCS.html (last accessed Jan. 4, 2001).
39. Cawley P., Hanlon P.: Hospital medicine programs add value to the throughput process. *The Hospitalist* 8:11–14, Sep. 2004.
40. Rozich J.D., Resar R.K.: Using a unit assessment tool to optimize patient flow and staffing in a community hospital. *Jt Comm J Qual Improv* 28:31-41, Jan. 2002.
41. Shea S.S., Senteno J.: Emergency department patient throughput: A continuous quality improvement approach to length of stay. *J Emerg Nurs* 20:355–360, Oct. 1994.
42. Murray M.: Answers to your questions about same-day scheduling. *Fam Pract Manag* 12:59–64, Mar. 2005.
43. Plauth A., Pearson S.D.: Discontinuity of care: Urgent care utilization within a health maintenance organization. *Am J Manag Care* 4:1531–1537, Nov. 1998.
44. Raddish M., Horn S.D., Sharkey P.D.: Continuity of care: Is it cost effective? *Am J Manag Care* 5:727–734, Jun. 1999.
45. Petitti D.B., Grumbach K.: Variation in physicians: recommendations about revisit interval for three common conditions. *J Fam Pract* 37:235–240, Sep. 1993.
46. Schwartz L., et al.: Setting the revisit interval in Primary Care. *J Gen Intern Med* 14:230–235, 1999.
47. Grandinetti D.A.: Make the most of your staff. *Med Econ* 8:56, Apr. 2000.
48. Grumbach K., Bodenheimer T.: Can health care teams improve primary care practice? *JAMA* 291:1246–1251, Mar. 10, 2004.
49. Patel V., et al.: The collaborative health care team: the role of individual and group expertise. *Teach Learn Med* 12:117–132, Summer 2000.
50. Weymier R.E.: Ideas for optimizing your nursing staff. *Fam Pract Manag* 10:51–52, Feb. 2003.
51. Wagner E.H.: The role of patient care teams in chronic disease management. *BMJ* 320:569–572, Feb. 26, 2000.
52. Hall R.: *Queuing Methods for Services and Manufacturing.* Englewood Cliffs, N.J.: Prentice Hall, 1991.
53. Carlson B.: Working too hard, doctor? Poor work flow could be to blame. *Manag Care* 11:48–49, Jul. 2002.
54. Endsley S., Magill M.K., Godfrey M.M.: Creating a lean practice. *Fam Pract Manag* 13:34–38, Apr. 2006.

Journal on QUALITY and PATIENT SAFETY

Organizational Change and Learning

Using a Framework for Spread:
The Case of Patient Access in the Veterans Health Administration

Kevin Nolan, M.A.
Marie W. Schall, M.A.
Fabiane Erb, R.H.I.A.
Thomas Nolan, Ph.D.

The experiences of four Veterans Health Administration (VHA) clinics in spreading operational changes and achieving improved access for veterans are discussed in detail elsewhere.[1] Much has been written about the problem of and reasons for the lack of widespread implementation of evidence-based innovations in health care.[2-4] Such innovations would include not only new drugs or equipment but an operational system, such as one that orders, dispenses, and administers medications. The lack of implementation makes it clear that strong evidence for an innovation is necessary but not sufficient to result in its adoption.

Experience indicates that an effective operational system, such as those suggested above, will spread much more slowly than, for example, a new antinausea drug. No press releases will announce the approval of the medication system by the Food and Drug Administration. Patients will not demand its installation. No army of persons knowledgeable of the system will be dispatched to explain it. The spread of operational systems presents significant challenges—not faced by a drug company spreading an antinausea drug—for the following reasons:

■ Operational systems are often large or complex and thus difficult to describe and communicate.

■ The systems are usually not services for sale. Thus, well-developed marketing and sales processes are not available to create demand for them.

■ Even if the new system was desired, the transition from the current system to the new system may be difficult.

Because these challenges seem difficult to overcome without purposeful leadership, we focus our attention on

Article-at-a-Glance

Background: Experience indicates that an effective operational system will spread much more slowly than, for example, a new antinausea drug. The Veterans Health Administration (VHA) used a Framework for Spread to spread improvements in access to more than 1,800 outpatient clinics between April 2001 and December 2003. The framework identifies strategies and methods for planning and guiding the spread of new ideas or new operational systems, including the responsibilities of leadership, packaging the new ideas, communication, strengthening the social system, measurement and feedback, and knowledge management.

Applying the Framework for Spread: Following a collaborative for reducing waiting times for patients without the large-scale addition of resources, each of the participating 22 Veterans Integrated Service Networks (VISNs) used the framework to expand improvements in access to care to six additional targeted clinics (for example, primary care, eye care, cardiology).

Results: During the VHA's spread initiative, waiting time for a primary care appointment decreased from 60.4 days at the end of fiscal year (FY) 2000 to 28.4 at the end of FY 2002. Results were sustained. Waiting time was < 25 days at the end of FY 2004.

Discussion: The Framework for Spread suggests areas that organizations should consider when developing and executing a strategy for a spread initiative. Further study is needed to determine the specific activities that should be emphasized to accelerate spread.

JOINT COMMISSION™ Journal ON QUALITY AND PATIENT SAFETY

A Framework for Spread

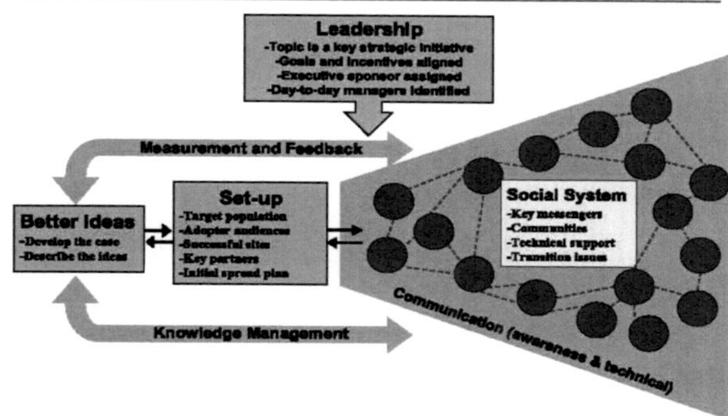

Figure 1. *This diagram illustrates the strategies and methods that have been shown to contribute to the effective spread of new ideas or operational systems both within and across organizations.*

spread within organizations. This does not preclude the spread of such systems between organizations if an appropriate umbrella organization such as a professional association exists.

In 1996, the Institute for Healthcare Improvement (IHI; Cambridge, MA) initiated the Breakthrough Series Collaborative in an attempt to reduce the gap between available knowledge and its use in practice in areas such as waits and delays, end-of-life care, and chronic disease care. A collaborative is an improvement method that brings together multiple similar sites with a common aim to adapt and spread existing knowledge.[5,6] Collaboratives are particularly useful to hone an operational system, to document its advantages, and to begin the spread process.

Although collaboratives proved successful,[7–11] a more general approach to the spread of operational systems was needed to reach a wider audience. In 1999, the authors began a literature review and conducted interviews with organizations successful in spread. In 2000, testing of an approach to spread began in projects in health care and in industries such as chemical, landscape maintenance, and building products. Figure 1 (above) presents the Framework for Spread that evolved. The framework is founded on Everett Rogers's[12] definition of diffusion and draws both from the literature and from the experience of organizations actively

involved in spreading improvements from a local site to their entire system.

The Framework for Spread identifies the following components for planning the spread of new ideas:

- The responsibilities of leadership (including set-up)
- Identification of better ideas
- Communication
- Strengthening the social system
- Measurement and feedback
- Knowledge management

The framework is not meant to be prescriptive nor considered as a specific intervention but rather it is meant to suggest some general areas to consider as a large spread project is undertaken. Factors such as an organization's infrastructure, culture, size, strength of its underlying social system, and the operational system being spread will influence how the components of the framework are applied. Check lists for spread appear in sidebars throughout the article to help in planning a strategy.

The section that follows describes the components of the Framework for Spread and the application of the framework in the VHA, which has attempted other spread projects with varying degrees of success,[13] as an example.

Applying the Framework for Spread to the VHA

The VHA partnered with the IHI to conduct a collaborative from July 1999 through March 2000 on reducing waiting times for patients without the large-scale addition of resources. The collaborative included teams from 134 facilities from the then 22 Veterans Integrated Service Networks (VISNs). Following the collaborative, each VISN was asked to expand the improvements in access to care to additional clinic sites within six performance clinics (primary care, eye care, audiology, cardiology, orthopedics, and urology) with large patient volumes and long waiting times for appointments. The clinics care for approximately 3.8 million patients per year in more than 1,800 sites (Figure 2, page 341). This strategic effort was referred to as the Advanced Clinic Access (ACA) initiative.

340

J̲O̲U̲R̲N̲A̲L̲™ ᴏɴ QUALITY ᴀɴᴅ PATIENT SAFETY

Veterans Health Administration (VHA) Organizational and Clinic Structure for Spread of Improved Access

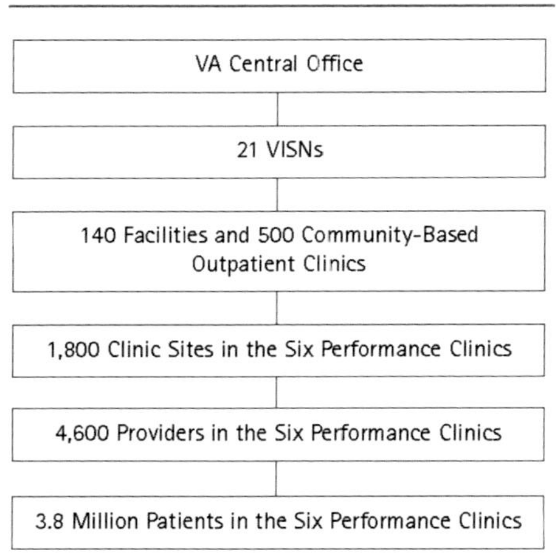

Figure 2. *This chart shows the multiple levels of the organization that were utilized by the VHA in building a plan to spread improved access across its system. VA, Department of Veterans Affairs; VISN, Veterans Integrated Service Network.*

Each of the then 22 networks (VISNs) within the VHA used the Framework for Spread to guide its efforts. VISN 2, the VA Healthcare Network of Upstate New York (VISN 2), consists of 5 medical centers and 27 community-based outpatient clinics (CBOCs) or access points for care. VISN 2's work in attempting to achieve the VHA standard of < 30 days average wait time for an appointment is presented in terms of the Framework for Spread components.

Leadership

Leaders at many levels in VISN 2—including the network director, chief medical officer, facility directors, and network and local care line managers—"set the agenda"[12] for change through the following actions:

■ Embraced improved access as a key strategic initiative and set waiting time goals. This was communicated through facility leadership meetings, the VISN 2 Web site, and publications. Leaders also committed funding and staff time.

■ Aligned goals for improved access with two existing incentive programs, the Provider Compact and Goal Sharing. The Provider Compact funded provider educational activities depending on the level of attainment of a set of measures. The Goal Sharing Program allotted dollar awards of graduated amounts to teams achieving certain levels of performance.

■ Established a multifunctional steering committee to lead the spread effort

■ Supported a VISN 2 point of contact (POC) and facility POCs to manage the day-to-day activities of the VISN spread strategy. One of the barriers faced was the time commitments required from the POCs and others to facilitate spread. VISN 2 staff members do this work in addition to their regular duties, which caused several to drop out over time. This required the VISN core group, which does remain intact, to develop a system to recruit and train staff members to support the work.

Better Ideas

A key attribute of ideas that influences their rate of spread is their benefit to all adopters relative to other ideas.[12,14] The concepts and ideas to improve access adopted in the VHA are consistent with the advanced or open access approach currently used with success in a number of health care settings.[15,16] The VHA assembled these ideas into an easy-to-use booklet and developed them into a Web format for the national VHA Web site (available at the IHI Web site[17]). Two primary care and three specialty care areas in VISN 2 demonstrated during the national collaborative that adopting these ideas to improve access can provide benefits not only for patients but also for providers.[18] It was determined that the ideas could be replicated in other primary and specialty care units.

Set-up for Spread

Once the better ideas are documented and successful sites identified, leaders should initiate the set-up for spread by identifying the target population. Consideration should be given to the different audiences (for example, physicians, nurses, technicians) within the target population. Leaders should also

Journal ON QUALITY AND PATIENT SAFETY

oversee the development of an initial plan for spread, which could include ways to attract those in the target population willing to adopt the improvements.[19,20] Ways to attract these early adopters might include the planning of broad-based communication about the new system's advantages, developing a process to identify persons influential with their peers, or developing a plan to share comparative data with adopters. The initial plan might also include the infrastructure changes, such as in information technology and distribution systems, and the realignment of functions within the organization needed to achieve the goals of the initiative.

VISN 2 used a general communication campaign to attract adopters, which was followed by a series of meetings to showcase the work of the successful clinics. VISN 2 focused on a group of clinics at a time. Clinics willing to be part of the initiative would constitute the initial waves. Improvement in the national scheduling system aided VISN 2 in its work.

General Communication and Knowledge Transfer in the Target Population

Because communication is at the heart of spread, the day-to-day manager of a spread initiative needs to organize a communication campaign.[21,22] Many different channels of communication can and should be used to raise awareness and share technical knowledge.[23,24] However, technical knowledge that focuses on the "how to" is best communicated through interaction with colleagues.[25-28] Persons who are influencers or opinion leaders in the social system serve as the best messengers.[29-32]

VISN 2 used a number of communication strategies to spread the ideas to improve access to the targeted clinics and strengthen the social system. Three successive "waves" of learning initiatives were launched in March 2000, March 2001, and January 2002. By making the successes of colleagues visible, the vast majority of clinics joined voluntarily. However, some staff members (physicians especially) refused to listen or to consider adopting the principles. Engaging them and spreading the access improvements to their clinics became a significant challenge for the access coaches and the leaders in VISN 2. It took extra effort to educate them and then have them put the concepts into practice and then see the benefits for themselves.

Sidebar 1. Checklist for Spread — Leadership, Better Ideas, and Set-up

- Is improvement in this area a strategic initiative within the organization?
- Is there an executive(s) who is responsible for the spread?
- How will this executive be involved on an ongoing basis?
- Is there a person or team who will manage the day-to-day spread activities?
- What are the positions of the key people who will make the adoption decision?
- Has the relative advantage of the changes been documented for all adopter audiences?
- Are the changes packaged so that they can be easily understood and tested by the adopters?
- Is there a successful site that has implemented the new system?
  - Are the changes implemented scaleable to the entire target population?
  - If there is no successful site, what is the strategy to create a good example?
- Has an initial plan for spread been developed? Consider:
  - Ways to attract early adopters
    - Planning broad-based communication
    - Developing a process to identify people in the target population who are influential with their peers
    - Developing a plan to share comparative data with adopters
  - Potential infrastructure changes needed

In 2002, VISN 2 also incorporated the use of "road shows"—events held at each of the five medical centers and at several large CBOCs. Physicians, nurses, and schedulers from successful sites met with staff. Part of the discussions were held in peer groups, for example, physicians meeting with physicians, schedulers with schedulers. In addition, articles about improving access and success stories appeared in VISN 2 newsletters.

Joint Commission™ Journal on QUALITY AND PATIENT SAFETY

Monthly video conferences, conference calls, team reports, and frequent e-mail exchanges were used to transfer knowledge. Personal coaching was available to sites that attended the VISN 2 meetings. In 2001, information was included on the VISN 2 intranet Web site. VISN 2 also communicated with patients. "No show" posters were designed to enlist patients' help in reducing the number of scheduled appointments cancelled.

VISN 2 took advantage of resources developed at the national level such as a theme ("Providing quality care when veterans want and need it"), a logo, a poster, messages for each adopter group, and information posted on the VHA national Web site. Other important resources for communicating both broad awareness and technical information about improving access included two nationally produced videos. One video, "The Time Has Come," showed patients, leaders, and providers from the VHA talking about the benefits of improving access. A second video featured Mark Murray, M.D., explaining the key ideas for improving access. Many providers also took part in national conference calls hosted by Dr. Murray and national e-mail groups.

Measurement and Feedback

Measurement is an integral part of improvement.[33] It provides information about whether the changes made in a system are having the desired effect. Two different types of measures are useful[34]: measures that demonstrate the extent of the spread of the recommended changes,[35] and a set of measures that demonstrate the outcome of the changes implemented.

A strong measurement system was in place in VISN 2 before the spread initiative began. Wait times data are now, however, included in the monthly VISN 2 report, reviewed at steering committee meetings, and used to give feedback to sites and to refine the VISN 2 spread strategy. The rate of spread (the percentage of clinics that have implemented the ideas to improve access) is also measured. A clinic using $\geq$ 75% of the 33 ideas to improve access for a period of $\geq$ three months is considered to have implemented the ideas. Clinics self-report these data quarterly on a standard data collection form. VISN 2 ACA coaches validate the data through observation within the clinics. The data are summarized and plotted twice a year with help from contacts at the facilities.

Sidebar 2. Checklist for Spread — General Communication and Knowledge Transfer

■ How will awareness of the initiative be communicated?
   – Have the benefits for different audiences been documented?
   – Have comparative data been shared?
   – What channels will be used to raise awareness in the target population?
■ How will technical knowledge be communicated to facilitate the adoption of the changes?
   – Are peer-to-peer interactions planned?
   – Are potential adopters influential in the social system willing to be involved?
   – How will successful units be involved to supply technical support?

Knowledge Management

As ideas are adapted to a local system during a spread initiative, adopters generate knowledge about the ideas and how best to improve outcomes.[36] Day-to-day managers need to develop systems to capture this knowledge and make it available to others on an ongoing basis. In VISN 2, knowledge was formally captured during face-to-face meetings and road shows. The day-to-day manager would make decisions on what information would be posted on the VISN 2 intranet Web site. The VHA national Web site also served as a mechanism to share tips, tools, success stories, and other information to assist others in making changes to improve access.

Results

During the spread initiative's time frame, the waiting time for a primary care appointment in the VHA decreased from 60.4 days at the end of fiscal year (FY) 2000 to 28.4 at the end of FY 2002. Waiting times at the end of FY 2004 were < 25 days (Figure 3, page 344). These results were based on waiting time data from all patients and are available from the VHA scheduling system. VISN 2 achieved similar results. The waiting time for all primary care patients decreased from > 50 days in April 2000 to < 20 days in April

343

122

Journal ON QUALITY AND PATIENT SAFETY

Sidebar 3. Checklist for Spread— Developing Measurement, Feedback, and Knowledge Management Systems

- How will outcomes be measured?
- How will the rate of spread be monitored?
- Who will be responsible for collecting, summarizing, and reviewing the data?
- What information/reports will be used as feedback to the sites and to monitor and refine the spread strategy?
- What systems will be used or developed to capture and share the new knowledge generated during the spread initiative?

2003 (Figure 4, page 345). Through the continued efforts in VISN 2, the waiting times in FY 2004 averaged approximately 16 days. In addition, all specialty care performance clinics were averaging < 30 days for their next available appointment. Figure 5 (page 345) shows the rate of spread in VISN 2. As of September 30, 2002, the ideas had spread to > 90% of the performance clinics and 78% of all clinics. The largest reduction in waiting times coincided with the successive waves. In VISN 2 during FY 2001 and FY 2002, there was a slight increase (5%) in the number of unique patients cared for and no increase in the overall and clinical FTEs. In addition, VISN 2 had no patients on waiting lists for entry into the system. The percentage of patients seeking primary care who were seen within 30 days increased from 74% in May 2002 to 92% in September 2004 (Figure 6, page 346).

Discussion

The work to spread improved access in each VISN within the VHA was guided by the Framework for Spread and supported by the infrastructure developed at the national level. Because this work was a strategic objective, many other areas, such as the scheduling system and referral guidelines, were focused on for improvement at the national level to support the spread initiative. Addressing issues—at the individual, unit, or organizational level[37]—that could inhibit adoption is essential to any spread effort.[38] One of the challenges faced by the national leadership in leading the spread of ACA was building leadership commitment and involvement at the VISN and facility levels. Tying ACA goals to annual performance reviews, using national meetings of VHA administrative and clinical leadership groups to build awareness as well as share effective leadership methods to support access improvement, and providing direction through the national steering committee all helped to guide, encourage, and acknowledge the role of regional and facility leaders.

The leaders in VISN 2 supported the day-to-day manager of the spread initiative in organizing a multifaceted communication campaign, allowing awareness

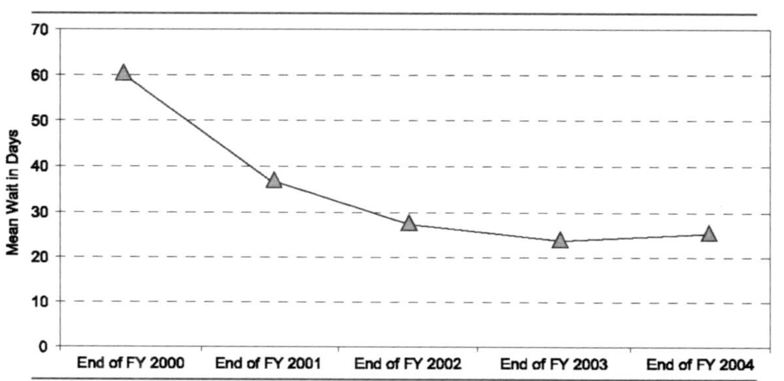

Figure 3. *This chart shows the national reduction in waiting time for a clinic appointment. FY, fiscal year.*

Journal ON QUALITY AND PATIENT SAFETY

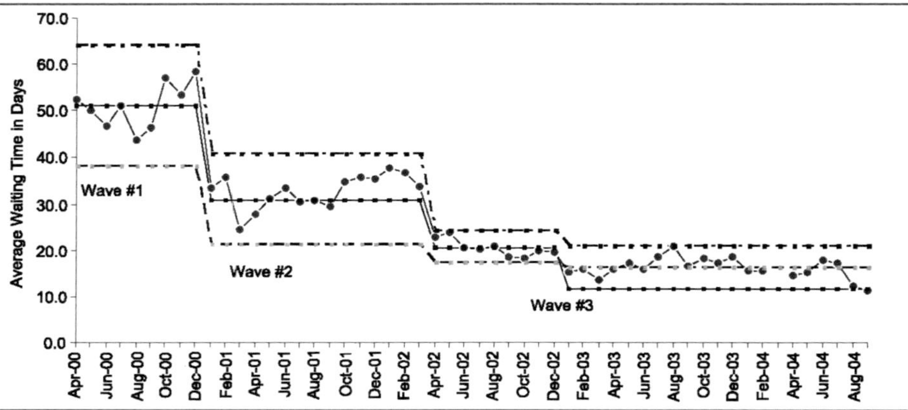

Figure 4. *This graph shows the reduction in waiting time for a clinic appointment in VISN 2 that coincided with the implementation of its spread plan.*

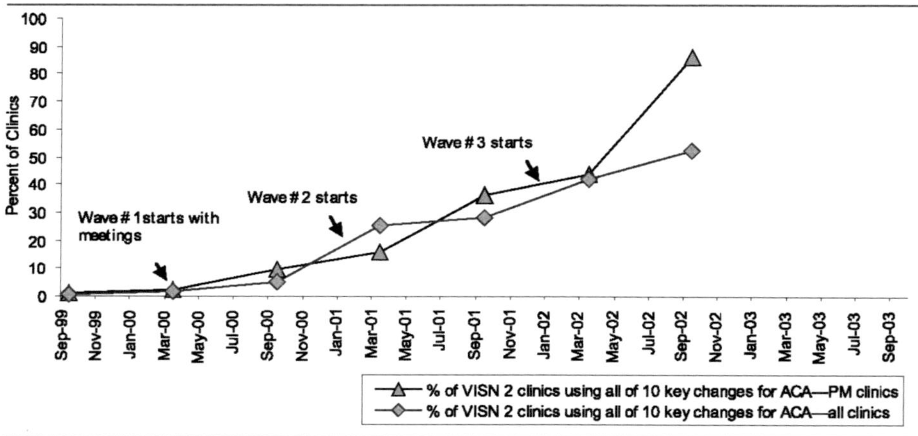

Figure 5. *This graph shows the increase in the number of clinics over time that implemented specific recommended changes to improve access as part of the Advanced Clinic Access project in VISN 2. ACA, Advanced Clinic Access; PM, performance.*

124

Journal™ ᴏɴ Quality ᴀɴᴅ Patient Safety

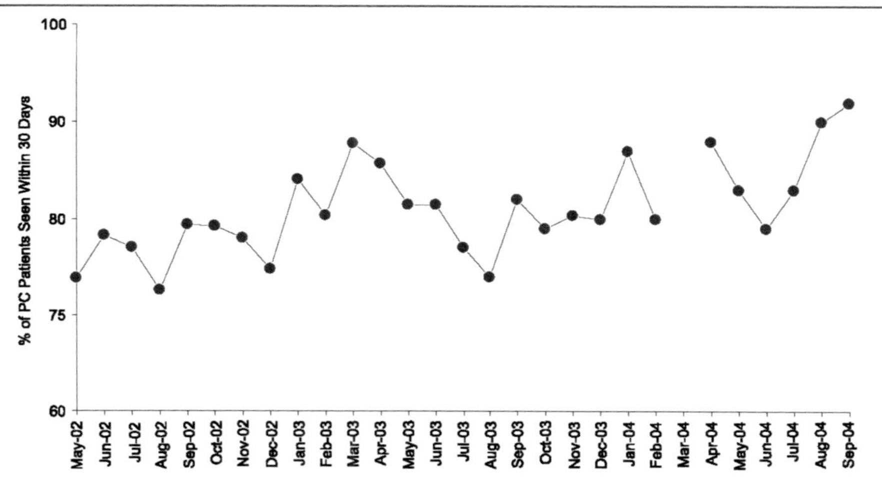

Figure 6. *This graph shows the increase in the percentage of primary care (PC) patients in VISN 2 who were seen within a 30-day time period from the request for an appointment to the clinic visit, as specified in the Veterans Health Administration access standards.*

and technical knowledge to improve access to be communicated throughout the VISN. Because of the succinct packaging of ideas and the coaching of their peers, clinics could readily test changes to their systems. The rate of spread accelerated as a new wave of clinics was reached in face-to-face meetings and follow-up. The social system strengthened as physicians, nurses, and schedulers interacted at meetings, road shows, and other scheduled VISN events. Celebrating successes and shining a spotlight on the top performers had a positive effect on participation levels and led to greater physician involvement. The VISN 2 and national Web sites continue to serve as key resources for information. Data on wait times, which are available from the scheduling system, continue to provide a key source of feedback.

The Framework for Spread suggests areas that organizations should consider to develop and execute a strategy for a spread initiative. VISN 2 undertook a certain set of activities within the framework. Other VISNs undertook some different activities to provide leadership for the project, communicate ideas, strengthen the social system, or provide feedback. Further study is needed to determine the specific activities that should be emphasized to accelerate spread. This might depend on the characteristics of an organization and the ideas being spread.

The VHA and VISN 2 are actively pursuing the initiative to improve access. The existence of a VHA systemwide database enables demonstration of sustained reduction of waiting time for an appointment. The veterans—and other patients—deserve no less. **J**

Kevin Nolan, M.A., is Statistician, Associates in Process Improvement, Silver Spring, Maryland. Marie W. Schall, M.A., is a Director, Institute for Healthcare Improvement, Cambridge, Massachusetts. Fabiane Erb, R.H.I.A, is Health Systems Specialist, VA Western New York Healthcare System, Buffalo, New York. Thomas Nolan, Ph.D., is Statistician, Associates in Process Improvement. Please address reprint request to Marie Schall, M.A., mschall@ihi.org.

Joint Commission on Quality and Patient Safety

References

1. Schall M., et al.: Improving patient access to the Veterans Health Administration's primary care and specialty clinics. *Jt Comm J Qual Improv* 30:415–423, Aug. 2004

2. Institute of Medicine. *Crossing the Quality Chasm: A New Health System for the 21st Century.* Washington, D.C.: National Academy Press, 2001.

3. Cabana M., et al.: Why don't physicians follow clinical practice guidelines: A framework for improvement. *JAMA* 282:1458–1465, Oct. 20, 1999.

4. Grimshaw J.M., et al.: Changing physicians' behavior: What works and thoughts on getting more things to work. *J Contin Educ Health Prof* 22:237–243, Fall 2002.

5. Kilo C.: A framework for collaborative improvement: Lessons learned from the Institute for Healthcare Improvement Breakthrough Series. *Qual Manag Health Care* 6:1–13, Sep. 1998.

6. Wilson T., Berwick D., Cleary P.: What do collaborative improvement projects do? *Jt Comm J Qual Saf* 29:85–93, Feb. 2003.

7. Lynn J., Schall M.W., Milne C., et al.: Quality improvements in end of life care: insights from two collaboratives. *Jt Comm J Qual Improv* 26:254–267, May 2000.

8. Flamm B., Berwick D., Kabcenell A., et al.: *Reducing Cesarean Section Rates.* Boston: Institute for Healthcare Improvement, 1997.

9. Lynn J., et al.: Reforming care for persons near the end of life: The promise of quality improvement. *Ann Intern Med* 137: 117–122, Jul 16, 2002.

10. Rainey T., et al.: *Reducing Costs and Improving Outcomes in Adult Intensive Care.* Boston: Institute for Healthcare Improvement, 1998.

11. Weiss K., et al.: *Improving Asthma Care.* Boston: Institute for Healthcare Improvement, 1997.

12. Rogers E.: *Diffusion of Innovations,* 4th ed. New York: The Free Press, 1995.

13. Mills P., Weeks W., Surott-Kimberly B.: A multihospital safety improvement effort and the dissemination of new knowledge. *Jt Comm J Qual Saf* 29:124–133, Mar. 2003.

14. Bandura A.: *Social Foundations of Thought and Action.* Englewood Cliffs, N.J.: Prentice Hall, Inc., 1986.

15. Murray M., Berwick D.: Advanced access: reducing waiting and delays in primary care. *JAMA* 289:1035–1040, Feb. 26, 2003.

16. Murray M., et al.: Improving timely access to primary care: Case studies of the advanced access model. *JAMA* 289:1042–1046, Feb. 26, 2003.

17. Institute for Healthcare Improvement: Primary Care Access. http://www.ihi.org/IHI/Topics/OfficePractices/Access/ (last accessed Apr. 21, 2005).

18. Sanderson J.: Waiting for care. *Vanguard.* U.S. Department of Veterans Affairs 48:16–18, 2002.

19. Prochaska J., Norcross J., DiClemente C.: *Changing for Good.* New York: William Morrow & Co., 1994.

20. Brown J., Duguid P.: *The Social Life of Information.* Boston: Harvard Business School Press, 2000.

21. Hirschhorn L.: Campaigning for change. *Harvard Bus Rev* 80:98–104, Jul. 2002.

22. Kotler P., Roberto E.: *Social Marketing: Strategies for Changing Public Behavior.* New York: Free Press, 1989.

23. Attewell P.: Technology diffusion and organizational learning: The case of business computing. *Organization Science* 3:1–19, Feb. 1992.

24. Fraser S.: *Accelerating the Spread of Good Practice.* Chichester, U.K.: Kingsham Press, 2002.

25. Avorn J., Soumerai S.: Improving drug-therapy decisions through educational outreach: A randomized controlled trial of academically based "detailing." *N Engl J Med* 308:1457–1463, Jun. 16, 1983.

26. Szulanski G., Winter S.: Getting it right the second time. *Harvard Bus Rev* 80:62–69, Jan. 2002.

27. Wenger E.: *Communities of Practice: Learning Meaning and Identity.* Cambridge, U.K.: Cambridge University Press, 1998.

28. Wenger E., McDermott R., Snyder, W.: *Civilizing Communities of Practice.* Boston: Harvard Business School Press, 2002.

29. Lomas J., et al.: Opinion leaders vs audit and feedback to implement practice guidelines. Delivery after previous cesarean section. *JAMA* 265:2202–2207, May 1, 1991.

30. Soumerai S.B, et al.: Effect of local medical opinion leaders on quality of care for acute myocardial infarction: A randomized controlled trial. *JAMA* 279:1358–1363, May 6, 1998.

31. Katz E.: The two-step flow of communication: An up-to-date report on an hypothesis. *Public Opinion Quarterly* 21:61–78, 1957.

32. Gladwell M.: *The Tipping Point: How Little Things Can Make A Big Difference.* Boston: Little, Brown, 2000.

33. Langley G., et al.: *The Improvement Guide.* San Francisco: Jossey Bass, 1996.

34. Dixon N.: *Common Knowledge: How Companies Thrive by Sharing What They Know.* Boston: Harvard Business School Press, 2000.

35. Bass F.: A new product growth model for consumer durables. *Management Science* 13:215–227, 1969.

36. Brown J., Duguid P.: Balancing act: How to capture knowledge without killing it. *Harvard Bus Rev* 78:73–80, May–Jun. 2000.

37. Cool K.O., Dierickx I., Szulanski G.: Diffusion of innovations within organizations: Electronic switching in the Bell System, 1971–1982. *Organization Science* 8:543–559, Sep.–Oct. 1997.

38. Grol R., Grimshaw J.: From best evidence to best practice: Effective implementation of change in patients' care. *Lancet* 362: 1225–1230, Oct. 11, 2003.

The Joint Commission Journal on Quality and Patient Safety

Performance Improvement

Implementing a Ventilator Bundle in a Community Hospital

Paul Youngquist, M.D.
Michelle Carroll, M.S.
Michelle Farber, R.N., C.I.C.
Deborah Macy, R.N., B.S.N.
Pamela Madrid, R.N., M.S., C.C.R.N., C.C.N.S.
Jeanine Ronning, R.N., B.S.N.
Amy Susag, R.N., M.S., C.C.R.N., C.C.N.S.

Ventilator-associated pneumonia (VAP) is the most common hospital-acquired infection among ventilator patients and has been associated with extended hospital lengths of stay (LOS) and higher rates of mortality for patients.[1] Average VAP rates in hospitals across the United States vary from 2.9 VAPs per 1,000 ventilator days in pediatric ICUs to 15.2 VAPs per 1,000 ventilator days in trauma ICUs.[2] Research has shown mortality rates ranging from 24% to 50%, depending on individual co-morbidities and pathogens involved.[3] Although some studies have not found VAP to be an independent contributor to intensive care unit (ICU) mortality,[3] hospital-acquired pneumonia increases complexity of care, ICU LOS by 6.1 days, and hospital LOS by 10.5 days.[4] Each VAP is estimated to add $40,000 to the cost of a patient's care.

Reductions of ventilator-associated pneumonia (VAP) associated with use of a bundle concept have recently been reported.[5] As a known complication with significant morbidity and mortality, VAP has also become one of the primary interventions for the 5 Million Lives Campaign, formerly known as the 100,000 Lives Campaign, initiated by the Institute for Healthcare Improvement (IHI).[6]

Mercy & Unity Hospitals of Minnesota implemented the IHI ventilator bundle concept as part of its participation in an IHI Breakthrough Series collaborative on improving care in the ICU, which was conducted from June 2003 through May 2004. This articles reports on the work that Mercy & Unity Hospitals conducted within the collaborative.

Article-at-a-Glance

Background: Mercy & Unity Hospitals of Minnesota implemented the ventilator bundle concept as part of an Institute for Healthcare Improvement (IHI) collaborative on improving care in the intensive care unit (ICU).

Methods: The two hospitals, which function as a single hospital, have a total of 450 beds, and each has a 20-bed ICU. The IHI bundle was composed of (1) head-of-bed elevation, (2) a daily "sedation vacation" along with a readiness-to-wean assessment, (3) peptic ulcer disease prophylaxis, and (4) deep vein thrombosis prophylaxis. Additional interventions likely complementary to the ventilator bundle were a hand hygiene campaign and an oral care protocol.

Results: Overall compliance with the four bundle elements reached 100% by January 2004. At the end of the collaborative, Mercy's VAP rate decreased from 6.1 to 2.70 per 1,000 ventilator days, and Unity's VAP rate decreased from 2.66 to 0 per 1,000 ventilator days.

Discussion: The all-or-none nature of the bundle may have helped multidisciplinary staff members perceive the project as a systemic change versus a one-time intervention. Staff members needed to implement both structural changes, such as preprinted order sets for ventilator management and sedation, and cultural changes, such as increased collaboration with respiratory therapy.

Conclusion: The decrease in VAP provides a promising example of the potential of intervention techniques and bundle implementation in a community hospital.

The Joint Commission Journal on Quality and Patient Safety

Methods

SETTING

Mercy & Unity Hospitals, located nine miles apart in the northern suburbs of Minneapolis, are part of Allina Hospitals & Clinics, a not-for-profit network of hospitals, clinics, and other health care services, that provide care throughout Minnesota and western Wisconsin. The hospitals function as a single hospital with two campuses and have a combined total of 450 beds. Intensive care beds include a 20-bed unit at Mercy, which combines a medical-surgical unit with cardiovascular surgery, and a 20-bed combined medical-surgical unit at Unity.

Ventilator Bundle

One of the key change concepts offered in the IHI collaborative was implementation of a ventilator bundle. The IHI bundle was composed of the following four elements[5]:
1. Head-of-bed (HOB) elevation
2. Implementation of a daily "sedation vacation" along with a readiness-to-wean assessment
3. Peptic ulcer disease prophylaxis
4. Deep vein thrombosis prophylaxis

Additional interventions that were likely complementary to the ventilator bundle were a hand hygiene campaign and an oral care protocol (which included oral care every two hours with swabs and a peroxide-based solution, teeth-brushing every 12 hours and a subglottic secretion removal every 6 hours.)

Several written communications were important in reminding and motivating ICU staff members about bundle implementation. Data on VAP rates were posted near nurse break rooms with initials of the patient included on the posters to help maintain motivation and focus on the fact that each complication happens to a real patient. Fact sheets and in-services were provided to bedside providers about the ventilator bundle. Compliance with the bundle was tracked in visible ways, including a goals sheet used during daily, multidisciplinary rounds.

The implementation of the ventilator bundle elements is now described.

1. HOB ELEVATION

As a compromise between literature that recommends an angle of 45 degrees[7] and staff members' concern about possible pressure ulcers and patients sliding down in bed, a 30-degree angle was selected as the minimum HOB elevation. The unit clinical nurse specialist performed daily written assessments to determine whether the practice was being followed. If not, the assessment became an opportune time to teach about the benefits of HOB elevation and to discuss options for patients who could not tolerate a 30-degree elevation but may be able to tolerate a lesser elevation.

In the beginning, the clinical nurse specialist and two nurse champions performed multiple informal assessments in addition to the daily written assessments. Their constant presence was key to spreading the practice throughout the unit. Other tools were helpful as well. For example, reminder signs were placed in rooms where 30-degree HOB elevation was applicable. Nurses and respiratory therapists were jointly responsible to ensure a minimum HOB elevation in all patients without contraindications. Monthly compliance audits were completed by the unit clinical nurse specialists, and the data were fed back to clinical staff.

2. DAILY SEDATION VACATION AND READINESS-TO-WEAN ASSESSMENT

The Mercy & Unity team implemented the sedation vacation through the use of rapid-cycle change methodology whereby several physicians and registered nurses (RNs) were selected to develop and test a revised order set for ICU sedation. Reduction in sedation occurred on a daily basis unless medically contraindicated. The interventions were reinforced by daily multidisciplinary rounds.

Each shift, a patient care nurse (RN) and a respiratory therapist jointly evaluated each ventilator patient's readiness-to-wean through the use of a well-established weaning parameter, the rapid shallow breathing index[8] and by reviewing medications, hemodynamic stability, and alertness. If the patient met the criteria for readiness to wean (Table 1, page 221), then a weaning trial could be implemented. In some instances, the physician chooses to play a more active role in the weaning process and is contacted for input before a weaning trial is undertaken.

3. PEPTIC ULCER DISEASE PROPHYLAXIS

Famotidine (Pepcid) 20 milligrams twice per day was used as the standard prophylaxis unless modified because of concurrent medications, renal status, and mental status.

The Joint Commission Journal on Quality and Patient Safety

Table 1. Readiness to Wean Criteria*

First Assessment Upon Admission to ICU

For neurosurgical patients do not assess weaning readiness or attempt weaning trial until direct physician order.

- Alertness to voice
- Hemodynamic stability: BP controlled, rhythm stable (may be on continuous IV medications for control) Exclude: Dopamine/Dobutamine $\geq$ 6 mcg/kg/min, Diltiazem $\geq$ 10 mg/hr
- Temperature < 101 degrees F
- Oxygen saturation $\geq$ 90% on < 60 FIO_2 and < 5 cm PEEP

Failure to Wean Criteria

- RR < 6 or RSB index > 100
- HR increase of > 20% baseline, ventricular ectopy or SVT
- Change in mental status
- Worsening clinical status
- If wean failure X 2 or patient on ventilator > 72 hours, obtain a pulmonary consult.
- HR > 130 bpm
- O_2 saturation < 90%
- Increased agitation
- Worsening of secretions

*ICU, intensive care unit; BP, blood pressure; IV, intravenous; FIO_2, forced inspiratory oxygen; PEEP, positive-end expiratory pressure; RR, respiratory rate; RSB, rapid shallow breathing; HR, heart rate; SVT, sinoventricular tachycardia; BPM, beats per minute.

Stress ulcer prophylaxis was discussed daily in multidisciplinary rounds as a redundancy to assure compliance with this element of the bundle.

4. DEEP VEIN THROMBOSIS PROPHYLAXIS

Several treatment options were developed. Unless contraindicated, elastic compression stockings with pneumatic compression devices were automatically applied to each patient.

CHART REVIEWS

Retrospective chart reviews for January 2003 through June 2003 were completed by clinical nurse specialists, who used the revised Centers for Disease Control & Prevention (CDC)–National Nosocomial Infections Surveillance System (NNIS) definitions for VAP were used.[9] VAP rates were calculated by using the number of ventilator hours divided by 24, with a denominator of 1,000 ventilator days.

Clinical nurse specialists coordinated completion of the surveillance check list for every ventilated patient. Questions were discussed with the infection control practitioner, and all "possible pneumonia" charts were reviewed by the infection control practitioner for the final determination.

ICU patients' charts were reviewed for the duration of their ICU LOS for the presence of symptoms developing 48 hours after intubation that were not incubating or present on ICU admission. These patients' chest x-rays and other CDC criteria were reviewed until 48 hours after the ventilator was discontinued or the patient was transferred out of the ICU.

Prospective chart reviews since July 2003 have been completed using slightly different methodology at the two campuses. At the Mercy campus, they are completed by the respiratory care advisory team in a group setting with the infection control practitioner. At the Unity campus, the clinical nurse specialist prospectively completes the chart reviews and discusses possible cases with the ICU medical director and the infection control practitioner. At both campuses, the infection control practitioner reviews all "possible pneumonia" charts for the final determination.

On both campuses, the infection control practitioner conducts inter-rater reliability testing on a random basis for all patients with abnormal chest x-ray presentation. Each surveillance checklist is completed for each ventilated patient who has been on the ventilator for 24 hours. To explore whether any pneumonia cases were missed, the infection control practitioner reviews the *International Classification of Diseases,* 9th revision (ICD-9) code for pneumonia, electronic reports of temperature, elevated white blood counts, and mentation changes in patients older than 70 years of age.

Beginning in July 2004, at the end of the collaborative, ventilator days were collected by the ICU staff at midnight to include each patient that was on a ventilator as a ventilator day. The number of ventilator infections was divided by the number of ventilator days and multiplied by a constant value, 1,000, to report rates as the number of ventilator pneumonias per 1,000 ventilator days.

The Joint Commission Journal on Quality and Patient Safety

Ventilator Bundle Compliance During IHI Collaborative

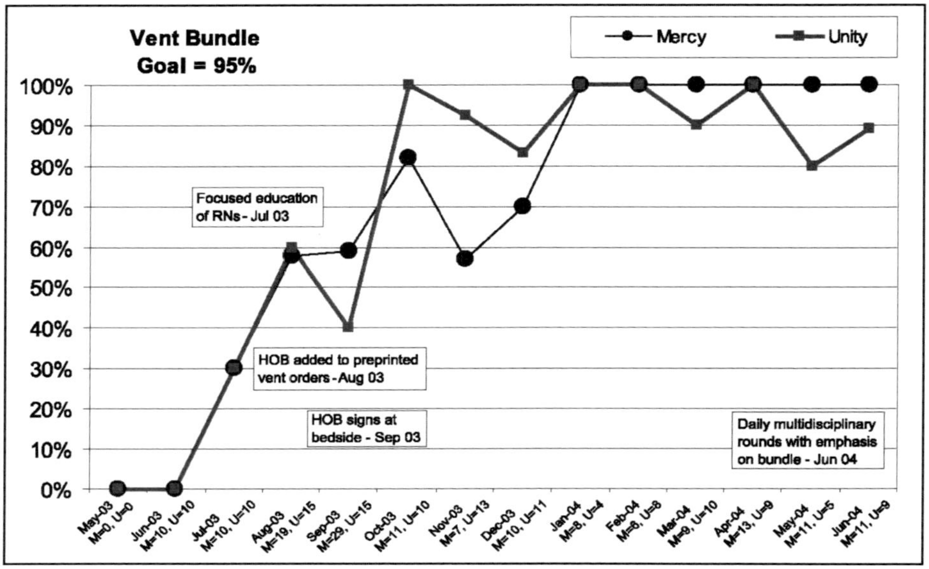

Figure 1. *Compliance of 100% was reached by January 2004 after focused RN education about the bundle, addition of head-of-bed (HOB) orders to preprinted ventilator order sets, and placement of the HOB elevation reminder signs in rooms of patients when it was not contraindicated. The number of ventilator patients audited each month is shown for Mercy (M) & Unity (U) Hospitals.*

Results

Data collected for the VAP bundle included one process measure, which identified overall compliance to the four bundle elements. Outcome measures included the total number of ventilator days, the frequency of VAP, ICU average LOS, and ICU mortality. The initial process goal was to implement all bundle components within 24 hours of admission in 95% of patients. Compliance of 100% was reached by January 2004 after focused R.N. education about the bundle, addition of HOB orders to preprinted ventilator order sets, and placement of the HOB elevation reminder signs in rooms of patients where HOB elevation was not contraindicated (Figure 1, above).

The baseline VAP rate from January 2003 to June 2003 for the Mercy campus was 6.01 per 1,000 ventilator days

and 2.66 per 1,000 ventilator days at the Unity campus. At the end of the collaborative (June 2004), Mercy's VAP rate decreased by 55% to 2.70 per 1,000 ventilator days, and Unity's VAP rate decreased to 0 per 1,000 ventilator days (Figure 2, page 223). The VAP rate at Mercy continued to decrease—to 2.20 per 1,000 ventilator days. Unity experienced one VAP case, which brought its rate to 1.47 per 1,000 ventilator days. In 2006, Mercy's VAP rate was 0 per 1,000 ventilator days and Unity's VAP rate was 1.69 per 1,000 ventilator days.

Both campuses' rates are below the published CDC pool mean rates for non-teaching medical-surgical ICUs of 5.1 per 1,000 ventilator days.[1] In addition, there has been a statistically significant reduction (p = .02) in average LOS for ventilator patients at the Unity campus between 2003 and

The Joint Commission Journal on Quality and Patient Safety

2004 (Table 2, page 224). At Mercy, there was not a statistical difference in LOS for ventilator patients, although the LOS was already low (9.0 days).

Discussion

Bundles, as defined by IHI, are a cohesive unit of evidence-based interventions that should be implemented as a set[6] as a strategy to help reduce inpatient mortality. Bundle theory posits that a set of practices implemented all at once improves reliability because it demands a high level of teamwork and fundamental changes in how work is performed.[5] Experiences with the VAP bundle have shown that use of the bundle is correlated with significant decreases in VAP rates, despite the fact that two of the four bundle elements (deep vein thrombosis

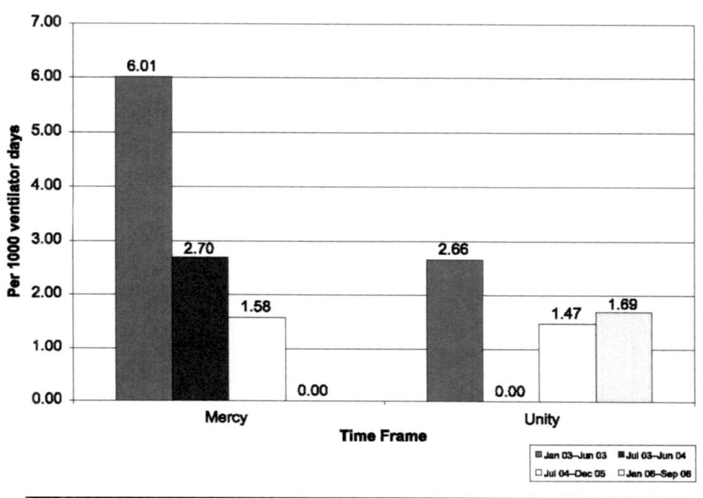

Figure 2. *At the end of the collaborative (June 2004), Mercy's VAP rate had decreased by 55% to 2.70 per 1,000 ventilator days, and Unity's VAP rate had decreased by 100% to 0 per 1,000 ventilator days.*

prophylaxis and stress ulcer prevention) have not been correlated specifically with VAP reduction.[5]

We believe the all-or-none nature of the bundle helped multidisciplinary staff members perceive the project as a systemic change versus a one-time intervention. To meet the all-or-none compliance goal, staff members needed to implement both structural changes, such as preprinted order sets for ventilator management and sedation, and cultural changes, such as discussion of VAP at multidisciplinary weekday rounds and increased collaboration with respiratory therapy. The immensity of the change required staff members to approach the project as a team, keep a constant focus on the topic, and develop new relationships and processes.

One particularly challenging culture change was implementation of HOB elevation. The challenge was to keep staff members focused on HOB elevation throughout the day as patients were moved or manipulated in the

process of care. In the first few months, the clinical nurse specialist and two nurse champions on the unit each performed informal assessments multiple times a day, in addition to one daily written assessment of HOB elevation. Their presence served as a reminder to nursing staff and also generated productive discussions about elevations of less than 30 degrees that might be tolerated by patients with contraindications to a full 30 degrees. The "constant drumbeat" about HOB elevation in the beginning of the campaign solidified the change in the patient care environment.

Although the IHI collaborative promoted implementation of all bundle elements unless they were medically contraindicated, it recommended that hospitals implement the bundle according to each organization's unique needs.[6] We believe that such flexibility hastened implementation by allowing adaptation of the initiative to pre-existing structures in our individual environments. For

The Joint Commission Journal on Quality and Patient Safety

example, prospective chart reviews for "possible pneumonia" cases were completed with slightly different methodology on our two campuses. On the Unity campus, such cases were flagged by a clinical nurse specialist, then discussed with the ICU medical director and infection control practitioner. On the Mercy campus, staff members folded chart review work into the pre-existing respiratory care advisory team.

Although the all-or-none bundle sparked systemic and cultural changes, measurable outcomes appeared to be a more significant motivating factor for continued focus on VAP rates once the collaborative was over. When frontline staff members realized during the collaborative that VAP rates were falling, they began questioning how they could build on their successes after the collaborative. Analysis of VAP events and efforts to encourage bundle compliance remained in place. The campuses' joint multidisciplinary critical care quality improvement committee took on the task of pursuing other opportunities to affect VAP rates. Because the two campuses function as one hospital, with mostly the same policies, procedures, and equipment, the committee determined that further analyses could help target small differences in practices that could affect VAP rates. Analyses on each campus revealed differences in endotracheal saline instillation protocols and identified several better practices, which were subsequently implemented systemwide:

■ Limiting of saline instillation because of a lack of supporting evidence[10]

■ Use of a inline-catheter to maintain the closed suction system

■ Documentation of in-line suction catheter changes every 72 hours per the manufacturer's recommendations

■ Use of a new device for removal of condensation in ventilation tubing to prevent accidental patient lavage

■ Locking of suction port when not in use to prevent accidental patient lavage

Education was undertaken on these practices, as well as on the following:

■ The importance of not leaving saline bullets attached to suction catheters and also to announce a transition to the use of 5-ml sterile saline bullets

■ Proper endotracheal and subglottic suctioning techniques to help reduce migration of oral secretions past the endotracheal tube

	Table 2. Length of Stay (LOS) for Intensive Care Unit Ventilator Patients, Unity Campus, 2003–2004*			
Year	Total Number of Patients	LOS Hours	ALOS	S.D.
2003	205	65,342.0	13.3	12.34
2004	224	58,165.0	10.8	10.50

* S.D., standard deviation; p = .02.

■ Use of the correct port for saline lavage.

An initial audit performed in June 2004 at the conclusion of the collaborative revealed a compliance rate for all eight practices of 74%. In August 2004, after education (which included one-on-one sessions, staff in-services at shift change, and a display), a repeat audit showed a compliance rate of 93%. Currently, random audits are completed to monitor compliance. Other activities undertaken during the same postcollaborative time period included review and implementation of recommendations from evidence-based guidelines. For example, the team standardized time intervals for changing heat-moisture exchangers and closed suction catheters. They also performed a gap analysis using the 2003 CDC Guidelines for Preventing Health-Care Associated Pneumonia (published in March 2004[11]). These additional interventions relied on the platform of multidisciplinary teamwork and focus established during the IHI collaborative.

Some limitations of the study should be noted. Statistical significance in the VAP rate decrease was not established because of low rates at project commencement. A full accounting of patient status before and after bundle interventions would involve a detailed analysis of the patient population (including reasons for mechanical ventilation, ages, proportion of medical versus surgical patients) and a multivariate analysis to demonstrate the effect of the bundle on VAP rates; such an analysis was not undertaken. In addition, although steps were taken to avoid bias in the retrospective chart reviews, those reviews are inherently subject to human bias. At Mercy & Unity, several non-bundle initiatives undertaken before, during, and after bundle implementation were not analyzed for their effect on VAP rates, including the hand hygiene campaign, refinement and relaunching of oral care practices,

The Joint Commission Journal on Quality and Patient Safety

and the initiatives undertaken, as noted, by the critical care quality improvement committee.

Conclusion

Although further study is needed on the ventilator bundle and the additional interventions conducted at Mercy and Unity, the reported decrease in VAP provides a promising example of the potential of VAP intervention techniques and bundle implementation in a community hospital setting.

The authors acknowledge Dennis O'Hare, M.D., Gloria O'Connell, Kathy Wilde, and Linda Zespy for their support and assistance in the preparation of this manuscript.

Paul Youngquist, M.D., is a Physician in Critical Care Medicine at Mercy & Unity Hospitals, Coon Rapids, Minnesota. **Michelle Carroll, M.S.,** is a Data Analyst/Statistician, Allina Hospitals and Clinics, Minneapolis. **Michelle Farber, R.N., C.I.C.,** is an Infection Control Specialist; **Deborah Macy, R.N., B.S.N.,** is Director of Emergency, Trauma, and Critical Care Services; **Pamela Madrid, R.N., M.S., C.C.R.N., C.C.N.S.,** is a Clinical Nurse Specialist, Emergency and Critical Care; **Jeanine Ronning, R.N., B.S.N.,** is a Quality Case Consultant Supervisor; **Amy Susag, R.N., M.S., C.C.R.N., C.C.N.S.,** is a Clinical Nurse Specialist, Emergency and Critical Care, Mercy & Unity Hospitals. Please address reprint requests to Paul Youngquist, p_youngquist@msn.com.

References

1. Richards M.J., et al.: Nosocomial infections in medical intensive care units in the United States: National Nosocomial Infections Surveillance System. *Crit Care Med* 27:887–892, May 1999.
2. National Nosocomial Infections Surveillance (NNIS) System Report, data summary from January 1992 through June 2004, issued October 2004. *Am J Infect Control* 32:470–485, Dec. 2004.
3. Bregeon F., et al.: Relationship of microbiologic diagnostic criteria to morbidity and mortality in patients with ventilator-associated pneumonia. *JAMA* 1997 Feb 26; 277:655–662, Feb. 26, 1997. Erratum in: *JAMA* 1997 Jul 2;278:25, Jul. 2, 1997.
4. Rollo J., et al.: Epidemiology and outcomes of ventilator-associated pneumonia in a large U.S. database. *Chest* 122:2115–2121, Dec. 2002.
5. Resar R., et al.: Using a bundle approach to improve ventilator care processes and reduce ventilator-associated pneumonia. *Jt Comm J Qual Patient Saf* 31:243–248, May 2005.
6. Institute for Healthcare Improvement: *Protecting 5 Million Lives from Harm Campaign.* http://www.ihi.org/IHI/Programs/Campaign/Campaign.htm?TabId=2#PreventVentilator-AssociatedPneumonia (last accessed Feb. 7, 2007).
7. Drakulovic M.G., et al.: Supine body position as a risk factor for nosocomial pneumonia in mechanically ventilated patients: A randomised trail. *Lancet* 354:1851–1858, Nov. 27, 1999.
8. Manthous C.A., Schmidt G.A., Hall J.B.: Liberation from mechanical ventilation: a decade of progress. *Chest* 114:886–901, Sep. 1998.
9. Horan T.C., Gaynes R.P.: Surveillance of nosocomial infections. In Mayhall C.G. (ed.): *Hospital Epidemiology and Infection Control* 3rd ed. Philadelphia: Lippincott Williams & Wilkins, 2004, pp. 1659–1702.
10. Kinloch D.: Instillation of normal saline during endotracheal suctioning: Effects on mixed venous oxygen saturation. *Am J Crit Care* 8:231–242, Jul. 1999.
11. Centers for Disease Control & Prevention: Guidelines for Preventing Health-Care-Associated Pneumonia, 2003. Recommendations of CDC and the Healthcare Infection Control Practices Advisory Committee. *MMWR* 53:RR-3, Mar. 2004.

Journal Reference Resources

Acute Heart Failure

Bradley E.H., et al.: Strategies for reducing the door-to-balloon time in acute myocardial infarction. *N Engl J Med* 355:2308–2320, Nov. 30, 2006.

Henry T.D., et al.: Design of a standardized system for transfer of patients with ST-elevation myocardial infarction for percutaneous coronary intervention. *Am Heart J* 150:373–384, Sep. 2005.

Henry T.D., et al.: ST-segmented elevation myocardial infarction: Recommendations on triage of patients to heart attack centers: Is it time for a national policy for the treatment of ST-segment elevation myocardial infarction? *J Am Coll Cardiol* 47(7):1339–1345, 2006.

Keeley E.C., Grines C.L.: Primary percutaneous coronary intervention for every patient with ST-segment elevation myocarcial infarction: What stands in the way? *Ann Intern Med* 141(4):298–304, 2004.

McNamara R.L., et al.: Hospital improvement in time to reperfusion in patients with acute myocardial infarction. *J Am Coll Cardiol* 47:45–51, Jan. 3, 2006.

Stroke

Moser D.K., et al.: Reducing delay in seeking treatment by patients with acute coronary syndrome and stroke: A scientific statement from the American Heart Association Council on Cardiovascular Nursing and Stroke Council. *Circulation* 114:168–182, 2006.

Ventilator-Associated Pneumonia

Iregui M., et al.: Clinical importance of delays in the initiation of appropriate antibiotic treatment for ventilator-associated pneumonia. *Chest* 122(1):262–268, 2002.

Tuberculosis

Pascopella L., et al.: Laboratory reporting of tuberculosis test results and patient treatment initiation in California. *J Clin Microbiol* 42(9):4209–4213, 2004.

Transfer Delays

Berns K.S., Hankins D.G., Zietlow S.P.: Comparison of air and ground transport of cardiac patients. *Air Med J* 20:33–36, Nov.–Dec., 2001.

Nallomothu B.K., et al.: Times to treatment in transfer patients undergoing primary percutaneous coronary intervention in the United States: National Registry of Myocardial Infarction (NRMI)–3/4 analysis. *Circulation* 111:761–767, Feb. 15, 2005.

Young M.P., et al.: Inpatient transfer to the intensive care unit: Delays are associated with increased mortality and morbidity. *J Gen Intern Med* 18:77–83, Feb. 2003.

Care Coordination

Mosenthal A.C., Murphy P.A.: Interdisciplinary model for palliative care in the trauma and surgical intensive care unit: Robert Wood Johnson Foundation Demonstration Project for improving palliative care in the intensive care unit. *Crit Care Med* 34(suppl. 11):S399–S403, 2006.

Emergency Department

Chan T.C., et al.: Impact of rapid entry and accelerated care at triage on reducing emergency department patient wait times, lengths of stay, and rate of left without being seen. *Ann Emerg Med* 46:491–497, Dec. 2005.

Appointment Delays in Physician Offices

Murray M., Berwick D.M.: Advanced access: Reducing waiting and delays in primary care. *JAMA* 289(8):1035–1040, 2003.

Timing Is Everything: Strategies for Reducing Delays in Patient Care

INDEX

A

B

C

D

E

I

Q

R

S

T

U

V

W

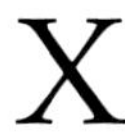

X

The Practical Book of
REIKI

Healing Through
Universal Lifeforce Energy

Mrs. Rashmi Sharma

Herbal Beautician

Founder
RASHMI CAVES HERBAL EDUCATIONAL SOCIETY (R)

&

Maharaj Krishan Sharma

Master Reiki Healer

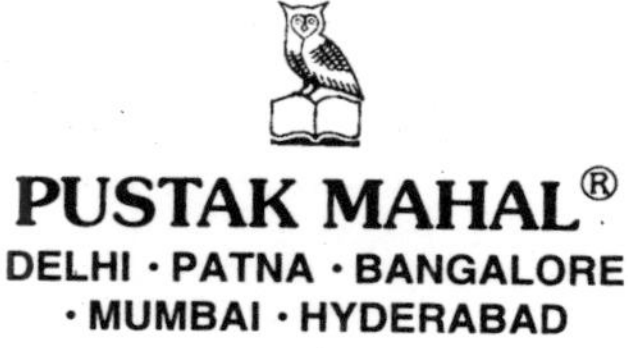

PUSTAK MAHAL®
DELHI · PATNA · BANGALORE
· MUMBAI · HYDERABAD

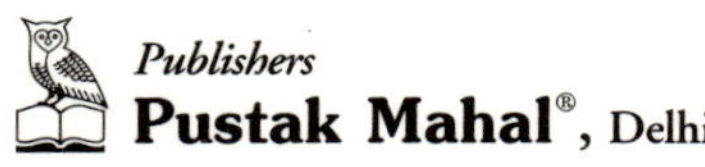

Publishers
Pustak Mahal®, Delhi

J-3/16, Daryaganj, New Delhi-110002
☎ 23276539, 23272783, 23272784 • *Fax:* 011-23260518
E-mail: info@pustakmahal.com • *Website:* www.pustakmahal.com

London Office
51, Severn Crescents, Slough, Berkshire, SL 38 UU, England
E-mail: pustakmahaluk@pustakmahal.com

Sales Centre
10-B, Netaji Subhash Marg, Daryaganj, New Delhi-110002
☎ 23268292, 23268293, 23279900 • *Fax:* 011-23280567
E-mail: rapidexdelhi@indiatimes.com

Branch Offices
Bangalore: ☎ 22234025
E-mail: pmblr@sancharnet.in • pustak@sancharnet.in
Mumbai: ☎ 22010941
E-mail: rapidex@bom5.vsnl.net.in
Patna: ☎ 3294193 • *Telefax:* 0612-2302719
E-mail: rapidexptn@rediffmail.com
Hyderabad: *Telefax:* 040-24737290
E-mail: pustakmahalhyd@yahoo.co.in

© **Pustak Mahal, Delhi**

ISBN 978-81-223-0110-6

Edition : 2008

Printed at : Param Offsetters, Okhla, New Delhi-110020

PUBLISHER'S NOTE

We all are aware of the fact that we continue to move steadily towards the 21st Century. In our present time, our spiritual awareness is evolving at a swift pace. In modern living, more and more people are opening up in their consciousness to alternate natural methods of healing for the mind and body. Modern Science acknowledges the relation between mind and body. Physicians advocate relaxation techniques, and an increasing number of people are finding themselves drawn to working with healing energies.

Among many methods of natural healing, Reiki is one of the prime and effective methods that is being practised world over. The word "Reiki" is a Japanese one meaning Universal lifeforce or the energy of healing which works on physical and mental level. **Reiki is neither a religion nor a cult. It does not involve faith healing or black magic. It is a natural method of healing, using Universal healing energy.**

The Practical Book of Reiki tells all about Reiki. Reiki — in its current form is a new concept — but we may find some *Shlokas* in *Atharvaveda* which refer to such spiritual healing energy as we now call it Reiki.

And what does Reiki heal? The author answers this question in a very lucid and simple language, ranging from mental to physical body and to remove blocks of negativity and allowing the release of destructive emotional patterns which manifest as pain and other serious ailments in the body.

Through this wonderful concept — as explained in this book, accompanying with many lively illustrations, anybody can continue to increase his/her vibratory level and healing capacity by self-treatment.

This book is for those who are looking for such a useful treatise on self-transformation with principles that actually work. It is a practical, powerful guide that tells you in a plain language exactly what you need for leading a joyful and better life.

Spend everyday casually, but industriously — in a series of moment-to-moment victories.

— Publishers

CONTENTS

PART II

11. KEEP YOUR HANDS ON PRACTICE 80

12. ENERGY FIELD 90

A TRIBUTE

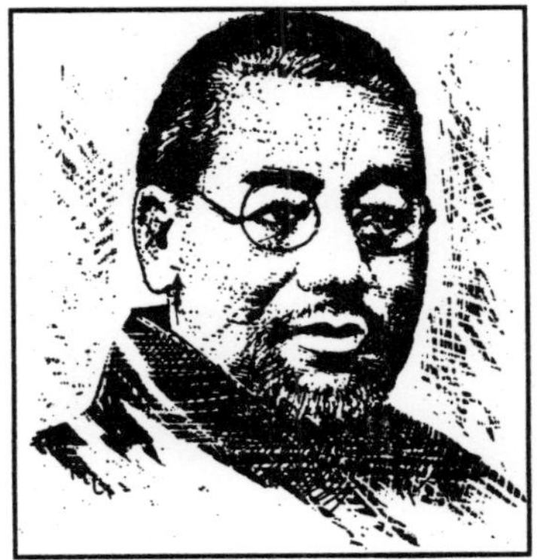

Dr Mikao Usui

*We are deeply grateful to Dr Mikao Usui for showing us the hidden path of the Universal Lifeforce Energy—**Reiki** in this jet-age of our world. We honour and respect this unconditional divine healing energy—**REIKI**. It always went for the welfare of all without the discrimination of the state of health or sickness, conditions of religion, belief and birth. We pay our affectionate homage from the core of our hearts to this great reoriginator of the Divine Power—**REIKI**.*

INTRODUCTION

In the discovery from the experiences of Yogis, *Purohits* and *Atharvaveda* shastra we have concluded that the Birth, Sickness and Reappearance are the processes of rediscovering the wiser parts of ourselves.

We are parts of the Earth

We are parts of the Water

We are parts of the Fire

We are parts of the Air

We are parts of the Metal

(All these are called as panch Tatva)

and experiences show:

I am not this Body

I am not this Life

I am not this moment of Today

I am a moment of Memory

Love me — Love all

One is Everywhere

Supreme Power

A Divine Power

Whole, Holy and Complete

The highest empowerment referred to our ancient is from *Atharvaveda*, which was only available with *Vaids*, *Purohits* and Gurus. Today the system known as Reiki — a Divine Healing Power has this same capacity of healing.

THE DIVINE POWER

The Divine Power Reiki works to heal on the physical, subtle and casual levels. When one begins to see the important links, he can make between Reiki and all other forms of healing and spiritual unfoldment. Our understanding is that we are composed of more solid energy fields, which we call the physical body and less dense fields which we call subtle organizing energy fields (SOEFs). These SOEFs are moving faster than the speed of light and also simultaneously slower than the speed of high reflection of the multidimensional human conditions. These SOEFs, act as vortexes for the faster than the speed of light cosmic energy to come into the body, which is slower than the speed of light dimension and also acts as templates for the structure and the function of the emotional, mental and physical body. On the physical level these SOEFs are filled with energy and then they become well organised DNA/RNA system, which, in turn creates well functioning enzymes, protein synthesis and cell divisions. When the cells divide and function well, then the glands, organs and tissues also function well and we have sound health.

Conversely, when the SOEFs lose energy and become disrupted through the stress of emotional, mental, spiritual, or poor lifestyle imbalances, they act as poor templates for the physical functioning and we get disease. The process of SOEFs, loss of energy and disorganisation is the process of aging or in terms of second law of thermodynamics, it is an increase in entropy. The process of increasing the energy and therefore the organisation of the SOEFs, is the process of growing younger. It is a process of healing.

According to the second Law of thermodynamics, it is reversing entropy. Reiki directly brings in the universal lifeforce to the SOEFs which directly energizes them and consequently organizes them. In other words, Reiki reverses the aging process by reversing the increase in entropy. It does this directly and also indirectly by rebalancing the subtle bodies and chakras. When the subtle bodies and chakras are not aligned, they block the incoming universal lifeforce into the human system. Once aligned, the energy flows freely. This results in a reversal of entropy and therefore undergoes healing on an emotional, mental and spiritual level. Once, if the reader understands this simple concept, it is easier to appreciate the depth of the writer.

If one understands as explained above, we humans are human crystals made of a series of oscillating solid and liquid crystals. Dissonant thoughts and negative thoughts or emotions have a lower vibration in our crystalline structure, with Reiki — a Divine Power, the vibration rate is raised towards our full potential. It becomes so strong that the crystallized denser thought forms are not able to sustain their local locus of dissonance and become broken up and released from our physical or subtle bodies. If we are just able to observe them and release them, rather than get involved with them they leave our total system. It is also observed that this same process happens for meditators as well. The overall crystalline structure of our system becomes more resonant and the universal lifeforce moves more freely. The more the life energy is free to move in the body, the easier it is for "KUNDALINI", the spiritually transformative energy, to be awakened. Once KUNDALINI is awakened, the release of emotional and mental blocks are even more accelerated.

Reiki is not only a democratization of the ability to heal, but also it makes a level of spiritual transformation available to non-meditators, that is usually reserved for those with a meditative path.

1. DESCRIPTION OF REIKI

THE DEFINITION

Reiki is a Japanese word for universal lifeforce energy. When the Rei and Ki are broken down into their two component parts, the definition for "Rei" is universal transcendental spirit, mysterious power essence and "Ki" is described as the vital force energy. Reiki energy is available to all of us from the beginning of our birth. What makes Reiki different from other **healing methods, is the "attunement"** (also known as initiation) process which the student experiences in the various levels of Reiki. Any one can lay his hands on another person and help to accelerate the healing process by transferring magnetic energy. A person who has been through the process of Reiki attunements, however has experienced a very ancient technology for fine tuning the physical and ethnic bodies to a higher vibratory level. In addition, certain energy centres, also known as chakras are opened to enable the person to channel (and vibrate) higher amount of universal lifeforce energy.

APPLICATIONS AND BENEFITS

Reiki is never sent. It is drawn through the channel, for example, I lay my hands on you to do the treatment, you will draw appropriate amounts of energy to which every area of your body needs it. I am never drained in the process, as I am too treated when I give a treatment. The energy enters my crown chakra and passes through the upper energy centres to my heart and solar plexus. The rest then passes through my arms and hands to your body. I am thus never drained in the process, because a certain amount of energy is stored in me. However, at the sametime, you do not take any of my stuff (negative energy or blocks) as, the Reiki passes through a purified channel in my body opened by the attunement.

One of the greatest benefits of Reiki is the possibility of self treatment. Once a person is attuned he or she needs only to have the intention to do Reiki on himself/herself or others and the energy is immediately drawn through. Self treatment is an extremely effective technique for total relaxation and stress release. It amplifies the lifeforce energy in our body which then helps to create balance in the physical and etheric bodies. Treating oneself also helps to release withheld emotions and energy blocks.

REIKI—THE HIDDEN ANCIENT SCIENCE

Reiki is not a religion as it holds no creed or doctrine. Indeed, it is a very ancient science hidden for thousands of years until Dr Usui rediscovered this very old technology hidden in Tibetan sutras. Researchers using highly sensitive instruments, vrhich measure the flow of energy forces entering the body determined that the Reiki Energy enters the healer through the top of his head (crown chakra) and exits through the hands.

The Energy Force not only comes from a northerly direction but also from the south when it is below equator. In addition once the Reiki energy is activated it seems to flow in a counter clockwise spiral motion, much like the double helix in DNA.

THE TOOL OF SELF-CONSCIOUSNESS, ENLIGHTENMENT AND JOY

The evidences show very clearly that there is indeed a plasmatic streaming — a release of energy through the bodily system — when blocks are released. All outcomes are different for every treatment, as the healer being the determining factor in the net result. Each person draws in just the right amount of lifeforce that he or she needs to release, activate or transform the energy of the physical and etheric bodies. Reiki not only can effect change in the chemical structure of the body by helping to regenerate the organs and rebuild tissues and bones, it also helps to create balance on the mental level. Reiki is not a belief system, therefore no mental preparation or direction is needed to receive a treatment. Only need is a desire to receive and accept the energy. On the other hand, from the standpoint of the practitioner, since it is not a belief system, once the intention is clear to start a treatment it will always be activated when used as instructed. Reiki is a wonderful tool to help one to develop conscious awareness, the very key to enlightenment.

2. THE HISTORY OF REIKI

THE BACKGROUND

Dr Mikao Usui was the Dean of a small Christian University in Kyoto, Japan in mid 1800s. This was an exciting period in Japan's history and many changes were occurring throughout the society. The Japanese had only recently opened their shores to the foreigners and were quickly adopting all the new technology of Industrial Revolution. Dr Usui, however had adopted Christianity whole-heartedly, becoming a minister and then finally the Dean of Christian seminary.

One day, during the discussion with some of his students, Usui was asked if he believed literally in the Bible. When he replied in affirmative, his students reminded him of the instant healings of Christ. The students mentioned that in the Bible Christ states, " **You will do as I have done and even greater things if this is so".** They asked, "Why are not there many healers in the world now performing the same act as Christ?" In addition, Chirst also asked the apostles to heal the sick and raise the dead. "If this is true", the students said, "please teach us the methods". Usui was stunned. In traditional Japanese style, he was bound by his honour as Dean, to be able to answer their questions. On that day Usui resigned his position and determined to find the answers to this great mystery. As most of his teachers had been American Missionaries and America was predominantly a Christian country, he decided to begin his studies at the University of Chicago in the theological seminary. After a long period of study in which he did not find his answers, Usui resolved to continue his research elsewhere.

IN SEARCH OF THE GREAT MYSTERY

Dr Usui realized that Buddha was also known to have performed incredible healings. So he determined to return to Japan and see if he could indeed find some "new" old information about more of the instantaneous types of physical healing. Even if all records of the "how and wherefore" of Christ's healings had been lost, perhaps he might find information about Buddha's healings in Japanese "LOTUS SUTRAS". After his return, Usui began his investigations in several Buddhist monasteries. Each time he approached the abbots of various monasteries asking, "Do you have any record of Buddha's healings of the body?" He received a similar reply that all focuses were now placed on the healing of the spirit. Usui was determined in his search and after many trials he came upon a Zen monastery, where for the first time he was encouraged to continue his search by an old abbot. The latter agreed that it must be possible to heal the body, as Buddha had indeed done, but for centuries all concentration had been focused on healing the spirits. He said that whatever was possible at one time, could be accomplished again, perhaps he should stay there and continue his quest for it. Usui was greatly inspired by the abbot's enthusiasm and began a long study of the Sutras in Japanese. When the results were not forthcoming, he began an in-depth study of Chinese and later covered as much of the Chinese sutras as he could find.

Once again with little new information being revealed, Usui determined to study the sutras of Tibet. To do this, he required a knowledge of Sanskrit, the next study, which was gladly pursued. It is very likely that shortly after this time he made a trip to Northern India and Himalayas during the last century. Tibetan scrolls found were the documents of the travels of St. Isa. Many scholars believed that it was really Jesus. Whether Usui found these same scrolls or perhaps some other ancient scrolls with the recording of certain healings, are not known. What we do know that after completing his studies of `Tibetan Lotus Sutras', Usui felt that he had found the intellectual answer to the healing of Christ. What he needed then was empowerment.

KEY TO SUCCESS: EMPOWERMENT AND VISION

Realizing that he had found the key to healings, Usui went back to his friend abbot to ask for advice on how to receive empowerment. They both began to meditate and together came to the conclusion that Dr Usui should proceed to a sacred mountain about 17 miles from Kyoto **"Mount Kuri Yama"** and commence a 21 day fast and meditation, very much like an American-Indian vision quest.

Soon after Usui began his pilgrimage up the mountain, he came to a specific spot facing east and gathered up a pile of 21 stones which would be his calendar. After 20 days of fasting he arrived at the pre-dawn of 21st day. As it was the time of new moon, it was quite dark when he felt around for his last stone. Nothing out of ordinary had occurred upto this point. He prayed for the answer to come. Out of the sky he saw a flicker of light began to move very rapidly towards him. He felt like getting up and ran away, but finally he realized that this must be some sort of sign, he had sought so long and heard all those years. He girded himself for whatever might come and momentarily the light struck him in the centre of his forehead. Usui thought he had died. Millions of rainbow coloured bubbles appeared before his eyes and soon they became white glowing bubbles each one containing a three dimensional Sanskrit character in gold.

MIRACLES OF THE MORNING

The bubbles appeared one by one, just slowly enough for Usui to register their characters. Finally when it felt complete he was filled with gratitude as he had been in a trance-like state. He was surprised when he awakened as it was broad daylight. In his excitement to share his experience with his old friend the abbot, Usui began to run down the mountain. He was amazed to find himself so strong and rejuvenated after considering the long fast he had just completed.

This was the first "MIRACLE" of the morning. Suddenly in his haste, he tripped and stubbed his toe. As he instinctively reached down to grab it, he was amazed to see that within a few minutes the bleeding had stopped and it had been completely healed. It was the second MIRACLE of the morning. As he was climbing down the mountain he came to a typical roadside stall (eating place) and proceeded to order a full breakfast.

As any one knows who is acquainted with fasting procedures, it is quite dangerous to break a long fast with a heavy meal. The proprietor of the eating house could make out Usui in monk's grab and unkempt beard that he had been fasting and meditating, and encouraged him to have some special broth. Usui declined and ordered the full breakfast. The third MIRACLE of the morning occurred when he ate it without indigestion.

As he turned out, the old man's granddaughter who served Usui was in dire pain. She had a severe toothache and her jaw had been swollen for days. Her grandfather was too poor to take her to the dentist in Kyoto. So when Usui offered to try and help, she gladly accepted. After he put his hands on the sides of her face the fourth MIRACLE of the day occurred as the pain and swelling began to disappear.

Dr Usui then continued on his way back to the monastery. He found the abbot in great pain with a bout of arthritis, while Usui shared his experiences with the monk. He laid his hands on the arthritic areas and very quickly the pain disappeared. The old abbot was truly amazed. Usui sought his advice as to what he should do with his new found ability. He was again encouraged to meditate and finally after some discussion he decided to go and work in the beggars' quarters of Kyoto. He hoped to heal the beggars so that they could receive new names at the temple and thus be reintegrated into society.

When Usui entered the beggars' quarters he set about immediately healing young and old alike. The results were remarkable and many received complete healings. However, after about seven years of his experiences there, Usui began to notice the familiar faces and was disappointed and left that place.

By this time, the importance of an exchange of energy became clear to him; people needed to give back for what they received. Dr Usui laid down five Principles of Reiki and began to teach throughout Japan. It was also at this time that the purpose of the symbols he had experienced in his vision became clear. He would use them to attune people so that they could take responsibility for their own well-being. By helping them and amplifying their energy they could take a bigger step towards their own mastership. As the old dross was cleared away, Usui began to train other teachers/young men who would join him in his travels shortly before his death around the turn of the century.

THE FIRST REIKI CLINIC

Dr Chujiro Hayashi (the nearest loving student of Dr Usui), a retired naval officer founded the first Reiki Clinic in Tokyo, the taking up the responsibility to carry on the traditions of Reiki. In 1935 Hawaya Takata, a young Japanese-American woman from Hawaii appeared in Hayashi's clinic. She was very ill with a variety of organic disorders and also locking the energy due to depression over the death of her husband a few years earlier. Having been on the verge of surgery while visiting her parents who had returned to Japan, she heard the voice of her deceased husband urging her emphatically to avoid the operation. After conferring to the doctor her reservations about the upcoming surgery, he recommended that she could try the Reiki clinic and later she began to receive treatments and was finally healed.

Takata was impressed with Reiki healing and decided to learn it herself. Reiki had become a man's domain and that meant hands-off to women. Takata was a typical determined woman and did not give up easily. Her persistence ultimately paid off and finally introduced in both first and second degree techniques, and started practising. Dr Hayashi finally decided to make Takata his successor and in 1930 when he consciously left his body, Mrs. Takata took over the charge of the clinic. In 1970 she began to train other masters, until her death in 1980. She trained about 300 Reiki masters teaching around the world.

3. HOW REIKI IS DIFFERENT FROM OTHER HEALING SYSTEMS

METHODS OF SIMPLICITY AND THE PROCESSES OF ATTUNEMENT

The first thing is its simplicity, where other forms of therapy may demand months and years of training for a healer, Reiki can be taught easily and comfortably to any person ranging from young to old, irrespective of sex and who is still very much attached to the intellect as a means of learning and also is conditioned that learning takes time. Reiki can be disconcerting. The real difference is in the attunement process which puts Reiki in the category of energy work. Reiki is a process of empowerment, something which western culture has had little acquaintance with since the age of knowledge and reason. After having been gone through the attunement process (which is based upon mantras/symbols) most medical persons, massage therapists and people well acquainted with the touch and feel of the human body, noticed immediate increase in the amount of energy or the feeling of heat emanating from healers' hands during the treatment. Thus, people with the prior experience of the body usually received immediate feed back of the change which occurs as a result of getting attuned from Guru/Master, not to mention the sensations sometimes occur during the actual attuning. People with less experience or sensitivity need time and practice doing treatments to learn to perceive the changes immediately. Actually most people do it, with too many preconceived notions. They need to learn how to listen to the body, because a successful treatment requires a clear listening process.

CHANGES IN MIND AND BODY— INTERESTING ENERGY WORK

My personal experience as a Neuro-massage therapist is the immediate and large increase of heat that sets on just after five minutes at the beginning of a Reiki treatment as compared to the minimum heat generated by giving ten full massage sessions in a row. Naturally this is most impressive. Having been trained in a variety of body work techniques, but being primarily interested in deep tissue work, Reiki came as quite a surprise. I was of the mindset that it was necessary to do deep work to bring about really profound changes in the mind/body structure. It came as quite a surprise to me as some of my clients whom I had started to introduce Reiki along with their regular massages began to ask me about that. It is an interesting energy work which I had added to their treatments. Old pains disappeared, and creative spurts from my clients began rolling in.

There are other interesting differences in this fascinating energy work that really struck my attention. Normally when a massage therapist works on a client, especially during deep tissue release work, has to keep the knees unlocked or slightly bent similar to *ti chi* stance. This is because the therapist acts as a grounding rod to the client. For example, if I am helping you release a large knot in your neck or shoulder, as I guide your breathing, you consciously release the lactic acid from the muscle. As long as my hands are on the knot, the negative energy being released runs into my hands, down my arms and out of my feet into the ground. If ever I keep my knees stiff or locked during the process, your energy runs down my arm and body does not make abrupt U turn of my knees and return to exact spots in my body which is being released in yours.

It all sounds very esoteric when you are first learning about the movement of energy in the body, but it only takes a few unconscious moments to learn the truth of this process. It was quite surprising to find that with Reiki this was not a problem or concern.

TURNING THE IDEAS FROM NEGATIVES TO POSITIVES

Reiki is drawn by the healee through the open channel of the practitioner. The practitioner never absorbs energy from the healee as the energy is always "outward bound" with the exception of what may be deposited and stored on the solar plexus--an added benefit. The healee on the other hand draws Reiki through a clear channel and thus does not absorb any of the personal energy of the practitioner/healer. In Reiki once the initial intention to treat has been completed and the hands have been placed on the body, the energy will then be drawn of its own accord with no further intense focus from the practitioner. Thus, if by any reason the patient starts to "process" some old memories and emotions and feels the need to share, you can actually hold a conversation and continue to treat at the same time. Although this is an added benefit, here it is important that the counsellor should be trained enough to help to turn negative ideas into positive ideas.

LETTING OUT THE EMOTION: BALANCING THE BODY, MIND AND SPIRIT

Another point about which it is necessary to be reminded is the importance of letting emotion go. I have experienced that a patient after a long period of depression finally moves to a stage where anger begins to be released. As anger is a higher vibratory energy than depression, the person may develop a tendency to enjoy the expression of anger without moving on to a higher level of expression. Anger can be very seductive, because all of the drama involved really stimulates the ego to a high pitch. Anger is a result of feeling out of control. It is a result of failing to realise and take responsibility for all that we have created in our lives.

It is so important to understand that you are only receiving what you have at sometime put it as:-
"The Divine Law of Cause and Effect."

Life is your mirror, thanks to that which comes along and releases it. It does not have to continue. You are a creator. Realising the importance of taking responsibility for all that you create in your life indeed is one of the keys of Reiki. Reiki does not end after first year degree training attuned by a well trained master. Each person should take self responsibility for continuing with self treatments or in other words clear the blockages and orientation of chakras. **You are indeed your own Master.** Only you can determine the commitment to rate the progress of yourself.

It is clear now that like other therapies, Reiki is to seek help to each individual, find balance and harmony in the body, mind and spirit. It is truely a gift to yourself.

❈

4. REIKI TREATMENT AND ITS EFFECTS

THE BASIC TREATMENT PATTERN

Reiki treatment affects each individual person in a very personal way. The results of every treatment are determined by the needs of patient's body (sometimes not always obvious). There are some common denominators which seem to result in most treatments.

The format of a Reiki treatment will vary somewhat with each practitioner, however the primary focus will be on both the painful or troublesome area of the body and the endocrine system. Mrs. Takata taught a basic treatment pattern which covered all of these hormones of the body. To orthodox medicine, these glands are stimulated by neurotransmitters. Our body communicates with the nervous system through the brain which then stimulates the glands to release hormones that are needed for homeostasis. On the etheric level, each of seven main chakras or in other words energy centres, corresponds to one of the endocrine glands and thus the endocrine system acts as a "transducer" of energy to the etheric end centres or chakras. And likewise chakras act as "transducers" of energy back to the physical system through the endocrine glands. All levels are in someway interconnected.

THEORETICAL METHODS ON THE FUNCTIONING OF MAN

To explain further this interconnection of different systems Dr William A Tiller, a professor at Stanford university in the department of Material Science and a research scientist for many years offers a new theoretical model on the functioning of Man. Upto the present, most of the medicines of biology and agriculture community have viewed living organisms as operating via the following sequence of reactions.

Function ↔ Structure ↔ Chemistry ↔ Electromagnetic energy thus describing interactions only at certain levels.

Usually flaws have been traced to structural defects that arose from chemical imbalance with the repair procedure, being an adjustment of the chemical environment (via drugs in man or fertilisers in case of agriculture). The dilemma that occurs is that both the organisms (body and plants) and their threatening invaders adapt to a new chemical complex, in turn becoming less sensitive to it, so that an escalation of the potency must continue. The unnatural chemical content of the organisms thus increases and begins to influence other levels of functioning, not only the one being "corrected", with often pernicious results.

THE OTHER OPINION: SEQUENCE OF REACTIONS

Dr Tiller questions the validity of this equation. He explained the potential for physical and non-physical energy procedures in the treatment of imbalance. Osteopathic physicians have had great success in treating human functions with direct physical manipulations. In addition, he observed the serious reports of various types of non-physical effects over the last two hundred years to suggest the naivete of this equation. Tiller proposes a reworking of old theoretical model to a more multidimensional mode of substance. He proposes that this equation be replaced by:

Function ↔ Structure ↔ Chemistry ↔ Positive Space Time Energies
(The Physical body)

↔ Negative Space Time Energies ↔ Mind ↔ Spirit ↔ Divine
(The Etheric Body)

He uses positive space time energy to describe the physical body and negative space time energy, the etheric body in order to illustrate their kindred or coupled nature as well as the algebraic sign of their respective mass and energy states. To illustrate some of the link-ups in this expanded model, Tiller points out the mind/structure link in hypnosis, the mind/structure/function in Yoga or Zen or Aikido, mind/ chemical and chemical/mind in psychiatry in addition to many others.

Dr Tiller states, "The foregoing leads quite naturally to a perspective on healing, what pathology can develop at a number of levels and that healing is needed at all of them to restore the system to a state of harmony. The initial pathology begins at the level of mind and propagates effects to both the negative space time and the positive space time levels."

Dr Tiller then proposes that the best healing mode is to help the individual remove the pathology at the cause level and bring about the correction by a return to "Right thinking". He states that the next best healing mode is to effect repair of the structure at the negative space time level (etheric body). The next best level of healing is to effect repair of the structure at the positive space time (physical body) which is practised by medicine today.

THE "LINK-UP": - ETHERIC AND PHYSICAL BODIES

Reiki practitioners have always recognised the "link-up" of the etheric and physical bodies through the connection of chakras and endocrine system. In addition, second degree of Reiki teaches us the additional knowledge to help dealing with mental level of disease, where the casual factor is found. It is quite obvious to Reiki practitioners as Dr Tiller mentioned that the casual level of disease rests with the mind. Personally I would take this one step further and state that the casual level is due to mind being out of synchronisation with spiritual or divine aspects of man. Thus, Reiki energy naturally works on physical, etheric and mental levels. Reiki helps each individual release energy blocks and the connected emotions, which in turn helps to release the casual level of disease.

THE FIVE REIKI PRINCIPLES

1

Just for today I will live with the attitude of gratitude

2

Just for today I will not worry

3

Just for today I will not anger

4

Just for today I will do my work honestly

5

Just for today I will show love and respect for every living thing

WHAT ARE THE ATTUNEMENTS IN REIKI?

The attunements are the very core of Usui method of natural healing. Reiki is the Japanese word for universal lifeforce energy, something **we all have as our birthright and** any one can lay hand on another person and transmit **Magnetic lifeforce Energy.** What makes Usui's system unique is the attunement process which may be described as a series of initiations wherein a Reiki master using a very ancient Tibetan technology transmits energy to the student in an amplified state with the help of SYMBOLS well known as MANTRAS. This energy acts in such a way that it creates an open channel for cosmic energy to flow in from the top of the students' head through the upper energy centres and out through the hands for use in future treatments.

TRANSMISSION OF THE ATTUNEMENTS

The attunements are very precise and can only be transmitted by a Reiki master who has been trained in Usui Methods. There are two main schools of Reiki. One is headed by the Phyllis Lei Furumoto who is Mrs Takata's granddaughter and is called the Reiki Alliance. Several of the original 20 Reiki masters trained by Takata are members of this group. The other organisation called the American International Reiki Association (AIRA) is headed by Dr Barbara Weber Roy and for the past couple of years has used the term "The Radiance Technique" for describing Reiki. Reiki masters from each group are fully qualified to give the attunements. It is simply a matter of finding one that you resonate with. There are also a few others like myself, who are indirect products of these both organisations. In fact my own Reiki masters got their mastership from William C.S. Hauw, the trained teacher from the group of Furumoto, are respectable **Dr N.K. Sharma & Dr Savita Sharma,** of Delhi. Many Reiki masters give introductory lectures at different places. It is wise to attend one or two of these lectures to find the teacher who suits your needs. All are qualified masters but like teachers in any field, each of them has his or her unique focus. So it is good to find one with whom you feel a mutual bond or resonance.

One thing I like to point out that the attunements affect each person differently depending on your vibratory level when you first receive them. In other words, if you have spent time doing work to expand your conscious awareness and have reached a high vibratory level the attunement will provide a very quick Quantum Leap to an even higher level. The wonderful thing about Reiki is that even after the QUANTUM LEAP which is caused by attunements, you can still continue to increase your vibratory level and healing capacity by treating yourself daily and others whenever possible.

THE DEGREES OF ATTUNEMENTS

The First degree attunements are focused mainly on opening up the physical body so that it can then accept (channel) greater quantities of lifeforce energy. The four attunements of first degree raise the vibratory rate of the four energy centres of the upper part of the body which are also known as chakras. **The first initiation attunes both the heart and the thymus while also attuning the heart chakra on the etheric level. The second attunement affects the thyroid gland and on an etheric level helps to open up the throat chakra, the third initiation affects both the third eye which corresponds to pituitary gland (our centre of higher consciousness and intuition) and hypothalamus which affects the body's mood and temperature. The fourth initiation further opens the crown chakra, our connecting link with spiritual consciousness and it is corresponding to the physical partner, the pineal gland. This final attunement completes the**

process by peeling the channel open so that you can maintain the accelerated ability to channel the Reiki energy for the rest of your life. Thus it is essential to complete all four attunements to keep the Reiki channel open throughout your entire life time. Once you are attuned to Reiki energy, you can never lose it even if you don't use it for years, the moment you decide to use it, it will be there for you.

The Second degree attunement process provides a 'Quantum Leap" in vibratory level, at least four times greater than the first degree. The three symbols which are taught in second degree to be used for sending distant healings also become activated at this point. Second degree has great emphasis on adjusting the etheric body rather than the physical body which is the primary focus of first degree. In addition, the third eye or sixth chakra is greatly affected which often heightens the intuitive abilities and specially during the 21 days cleansing process. People often feel a considerable amount of energy in their root chakras because their survival and sexual centres become very stimulated and amplified by what is known as Kundalini energy.

The third degree attunement is used to initiate a master. This attunement again amplifies the vibratory level and activates the master symbol so it may be used to help others to empower themselves.

This is an important point, because it is essential for people to realise that it is their choice to receive an attunement. A Reiki master holds no lordly power over his or her students. A Reiki master is someone who has chosen to accept greater responsibility for their lives by acknowledging that he or she is indeed the master of his or her destiny. A co-creator with the absolute he or she openly accepts the effects of causes which he or she has created by accepting this responsibility. The Reiki masters are empowered to use specific ancient Tibetan Technology to help others further to empower themselves. The attunement process of Reiki is really exceptional in that. It enables you to get a sense of your true essence. When you begin the attunement process, you take a positive step towards acknowledging your own mastership.

EXTRA TOOLS TO USE WITH REIKI

The mentioned systems/tools are not directly connected to Reiki. After completing second degree, many students receive very clear intuitive messages to guide them in healing process. Mrs. Takata herself added a variety of procedures to her treatments which were not passed down from Usui. Each one of us has our own unique talents, and should feel comfortable about experimenting and even expanding our own repertoire of healing methods, because Reiki treatments do not require a constant focus of attention on the channeling of energy to the healee. The healer is left with an opportunity to observe and concentrate his thought processes elsewhere while Reiki in itself is a complete healing modality. You may choose to investigate some of the following methods in combination with a Reiki treatment.

REMOVING ENERGY BLOCKAGE

Occasionally while giving treatments, you may notice that a particular area of the body seems to draw very little or no energy and perhaps even feels cold to the touch. When you are quite sure that you are feeling an energy block and that your hands don't feel cool because they are drawing enough energy to feel hot in comparison to the patient's body temperature, you may choose to utilise the following techniques:

After having laid your hands on a very cool area of the body for five to ten minutes, without any sensation of energy being drawn in a quicker fashion you may intuitively sense that an energy block is present. In order to remove it, you can scoop the energy into a light compressed ball at the surface of the skin, grasp it with your left hand and lift it away from the body. Sever it with your right hand by making a slicing motion next to the surface of the skin and then lift the right hand to the left using it to surround the left in white light and let the ball of energy go. When you return .your hand to the body you will generally feel a definite increase in the flow of energy because the person is now free to draw and accept more Reiki. One thing I must point out about this procedure is that it is possible to do entirely in the mind's eye. In other words at times when the personality or belief system of the patient is such that to move the hands as I have described, would seem like "Mumbo-Jumbo" on the other hand. There are times when certain people would benefit by visually seeing you, extract the energy as verification that something negative is indeed being removed.

Energy blocks themselves are created in a variety of ways, for the most part, they are the results of stored emotions which have not been able to be expressed. Another cause of energy blocks is due to negative thoughts, which when a person becomes obsessed with them seem to take on an energy of lifeforce of their own. These may eventually attach themselves to the body in a large mass.

An average person does not realise that thoughts are indeed very powerful. All our thoughts amass in the etheric or energy body of the earth, that is why it is so important that we become consciously aware of individuals. Thoughts which pass through us quickly do not generally take on a life force of their own and are soon dissipated. However, if a person becomes obsessed with a negative idea over a period of time, the force of these thoughts will create actual "little beings" called elementals, which will, in turn help perpetuate the same thoughts. Long standing family and national feuds are powerful examples of the life force in elementals. On the other hand positive thoughts, which are repeated over and over also create a lifeforce of their own and will perpetuate themselves.

It is very important for the people to understand this phenomenon. Because at the present time with the powerful love, energy entering the earth to create healing, many people are experiencing large awakenings which are affecting their intuitive faculties. Some are even developing the ability to see elementals, and begin to think that they are losing their mind due to the lack of cultural references to explain such occurrences.

Take the time to listen to your body and feel the areas which may be blocked. Daily self-treatments especially using the second degree mental healing technique, will help to release outmoded patterns of behaviour, you may experience long withheld emotion coming up in addition to interesting dreams. Using these tools with your own intuitive abilities, you will begin to formulate the appropriate programme of healing for yourself.

USING COLOUR AND SOUND

There are many instances available which discuss the powerful healing effects of colour. During the experiments, the subjects were monitored by a polygraph machine and feasted for galvanic skin response. When subject viewed a violet light, several of them eluded to drop in their pulse rates. On the other end of the scale, males were more susceptible to rise in pulse rate; when viewing red, than female. The list in the next page illustrates the qualities of each colour and their effects on the body.

It is advised and encouraged to use colour not only in healing but also in everyday dress. I encourage the recipient to wear the colour which corresponds to the chakra or energy centre where emotional release is needed. Use of the corresponding chakra colour of an emotionally blocked area of the body, during release work, helps to promote further healing.

RED	Energises the nervous system and stimulates the senses. Activates the circulatory system. Helps to heal infections, X-Ray damage and ultraviolet burns.
ORANGE	Helps to strengthen lungs and bronchial tubes, stimulates the thyroid and stomach, relieves cramps and helps to build bones.
YELLOW	Stimulates the lymphatic system, motor and sensory nerves, digestion and increases hormone production.
LEMON	Nourishes the body and brain, helps to clear lungs, stimulates overall body repair.
GREEN	Balances the physical body and cerebrum, stimulates pituitary and acts as a germicide.
TURQUOISE	Repairs acute problems and heals burned skin.
BLUE	Acts as a sedative, lowers fever, relieves inflammations, itching and irritations. Also stimulates the pineal gland.
INDIGO	Sedative, stimulates parathyroids, shrinks abscesses and tumours and acts as an emotional depressant.
VIOLET	Activates spleen and 'white blood cells', helps to reduce fever and relaxes muscles.
PURPLE	Lowers body temperature, heart rate and blood pressure. Also acts as a kidney depressant and controls lung haemorrhages.
MAGENTA	Balances emotions, adjusts blood pressure to perfect balance and stimulates adrenal and kidneys.
SCARLET	Stimulates adrenals and kidneys, emotions and reproductive organs and raises blood pressure.

5. CRYSTALS

CRYSTAL TECHNOLOGY

Quartz Crystal has become very popular in recent years as a tool which helps to amplify the quantum leap taking place in man's consciousness. Some of which is thought to be ancient crystal technology is now coming to light. In addition to the exploration of crystal healing methods, which are being conducted by many individuals, traditional science has also discovered the powerful properties of the crystalline structure. In recent years, science has begun to utilise crystal technology for solar power, communication and information storage. The Piezo-electric effect, which occurs when crystals are placed under pressure and as a result emits measurable electric voltage is one property which is now being utilised. In other words, by mechanically squeezing a quartz crystal, it begins to emit electrons, conversely applying an electric current to a crystal that causes mechanical movement. The regularity at which mechanical movement occurs is quite precise, which is the reason why Quartz crystals are so useful in keeping time.

THE REMOVER OF ENERGY BLOCKS AND NEGATIVE THOUGHTS

The interconnection of the different bodily systems and the extreme versatality of the Reiki energy which enables it to penetrate all of the various systems has been discussed in effect of Reiki treatments, whereas Reiki energy penetrates the physical and etheric bodies simultaneously as well as penetrates the mental level where the casual factor of a disease lies. Crystals seem to work primarily on the subtle energetic bodies. This is the inherent usefulness of crystals, which is to amplify and focus energy directly at specific areas of blockage in the etheric system. If the disease is already manifest in the physical system, the positive changes of the crystals help to make on etheric level and will eventually also effect the correction of physical level. Thus crystals are a great help in removing energy blocks and negative thought forms on the subtle energetic level. But they will not necessarily be able to release a long ingrained mental or emotional pattern which lies at the casual level of disease. From the above information it can be seen that the crystals provide us with a powerful tool to amplify and direct healing energy but they can't prevent the healee recreating the negative thoughts from which is the illness created in the first place.

Crystal charging is the renewal of a crystal's vibrational change whereas activation increases its overall charge capacity. My personal experience has shown that first degree Reiki charges a crystal and second degree tends to actually activate a crystal by increasing its overall charge capacity.

CHOOSING A CRYSTAL

The main factor in choosing a crystal is to find out one which resonates with your energy field. Just as people of different energy patterns, crystals have their own unique vibrations. The colour, size, shape and type are all important factors in crystal selection along with the intended use. Your best guide is your intuition. An expert in colour and gem therapy recommended that the following exercises would help to develop sensitivity to subtle energies.

EXERCISE TO FEEL ENERGY

Rub your hands briskly for about one minute. Move your hands (palms facing each other) slowly apart until they are around six inches apart, then slowly move them towards each other until they almost touch. Continue doing this as you try to feel any tingling sensation, heat changes or any other subtle energy change in your hands. Once you have developed this sensitivity, try moving your hands over the top of a group of crystals to feel a similar energy.

CLEANSING AND CLEARING OF CRYSTALS

After purchasing a crystal or receiving one as a gift, it is wise to clean it, as quartz crystal tends to absorb many vibrations which are (or have been) in its close vicinity. Crystals tend to absorb and store the energy and thought patterns of people who have held them or have been in close contact with them. Crystals which are worn or used daily should be cleaned on a regular basis (atleast once a week). Those which are generally kept in a harmonious environment need only periodic cleanings. Some of the various methods for cleaning crystals are:

Soaking them in a salt water solution for atleast twentyfour hours. Placing and covering them in dry sea salt for atleast twentyfour hours, cleansing them with running water and also by blowing on each of their facets while visualising them becoming clean and pure.

CHARGING OF CRYSTALS

In order to renew the vibrational charge of a crystal, several methods may be used. You can put the crystal in the centre of a crystal grid work or under a pyramid for a number of hours, surrounding crystals with colour gels and projecting light in one way to charge them with different vibratory rates of colour. Also leaving the crystals in a highly energised point on earth, such as in a vertex area or one with a low geomagnetic pressure will help to give a charge.

Finally Reiki is a very powerful tool for charging crystals. Charging can be accomplished by any Reiki practitioner who holds a crystal between his hands with the intention of charging it and then focusing on the purpose for which he wishes to use it.

ACTIVATING CRYSTALS

As mentioned earlier, the activation of a crystal involves expanding its overall energy capacity so that it may accept a greater charge. It is recommended to expose the crystal to very high and very low temperatures to induce activation. However, the temperature changes must be gradual to prevent any cracking of crystal by exposing them to extreme weather conditions. Meditation can also be applied to increase crystal power.

CRYSTAL PROGRAMMING (HEALING PURPOSE)

Your crystal can be programmed for specific health problems. Visualise the person's health problem (or any other kind of problem) getting better feel of the healing energy that flows into the crystal.

Visualise the problem as completely healed. Be as detailed as possible. After the programming process you can give the person a treatment by holding the crystal over his body and guiding the energy where you want it with your mind. Visualise the energy flowing from you through the crystal and into the person's body. You can also give and loan the crystal to the person and get him treat himself or just carry with him. After a few treatments it is advisable to cleanse and reprogramme the crystal.

COLOUR PROGRAMMING

Every colour has a certain vibrational quality that can be used for numerous purposes. Colour can be used to induce changes in personality, emotions, states of mind and physical disorders. The colour for the change that you desire is programmed into the crystal and can be used in the same manner. Coloured plastic gels or papers can be wrapped on the crystal and placed in front of light source (may be sunlight or any other white light source) to change the colour programming process. The neutral objects which emit energy (i.e crystals) and extend and amplify their programme in a highly concentrated form. Programming is the process of storing specific energy and thought patterns so that they may then be transmitted into the objects of people of will. It is important to note that persons choosing to work with crystals should exercise responsibility, because although they may be used for mind to mind communication, their higher purpose is in the service of humanity for the removal of pain and suffering. For those who are acquainted with the history of Atlantis, whether you take it as fact or myth, it stands as a powerful example of the need to take caution and exercise for increased individual and collective responsibility being developed. Crystals can be programmed as a powerful tool to help the individual to promote self-transformation and when it is used with Reiki (universal power) the possibilities are as limitless as human mind.

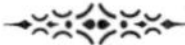

6. BALANCING BODY CHAKRAS

THE NATURAL HEALING -- THE LINE UP

Dr Usui's System of Natural healing has always been recognised as the "line up" of etheric and physical body through the connection between chakras and endocrine glands. Chakra is basically a Sanskrit word which means wheel. This term is appropriate, as the chakras appear to be spiraling disks of light to some one with clairvoyant abilities. The location of chakras in the etheric or energy body corresponds directly to the placement of the endocrine glands in the physical body. **The etheric body is an energy body of very fine vibration which totally envelops the physical body. Both are interconnected by currents of energy. The etheric body absorbs finer levels of energy from the enviornment and transduces this energy through the chakras into the physical body via the endocrine glands. The endocrine system controls the hormone balance in the body, which has a powerful effect on a person's mood and emotions.** Thus it can be gathered that if chakra system is out of balance, its counterpart, the endocrine system is also out. If an imbalance somehow occurs first in the endocrine system, it too will put the chakra system out of balance, because energy moves back and forth between the two. Reiki energy is absorbed by both systems simultaneously making it an excellent modality for creating balance in both the chakras and endocrine glands. Because the Reiki practitioner feels the energy being drawn in greater amount wherever it is needed in the body. There is a little guess work involved in trying to find the areas that are out of balance. The seven major chakras are shown in Fig. I. (see next page). A table is also provided subsequently to show the functions of seven major chakras.

As it can be seen in the diagram, not only are the endocrine glands effected by the chakras, but the surrounding organs and certain section of nervous system as well. Each chakra has also a specific function which corresponds directly to certain types of emotions and factors in human development. Some of the different purposes associated with each chakra are also explained separately. If one of the chakra is out of balance, its associated functions in the individual are also out of balance to some degree.

LOCATIONS OF CHAKRAS

Locations on the Physical Body are shown in Fig 2 (a, b), (next page).

- 2   There are two in front of the ears, close to where the jaw bones are connected.
- 2   There are two just above the two breasts.
- 1   There is one where the breast bone connects, close to the thyroid gland. This with the two breast centres, makes a triangle of force.
- 2   There are two, one each in the palms of the hands.

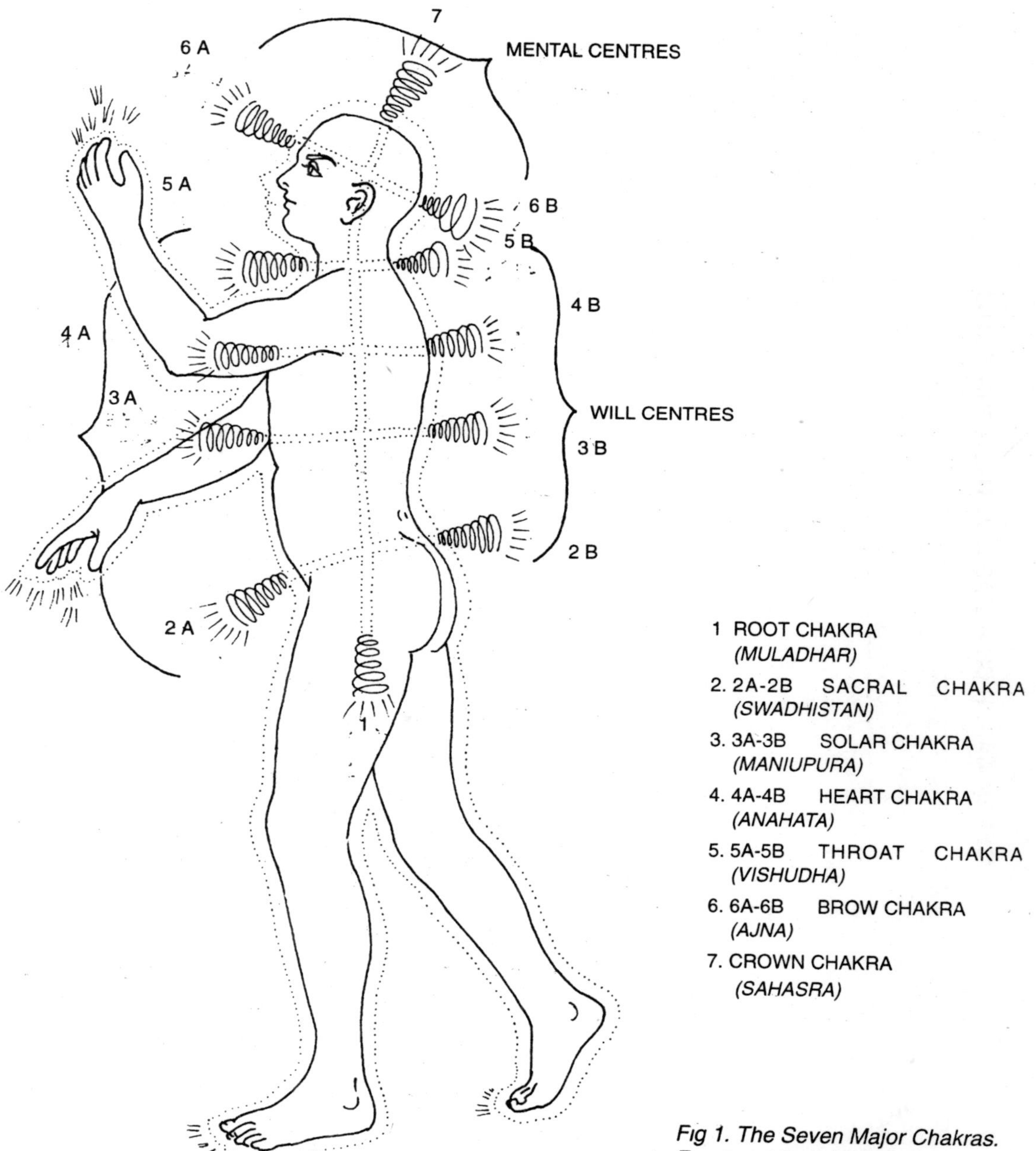

1 ROOT CHAKRA
   (MULADHAR)

2. 2A-2B   SACRAL   CHAKRA
   (SWADHISTAN)

3. 3A-3B   SOLAR CHAKRA
   (MANIUPURA)

4. 4A-4B   HEART CHAKRA
   (ANAHATA)

5. 5A-5B   THROAT   CHAKRA
   (VISHUDHA)

6. 6A-6B   BROW CHAKRA
   (AJNA)

7. CROWN CHAKRA
   (SAHASRA)

*Fig 1. The Seven Major Chakras.
Front and Back Views*

SEVEN MAJOR CHAKRAS AND THEIR FUNCTIONS

Chakra	App.Location	Gland	System	Organ	Function	Colour	Element	Mantra
1. CROWN CHAKRA (SAHASRA)	The top of head.	Pineal	Cerebro Spinal Nervous System	Upper Brain Right eye	Spiritual Vision enlightenment	VIOLET	Ether	OHM ॐ
2. BROW CHAKRA (AJNA)	Forehead between Eye brow	Pituitary	Autonomic Nervous System Nose & Ears	Hypothalamus Lower Brain Spine. Left Eyes Intelligence Light, Telepathy	Third Eye Intuition Clairvoyance	BLUE (Royal)	Ether	AUM अं
3. THROAT CHAKRA (VISUDHA)	Throat	Thyroid System	LYMPHATIC Upper Lungs Alimentary Canal Bronchianl & Vocal Apparatus	THROAT Self expression creative energy sound	Communication	SKY BLUE	Ether	GAM गं
4. HEART CHAKRA (ANAHATA)	Heart	Thymus	Circulatory System Vagus Nerve Arms	Heart, Lungs Blood, Liver Love Compassion Lifeforce	Group Consciousness	GREEN (grass)	Air	HAM हं
5. SOLAR PLEXUS CHAKRA (MANIPURA)	Stomach	Pancreas	Digestive System Spleen	Liver, Stomach Gall bladder Large Intestine Action	Emotion Power Wisdom	YELLOW	Fire	RAM रं
6. SACRAL CHAKRA (SWADHISTAN)	Below Navel	Gonads	Reproductive System	Sex Organs	Anger/Action Sexuality	ORANGE	Water	BAM बं
7. ROOT CHAKRA (MULADHAR)	Base of Spine	Adrenal Skeleton	Excretory System Muscle Spinal Column Legs	Peace Kidneys Bladder Survival Grounding Fear	Kundalini Security Fear, Physical energy	RED	Earth	LAM लं

2   There are two, one each in the soles of the feet.

2.   There are two, just behind the eyes.

2   There are two, also, connected with the gonads.

1   There is one close to the liver.

1   There is one connected with the stomach, it is related, therefore, to the solar plexus, but is not identical with it.

2   There are two connected with the spleen. These form one centre in reality, but such a centre is formed by the two being superimposed one on the other.

2.   There are two--one at the back of each knee.

1   There is one powerful centre which is closely connected with the vegus nerve. This is most potent and is regarded by some schools of occultism as a major centre; it is not in the spine, but is no great distance from the thymus gland.

1   There is one which is close to the solar plexus, and relates it to the centre at the base of the spine, thus making a triangle of the sacral cc-l-tre, the solar plexus, and the centre at the base of the spine.

All the chakras are of equal importance. This is very much necessary to know. It has been observed that many people only tend to focus solely on the development of the upper chakras because they are "More Spiritually" connected. The fact of the matter is that every thing is a manifestation of spirit and if one chakra is out of balance, they are all out of balance. The lower chakras tend to be more attuned to earthly energies, as can be seen by their connection to specific earth elements and upper chakras to more etheric or cosmic forms of energy. The heart which is the centre of the body is the meeting place of two energies. It is the place where the two polarities, spirit and matters meet in the expression of love. As heart is the element of air, it is truely the meeting place of heaven and earth. We need to focus a great deal of attention at this time at the development of lower four chakras, as growth in these areas will help to ground us to our mother earth and help in healing process. We must not forget that matter (earth) the female/mother polarity needs just as much recognition and love as (heaven) the male/father polarity.

In order to balance chakras and promote healing on all levels, full Reiki treatments are very much in order. If you desire briefer techniques the followings are also effective.

STANDING METHOD:- With the healee standing sideways, you place one hand a few inches in front of lower belly and other hand just a few inches away from the tip of sacrum where the root chakra is located. Hold your hand there for two to three minutes until you feel a wave like rise and fall of energy. Continue on up over each of chakras for a period of two to three minutes until you come to the crown chakra. Place your hand on top of the head leaving the fontanel uncovered. After some minutes bring the hands down over the chakras again ascending to foot chakra as you integrate the energies and close all of the centres.

BALANCING HEAVEN AND EARTH

With the person being supine, place one hand over the lower part (close to the table) of the top of the head and place your other hand under the coccyx (tip of the spine) wail until you feel the similar pulsation, tingling sensations or heat and then move one hand over the brow (Third Eye

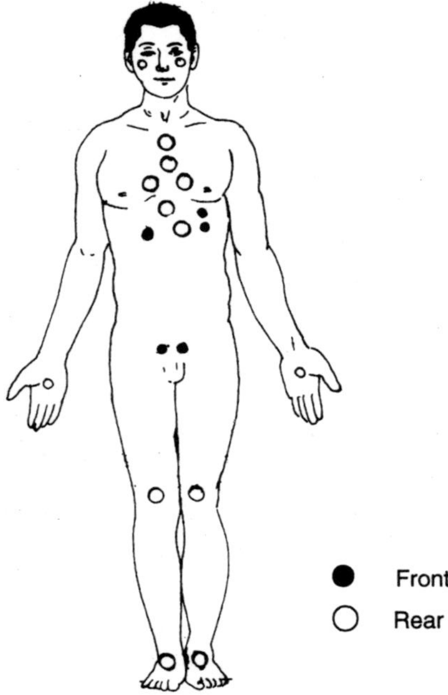

Fig. 2A. The Twenty one minor Chakras

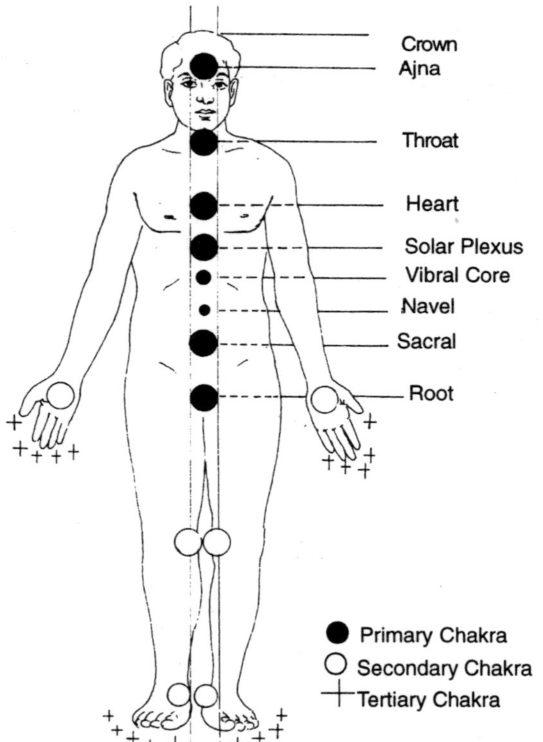

Fig. 2B. The Seven Major and other Chakras

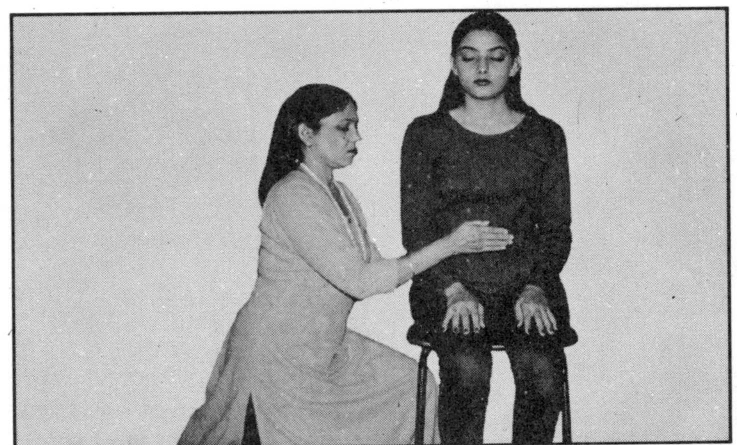

One hand in front of lower belly
and other hand on tip of sacrum
where the root chakra is located.

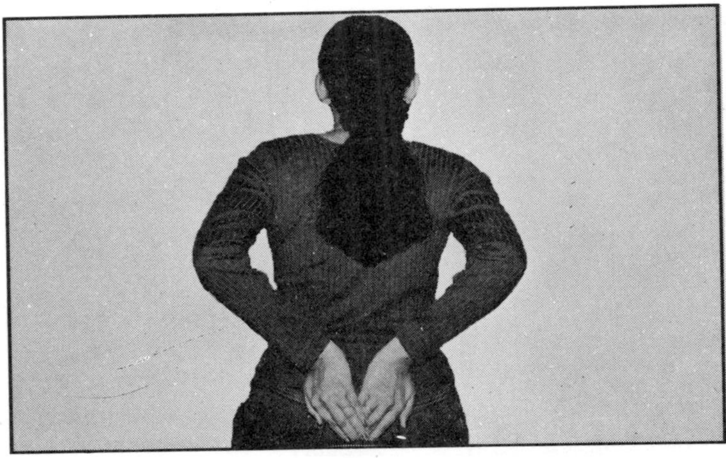

Position showing the tip of sacrum
where root chakra is located.

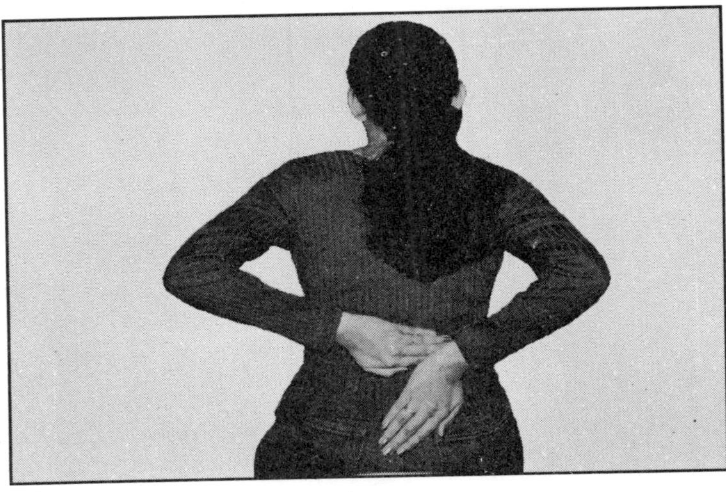

Position showing the back chakra
of sacrum.

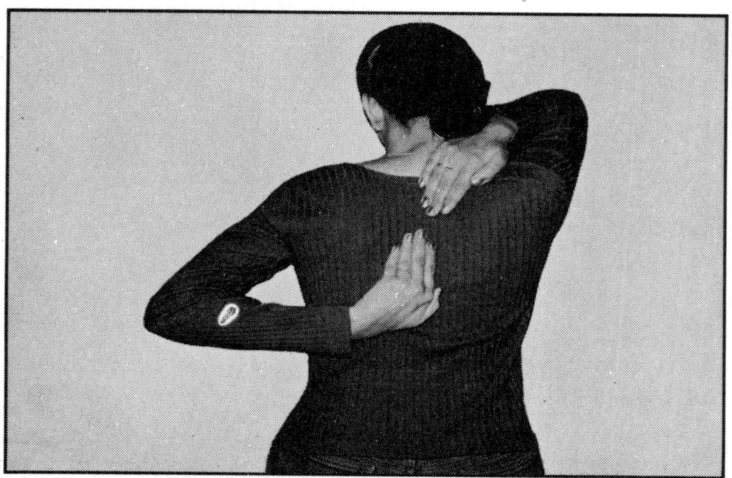

Position showing the back of heart chakra above sacrum.

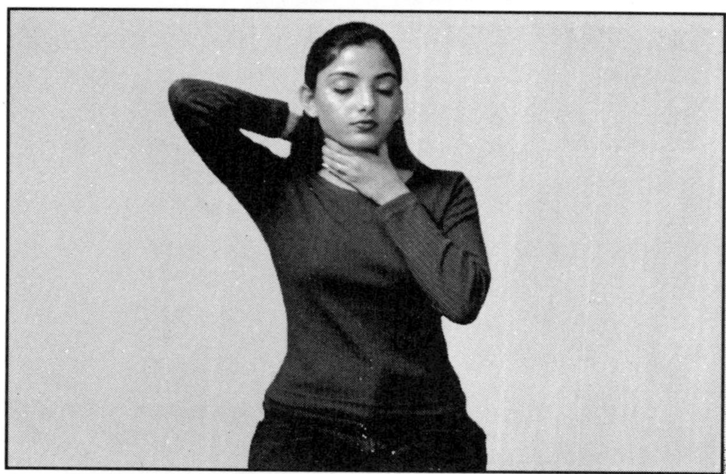

Position showing the front and back of throat chakra.

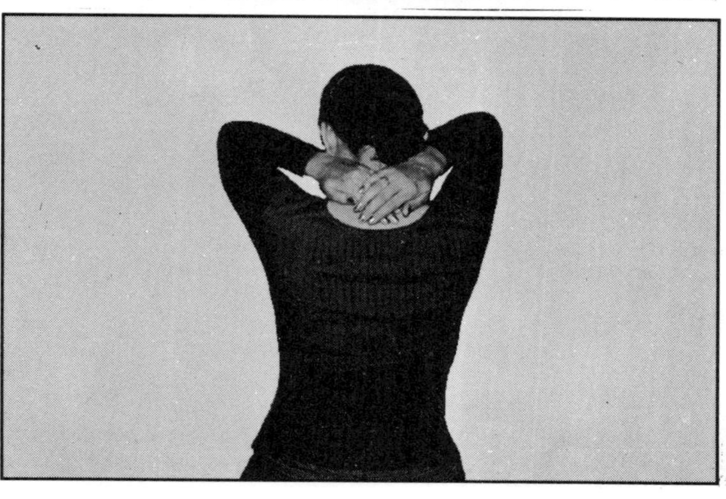

Position showing back of throat chakra on shoulders.

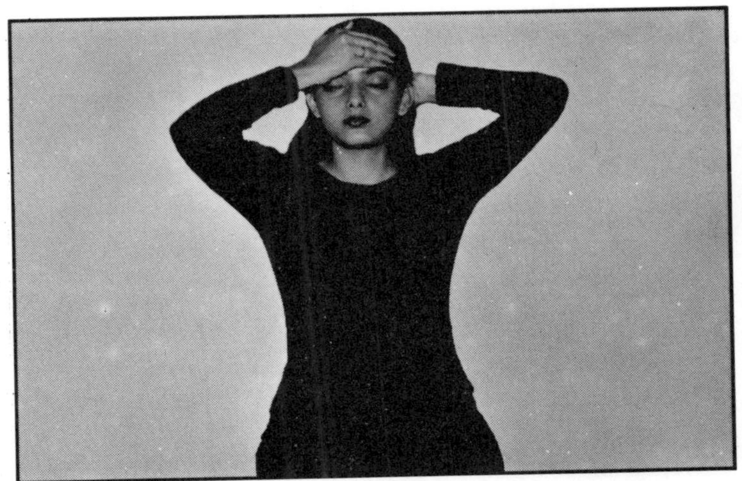

Position showing the front and
back of brow chakra.

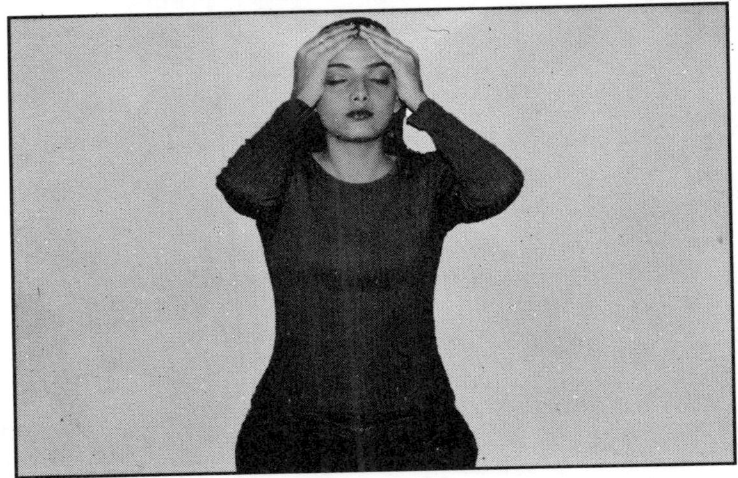

Position showing the front of
crown chakra.

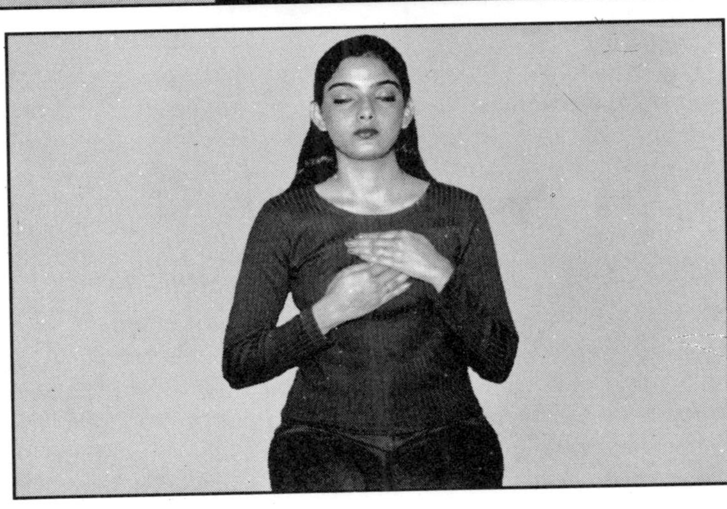

Position showing heart chakra.

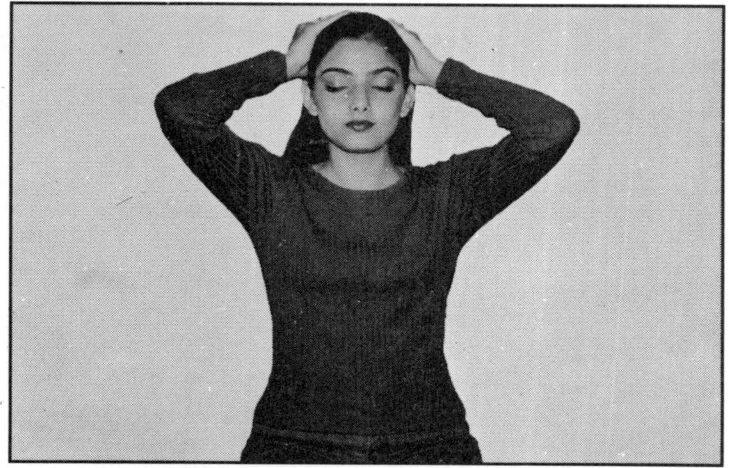

Position showing the crown chakra.

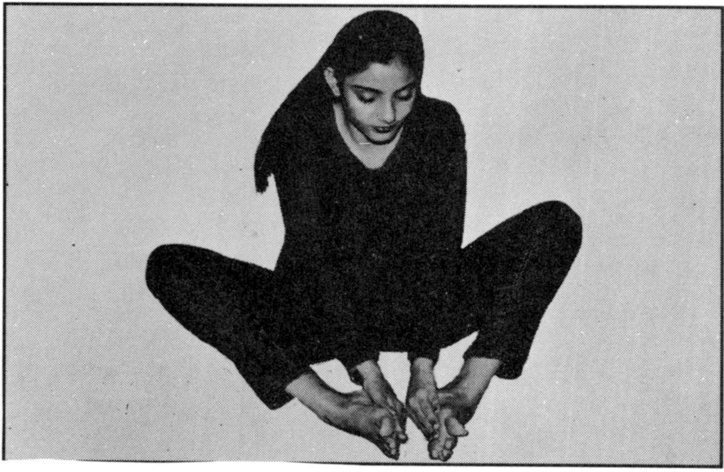

Position showing the feet chakra.

Chakra) and one hand upto the belly, (three fingers width below the navel). Again wait for the same sensation on both of your hands or an intuitive sense that they are balanced. Next place one hand gently over the throat and thyroid area (do not exert the pressure on the wind pipe) other on the solar plexus. Wait to feel a sense of balance between the two chakras and finally place both hands over the heart centre. When completed, gently and slowly raise your hands off the body, while taking into consideration the sensitivity of its Auric field (See Fig. 3 in the next page.)

CONSCIOUS AWARENESS

Be sure to engage your intuitive knowingness when balancing bodily energies. Feel free to connect different combinations of chakras as each person has different imbalances and might be aided in different ways. Balancing of chakras ultimately creates balance in all of the systems of the body. It is appropriate to focus on these energy centres when performing Reiki treatments. The endocrine system in the physical body will also benefit and the corresponding rise in the vibratory rate of the body will promote greater conscious awareness.

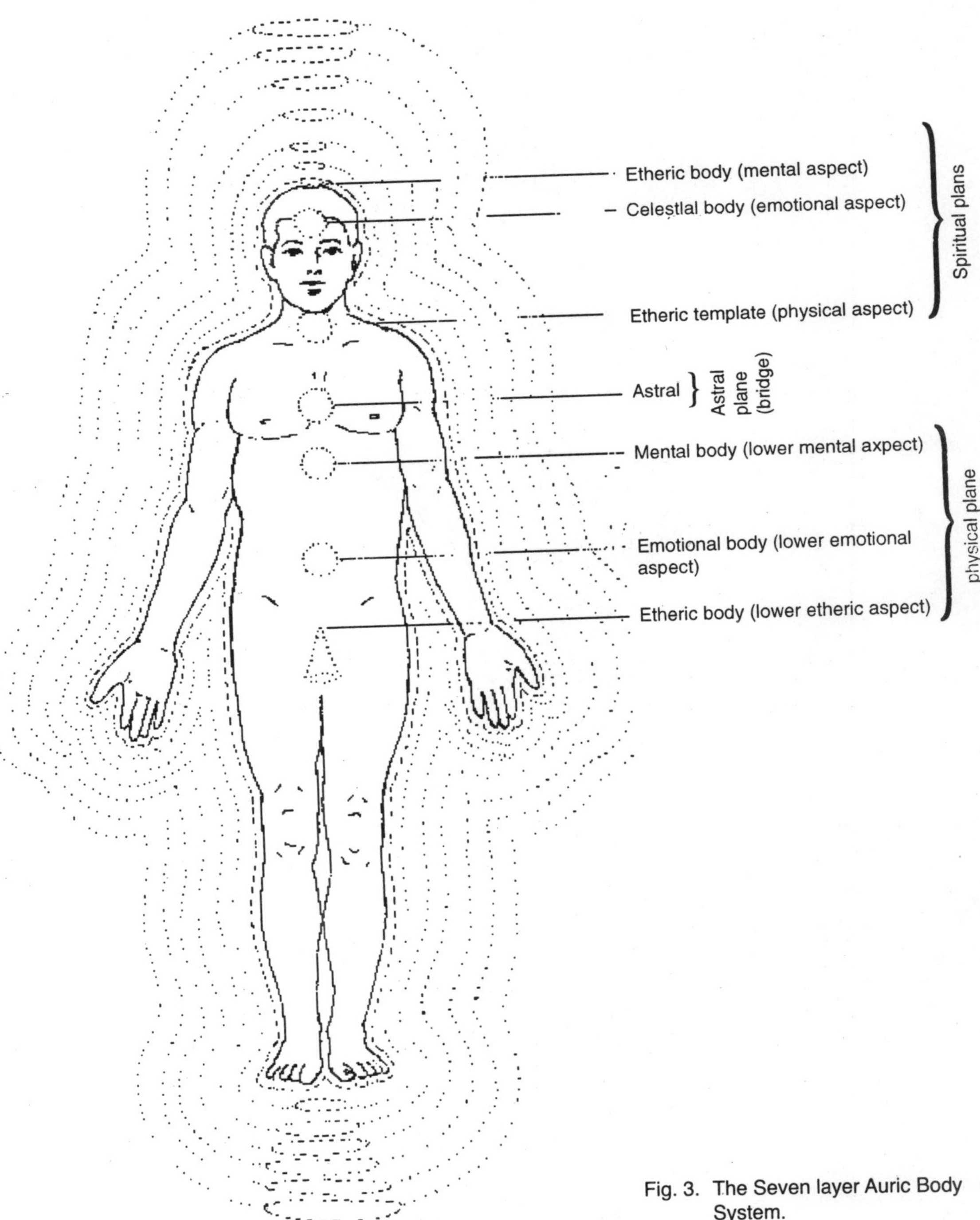

Fig. 3. The Seven layer Auric Body System.

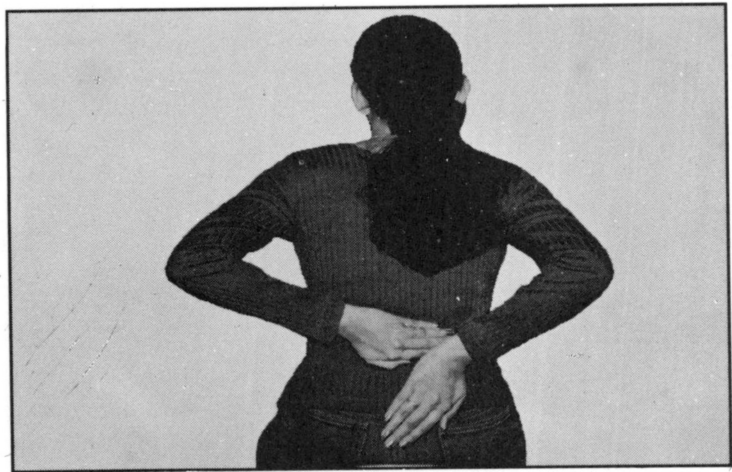

Position showing coccyx.

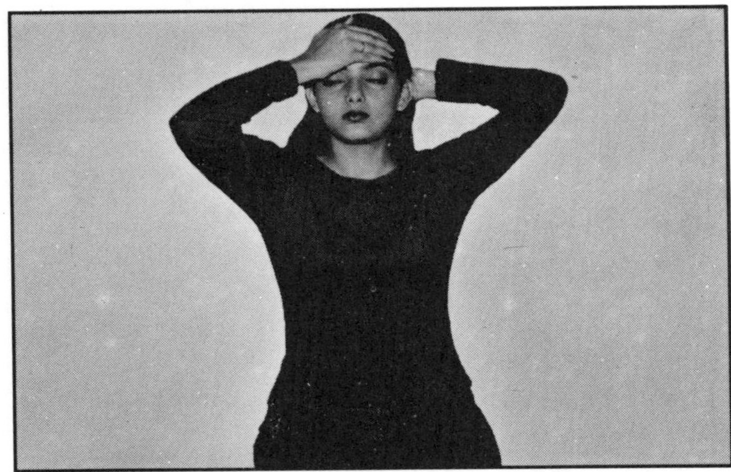

Position showing the brow crown chakra (third eye chakra).

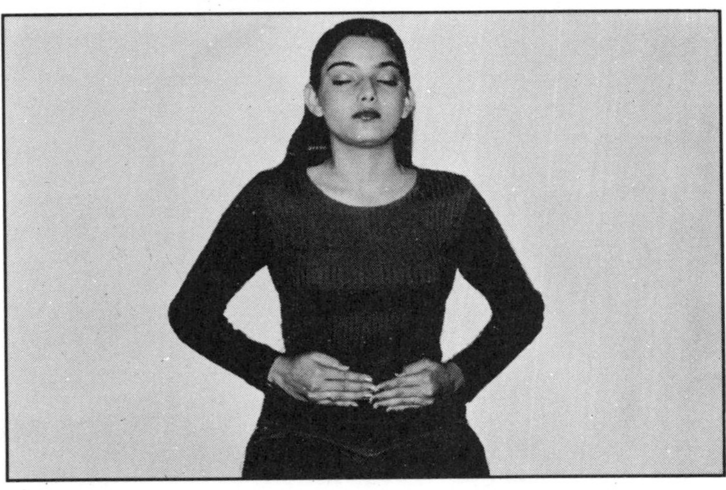

Position showing the Hara chakra.

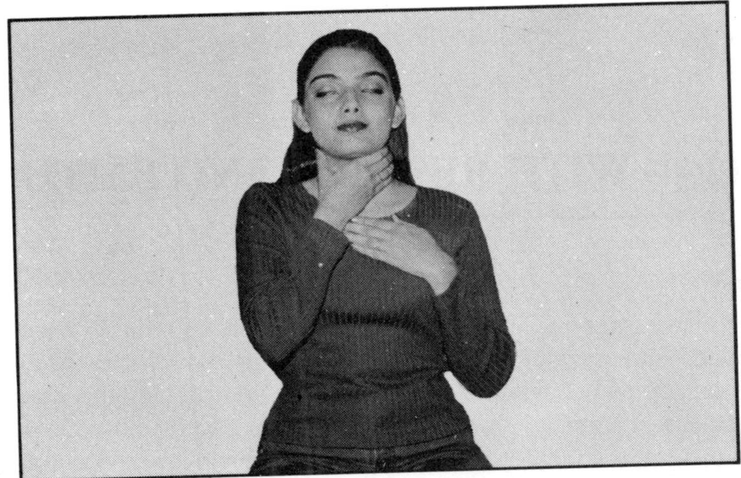

Position showing the throat chakra.

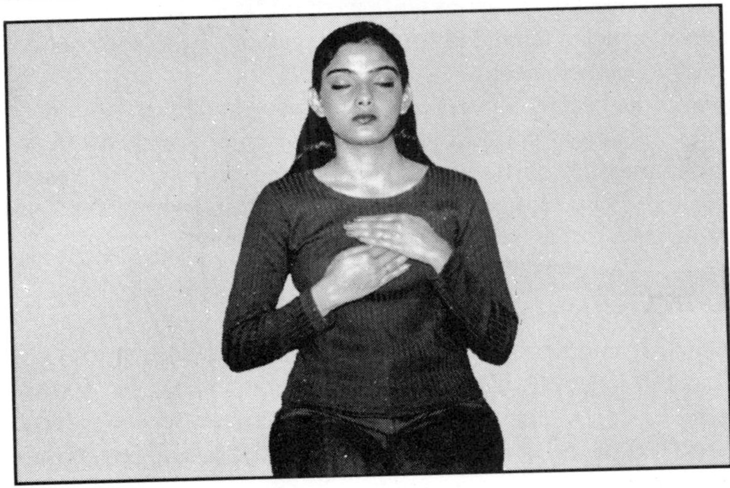

Position showing the heart chakra.

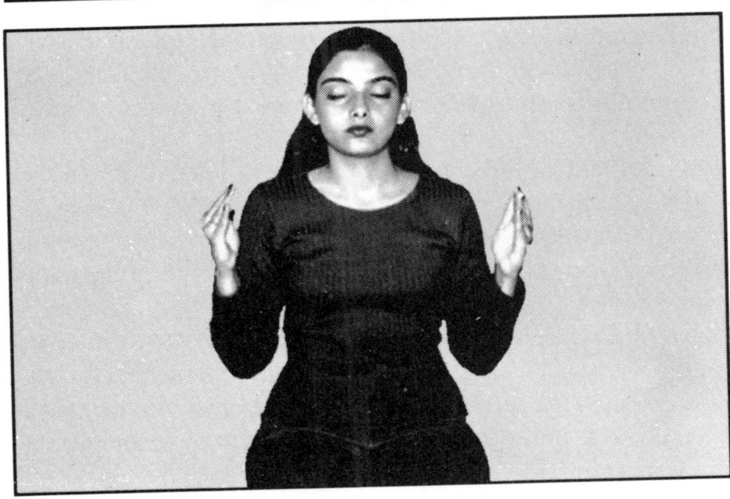

Position showing the rays of hands for taking into consideration the sensitivity of auric field.

7. HEALING — WITH RESPECT AND FAITH

THE SEEDS OF HEALING

During my many years of study, I have witnessed and helped to bring about many remarkable recoveries. I also learned the ways of understanding and sensing the energy or lifeforce that exists around all people. But what my teachers taught me first was the right attitude for approaching this practice. The healer does not heal, he/she facilitates a process that is active and implicit within all of us. The seeds of healing exist in the person in search of help. It is important that the recipient of healing touch be open and respectful of this healing process. In a certain sense we must be like children, open, receptive and ready to learn. By maintaining an open mind and spirit, the recipient allows the energy that flows to him or her to be taken in and utilized efficiently.

A reverential attitude towards the healing process is the basis of all traditional healing approaches and still is throughout the world. Healing is considered not as a lucky mix of chemical processes of most of the cultures, but as an expression of the harmonious joining of heaven and earth. Healing rituals are practised in many cultures to evoke greater faith which in turn triggers the healing forces within the person who is seeking help for himself, his family and community.

DRUGS/MEDICINES AND BELIEF

The scientific studies from which I report prove that the efficacy of therapeutic touch shows that people benefit from healing touch no matter what they believe. My experience has shown however, that those who are more open and receptive make quicker progress. For this reason I always maintain that "HEALING IS A GIFT OF NATURE WHICH YOU GIVE YOURSELF", because you must receive this enhanced life-energy and allow your body, mind and spirit to utilize it for whatever purpose you need. You can marshal these enhanced energies for your own purposes, something inside you accept and embrace the healing process.

As Norman Cousing wrote in **Anatomy of Illness,** *"Drugs* are not always necessary, belief in recovery always is."

We are living in a time where the bridge between ORTHODOX and ALTERNATIVE medicine must be built, if we are to have a truly humane and effective health care system. Medicine and health care are now in the throes of revolution. Today more and more people are seeking the counsel and treatment of alternative medical practitioners of acupuncture/acupressure/massage therapies/herbalism/diet and other traditional healing systems. Healing touch or Reiki is among those practices gaining credibility with both the lay public and medical professionals. Western society's world view is changing dramatically as science proves the wisdom and efficacy of the ancient healing approaches. This trend will continue as more and more people seek creative ways of healing old and intractable disorders. I hope that this book will inspire people to utilise this practice more and more in the process of healing themselves and others.

LEARNING THE SCIENCE AND LANGUAGE OF HEALING ENERGY

A healing power flows from your hands. This power can help people to overcome sickness, negative beliefs and old and useless habits. It can heal wounds, reduce pain, boost energy, improve psycho touch or what has been known as "Laying on of hands" has been used as a medical treatment technique in virtually every traditional culture. Healing touch can also serve as a powerful adjunct to conventional medical therapy. Today scientific study consistently prove its power to heal, though researchers still do not understand the way as to how the practice works.

In the broadest sense, healing touch is the act of consciously directing life energy from its infinite sources through the practitioner to the persons who are in need of assistance. It is done with the specific intention of giving love and support in overcoming a physical or psychological problem. This conscious transfer of energy can be facilitated and enhanced through an assortment of technique and by deepening your understanding of the practice.

Today, healing or therapeutic touch or Reiki is being taught at many places throughout the world. To understand the HOW and WHY of the healing touch can be utilised for its therapeutic value, we must open up to a larger view of ourself and of life.

In a sense, we must go beyond the restricted definition of life that is imposed upon us by our modern culture. We must view our lives in a more traditional way, that is in the way the people have seen life through the most of human history: as a physical, emotional and spiritual whole connected to other lives and to a greater understanding of our natural environment.

VIEWING THE LIFE IN A LARGER CONTEXT

We should also view health in a similar way. Rather than seeing health as merely the absence of symptoms, we must see it in a larger context, as a condition of wholeness or integration of body, mind and spirit with the greater cultural and natural environment. Each of us represents a vast potential to grow and develop emotionally, psychologically and spiritually. Our present world demands such growth and development. Indeed our health may be predicted on our ability to reach down continuously into the psyche and bring forth and develop the unique skills and characteristics that lie deep within us. Yet few of us realise our potential in part because many of our better characteristics are hidden within us, repressed or denied by fears and false beliefs. These repressive emotions act as energy blockages between our potential or true self and our own conscious mind. Thus we confront the world with only parts of our character, strength and spirit available to us.

BREAKING THE BARRIERS

Beside preventing self-realisation and self-understanding, energy barriers can also block life energy from flowing through the body. In the traditional, as well as the modern healing methods, the practitioners found that the optimal flow of life energy was the secret of health and the proper functioning of the entire body. When barriers to the lifeforce deprive certain parts of the body of the life energy, the cells, organs and tissues consequently become weak, sluggish and stagnant and gradually degenerate with time. These conditions can bring in some forms of diseases. The illness may be called one name or other but the true underlying source of the physical or mental problem is a diminution of the lifeforce flowing to that particular part of the body. Therefore, deep healing begins by a restoration of the lifeforce areas of the body that are deprived of life energy.

Healing touch/Reiki can assist us in dealing with all of these issues, by removing the blockages or respective barriers that prevent energy from flowing into body. Thus it can restore energy to the part of the body deprived of lifeforce. In the same way, healing touch can help us arrive at a deeper self-understanding and lead to a fuller expression of those talents and the creativity that lie within us.

After a single session of healing touch/Reiki the recipient invariably feels refreshed, stronger and cleaner as if he or she has just had a very restful nap. With repeated sessions, the health effect of healing touch is remarkable. Acute physical symptoms and long standing chronic complaints are reduced or disappeared.

One of the major goals of healing touch is to help people, become more aware of who they truely are and incorporate that awareness into daily life in practical ways.

In this book I am discussing about what scientific research has to say about the ancient practice of healing touch but for the most part I am approaching the subject with the same understanding, respect and spirit that traditional healers have applied since the birth of civilisation. No other explanation better articulates how the practice actually works and no other set of attitudes better prepares you to apply its principles.

Today, the practice of healing/Reiki is being restored to a place of respect, thanks largely to the many medical, scientific and lay practitioners who are using healing touch to help people overcome every sort of illness and problem.

My sincere efforts in this book will guide you how to use healing touch. It will show you how to make use of an energy that at this moment, is flowing through your entire being. To the extent that it is possible I will explain how this therapeutic touch works and why this book is intended for those of you, who want to rediscorer the healing power in your hands and utilise that power at whatever level you wish.

You can apply healing touch to yourself, your friends and your loved ones or with practice, study and continuous self refinement you can become a practitioner of this powerful healing tool.

BENEATH THE FLESH AND BONES THERE IS A LIVING ENERGY

Every traditional culture, be it Chinese, Japanese, Asian, Indian, Greek or native American, sees life as an Entity upto itself—a lifeforce—that resides in physical objects for a certain period of time. This lifeforce is actually a vast and limitless energy much like a river without beginning or end. This flow of energy manifests as individual people, animal, insects, plants and inanimate objects such as rocks.

The ancient Chinese called this infinite lifeforce "Chi", the Greeks called "PNEUMA", the Asian Indians "PRANA" and the Japanese "Ki" and the native Americans just referred to it as the flow of spirit.

Whatever be the name, the flowing of a universal lifeforce from the creator of the universe to each living thing is seen as the basis of physical, psychological and spiritual health in virtually every traditional culture. Your body is infused with this lifeforce. It surrounds, permeates every cell, organ and sense. It is life, a great ball of energy within which your body resides. As long as the lifeforce flows through the human body, all organs, systems and senses function optimally. Illness is caused by a diminution in the flow of lifeforce. Without a free flow of life energy, organs function at lower rates of efficiency. Blood and lymph flows stagnate, waste accumulates and illness manifest themselves.

THE TRADITIONAL WAY OF THINKING

No matter what therapies a traditional healer depends upon; he or she is essentially treating the lifeforce itself. Wherever the lifeforce is weak or deficient, the traditional healer attempts to make it strong, where it is too strong or excessive, the healer attempts to balance or modulate it. Restored to its optimal flow, the lifeforce will assist the body's natural healing functions to restore health.

According to the traditional way of thinking, a person's way of life affects the degree to which he or she absorbs the lifeforce and thus enriches or impoverishes his or her existence. Practices that strengthen the lifeforce within the individual, eventually form the basis for religious and spiritual life. For this reason virtually every religious tradition depicts its spiritual teachers as having a glowing countenance. **Evidences of powerful lifeforce emanating from spiritual figures abound: In Buddhism, the Buddha radiates a golden glow. In Christianity, Jesus is shown with a glowing halo around his head. In Bible and other religious books, these figures control the flow of that lifeforce to bring healing to others.** The same examples can also be seen in Hinduism i.e. Lord Rama and Lord Krishna, also Sikh Guru Nanak Devjee etc. They are always shown with glowing halos around their heads.

Archaeologists have also discovered in Dead Sea scrolls that the Asians formally trained people in the laying on of hands! Certain people within the Asian community possessed a marked ability of healing practices done by native Americans. Healing touch has been used throughout Asia. In fact all Taoist philosophy, acupuncture/acupressure and all martial arts are based on developing a mature understanding and utilisation of this underlying lifeforce for health, wisdom and personal power.

8. SCIENTIFIC SUPPORT TO HEALING TOUCH

REIKI—THE UNIVERSAL LIFEFORCE

The modern scientists are validating this ancient wisdom. When researchers examine the effects of healing touch in the laboratory, they report consistent and even remarkable results.

At Mc Gill University in Montreal, Canada, Dr Bernard Grad found that the wounds of laboratory mice that received healing touch healed faster than similar wounds on mice that did not receive therapeutic touch. Dr Grad also found that plants those received therapeutic touch grew faster and stronger and produced more chlorophyll than plants those did not receive such treatment. Dr Krieger reported that haemoglobin— the oxygen carrying substance in human blood increased in patients receiving healing touch. Since haemoglobin is essential to life and healing, this is suggested that healing touch enhances the body capacity to heal itself. Other studies have supported such conclusions. Doniel Win from California demonstrated increased wound healing in twenty two or forty four male student-volunteers who were given five minutes healing touch treatments after having surgical incisions.

In 1987 Dr Janet Quinn reported a significant improvement in immune function among the subjects receiving therapeutic touch. Among her findings was an enhanced ratio Between CD4 cells- the helper T cells that direct the immune response against the antigen and CD8 cells—the cells that shut off the immune system. (The enhanced ratio of CD4 and CD8 cells is particularly important for people of HIV and AIDS). These people typically suffer from a diminishing number of CD4 cells and a stabilising or increase in the number of CD8 cells. The drop of CD4 cells causes the immune system to rapidly decline while the increase in CD8 cells causes the System to shut off or to simply fail to respond in presence of pathogen or cancer cell.

Studies have shown that those people receiving healing touch have increased alpha brain waves, a characteristic of people in the meditative state. Such deep states of relaxation are associated with diminution of stress, improved respiration, better hormonal balance, enhanced bowel function, lower blood cholesterol levels and heightened immune response. It is important to note that healing touch works on plants, animals, and humans (both in infants and adults). It is a fact that weakens the argument that the whole phenomenon is caused by a placebo effect. Also there are no harmful side effects to such treatment. Healing touch/Reiki is safe and highly effective. These and other studies reveal that something more than nerve fibres is involved in the exchange between the practitioner and recipient.

Not only are researchers demonstrating in the laboratory that healing touch works, they are also finding the evidence for the underlying mechanism that may explain why it works. Scientists are proving in the laboratory that the human body is animated by a complex web of electrical energy and that this underlying energy can be enhanced to bring about healing.

MORPHOGENIC FIELD—THE LARGER ELECTRICAL BODY SYSTEM

Through a series of additional experiments, Becker discovered that there was indeed a larger intelligence that existed as an electrical field that surrounds and infuses the Salamander's body. Becker proved that this larger electrical body, a "MORPHOGENIC FIELD" actually organises and orders the DNA to produce whatever the body needs of a particular site. He proved that the information is passed from this morphogenic field to the animal's body which triggers the appropriate DNA response and in turn produces the appropriate organ.

ACUPUNCTURE / ACUPRESSURE AND ROLE OF THE MORPHOGENIC FIELD

The morphogenic field also plays a role in the healing power of Acupuncture/Acupressure and Healing touch, where it directs more life energy to specific parts of the body that needs healing. Becker demonstrated that whenever a person is injured or suffers from illness, the body increases the flow of direct electric current which provides the essential energy for healing to the injured or diseased site.

Acupuncture and therapeutic touch, to name just two forms of therapy, actually facilitate the focussing of additional energy to wounds and parts of the body that are diseased. Practitioners of healing touch perform this function by acting as conduits of life energy, which passes from the universal source through the practitioner of healing touch and performs the same function that the body itself is attempting to perform. The big difference is that, very often, the practitioner is able to boost the energy which helps to overcome blockages to the lifeforce and in many cases speed the healing process.

Scientists are on the threshold of learning a great deal about the electrical field or energy body that surrounds and infuses the physical form. But they have just scratched the surface. In order to have a working picture of this field we must rely on the model given to us by traditional healers and religious and spiritual teachers. This teaching which I use in my own practice, has not been proven by science and most likely never will be until we have some specific instruments/ equipments with the sensitivity to measure this very subtle energy. Even if science could analyse this energy, it could not measure the qualities of field, as it is only understood by traditional people. That understanding extends too far into the realm of spirit to be comprehended by the current scientific method. Nevertheless, we need a picture of energy body, by which this model provides to understand and perform this work. As you perform healing touch, Reiki, you will develop your own experiences.

THE ENERGY FIELD

The majority of us can sense another person's energy field. In fact very often the field is so palpable that most people perform mental and linguistic gymnastics in order to express in rational terms what we sense intuitively but can't adequately explain. Thus we refer to some people as having a strong presence or a weak presence. We describe people who are thin or frail as having "a delicate energy". "He is a light weight". Someone says of another, "She fills up the room when she enters it." We don't really mean that a person is so wide that he or she fills the room. We are talking about our clear perception of a person's energy field and all the information we derive from such perceptions.

Each of us senses the energy body and the consciousness that each energetic field contains. Some people radiate discipline, for example, wisdom, or power of danger, others appear bathed in shadows, no matter how much light is in the surrounding environment. Some people have a very stable energy; without saying a word they put you at ease, make you feel relaxed and calm.

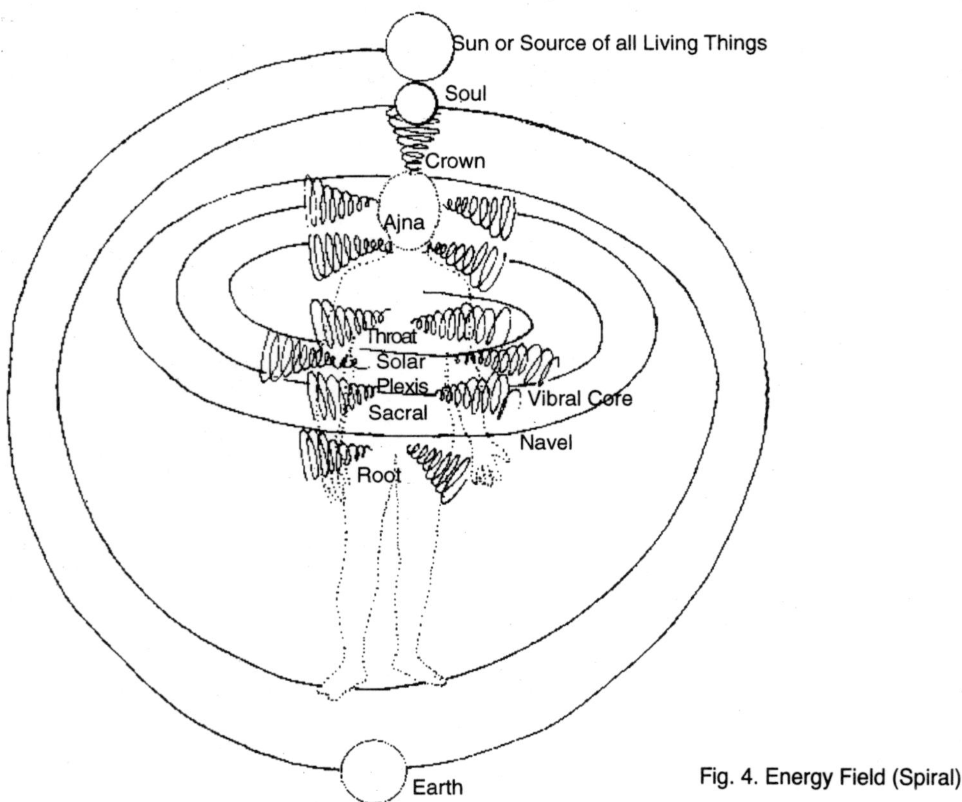

Fig. 4. Energy Field (Spiral)

Others have a very unstable field and within minutes, sometimes even seconds you feel the restlessness of their energetic body, their instability, their "static" electrical condition. "He was nervous." We might say to a colleague or friend later on. "How do you know?" "Did you see him shaking?", the friend might ask us. "No. But I could sense it.", we say Just as a lie detector works by measuring the electric fluctuations within the body, you and I react to the changes in another person's electric field. (Fig. 4)

GOOD AND BAD VIBRATIONS

We are taught from the childhood to censor such perceptions as irrational. Nevertheless, when someone sends out a powerful thought or feeling, you receive that thought or emotion and very often make it conscious. Someone's sexual energy—for example, can be very strong and palpable, even when that person has made so overt advances. Violence and danger are other powerful forms of energy that emanate from the field and affect us consciously. More subtle waves of energy also radiate from the field though we tend to reduce them to generalities. " I get good vibrations from this person", we sometimes say or "I got bad vibes". Yet, there is so much more to be gleaned from a person's field.

When we allow ourselves to observe the brightness of one person or the darkness of another, we recognise the relative amount of light emanating as nothing to do with his or her complexion or skin colour or hair or clothes.

SEEING THE AURA — THE RADIANT ENERGY

Think of the Aura of Nelson Mandela or Martin Luther King, both black men and note the kind of radiant energy that emanates from them. You just think of Pope John Paul, Mother Teresa or Margaret Thatcher, Dalai Lama—all of them are very different in colour, complexion and physical structure but all radiate a powerful light that seem shining far beyond their physical bodies, Fig. 5. The energy field gives us all our power, abilities and health.

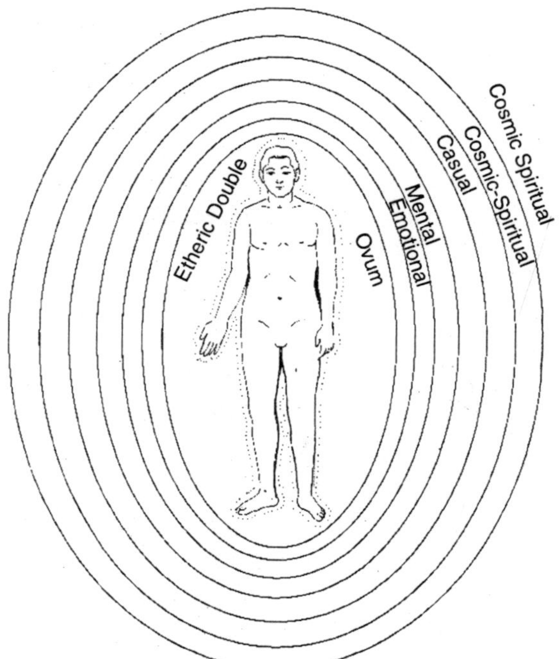

Fig. 5. Auric Field

Sometimes we can actually see wisps of this energy, especially if a person is sitting against a white wall in normal indoor light, in the form of little flames of light dancing around the person's head. If you allow your eyes to go slightly out of focus, when you look at someone, the energy body will become even more visible. This occurs in part, because letting the eyes go out of focus shifts the emphasis of sight to the rods on those cells within the optic nerve that perceive low intensity light. The counterpart to the rods are the cones, another group of cells within the optic nerves that perceive bright light and colour. The auric field is a low intensity light and consequently is more visible to the rods. Watch the energy more in flame like patterns around the head and shoulders. It appears very much like hot pavement emitting heat on a hot summer day.

Another way to see the aura is to note the fragments of light and colour that move around a hand or arm as the person makes a gesture. Sometimes, when the light is right, you can see the field chase after the hand like gossamer light, as the person raises the hand to his head or lower to the table or the arm of chair. The aura seems to be left behind as the hand moves, as if the hand were leaving a trail of light in its wake.

Your energetic field makes an impression on people too. Though it is impossible to know exactly how we affect others, we affect those with whom we interact. We also tend to attract similar kind of people into our lives over and over again. If you reflect on the similarities among the people you attract and the consistency of your certain experiences, you will begin to see that all these reactions are not coincidences but are responses to non-verbal energetic patterns if we regard them as positive or change behaviour and if we want to be free of them.

A MODEL FOR UNDERSTANDING

Think of the field as having the consistency of a big ball of cotton candy. In health, the field is very soft, pillowy and resilient. Each filament of energy within the field is like radiant spun sugar. Unlike the cotton candy, however the filaments in the field are uniform and in perfect relationship with each other. Shaped like an egg, the energetic 'you' is a sphere of energy that surrounds and fills every cell of your corporeal body. The energetic body also extends about three to five feet beyond your physical form. It is radiant with all the colours of rainbow. It is the energy that people are referring to when they use the word "Aura" or talks about the auric field. The **"energetic you"** maintain your physical health and indeed the life of your physical body for as long as you are on the earth. According to the healers and mystics of both East and West, the energy body does not die when the physical body dies. Just the opposite: when the energy body decides that its purpose on earth is complete, it leaves the physical body to return to the energetic or spiritual world. At that moment your physical body ceases to function and remains to the earth as disparate element. The consciousness that you know to be the real you, the "I" inside of you merges with the universal energy body which lives on eternally.

THE WHEELS OF ENERGY: CHAKRAS

Embedded within our field are seven wheels of energy, known as CHAKRAS. These chakras are arranged vertically in the centre of our body from the base of our pelvis to the top of our head. Each chakra provides the lifeforce to a specific set of organs, tissues and eventually to the endocrine gland. In addition each chakra is a centre of consciousness, providing emotional, psychological and spiritual capabilities to the body, mind and spirit. The chakras are energy tunnels that swirl uniformly like eddies of water. These perfect tunnels of energy are widest at the outside of the field and then funnel into the body to an endocrine gland. The point where the chakras intersect with the body is about the size of your palm. At the endocrine gland the funnel reverses itself, becoming larger and wider as it swirls from inside the body, out of the back and to the outer reaches of the field. The chakra tunnel does not disturb the uniformity and flow of energy fibres or filaments in the field but actually feeds and helps them to maintain balance and order within the field.

The seven primary chakras are located in the locations as shown in the diagram. The first chakra is found at the base of the pelvis and is known as ROOT CHAKRA. The second is located at the centre of the lower abdomen, about three or four fingers below the navel and is called the SACRAL CHAKRA. The third chakra viz, SOLAR CHAKRA is located at the solar plexus, the fourth chakra is located at the centre of the chest and is known as HEART CHAKRA. The fifth chakra is located at the throat and is known as THROAT CHAKRA. The sixth is found between the eyes just an inch above the eyebrows and is known as BROW CHAKRA, the seventh chakra is found at the top of the head and is known as CROWN CHAKRA.

In addition to these seven primary chakras, there are secondary chakras on the palm of hands, the backs of the knee, the soles of the feet and twenty tertiary chakras on the tips of fingers and toes.

9. THE SEVEN LAYERS OF LIFE

LAYERS OF LIFE

The energetic body is composed of seven layers. Each layer corresponds to specific aspect of consciousness. The Layers have a certain density that becomes more diffuse as you move away from your physical body. It is more dense as you move closer to physical body.

As corresponds to human health there is good communication among the layers of the field, so that each level influences the other six layers. All seven levels of the energy field are intimately connected and interdependent on each other. For example, thoughts create emotion and vice versa. Indeed one can't have a thought without the production of hormones which can trigger emotional changes. The quality of that thought will determine the character of the emotion and the physical response we experience. Memory can elicit compassion, fear or emotional pain, all having different effects on the physical body as well as on various layers of the field. Because of this interaction within the field, you and I are able to experience a wide array of information. At the same time, we can have an intuitive insight of it when we process that information intellectually and experience the joy such a revelation brings. In this way, insight and joy give us a true sense of our direction.

ETHERIC BODY: THE FIRST LAYER

Often referred to the aura, this layer of energy is joined directly to the physical body, and every cell, tissue and organ which are infused with the ovum of etheric body. Receiving the lifeforce from this most intimate part of the field, the ovum or etheric body is often depicted in spiritual art. Another image that I often use to describe the etheric body is the waves of heat that come off a road on a hot summer day. This ovum holds to the physical body and moves around in much the same way and is the easiest part of the field to perceive with four touches. All you have to do is hold your hands within few inches of a person's body and you can perceive its powerful radiant energy. Whenever you kiss a baby, your lips receive this layer in the field: often a baby's etheric body is so palpable that it seems to have an almost liquid quality.

The etheric body which extends between two and five inches from the body is often referred to as the "Etheric Double" because all the organs are replicated in the etheric form. Indeed your entire body is a physical manifestation of the etheric body.

Human beings are not the only living creatures with the etheric body. All plants and animals have the same corona or golden glow surrounding and permeating their every cell and fibre.

EMOTIONAL BODY: THE SECOND LAYER

From this level within the field, all our feelings, emotions, desires, joys, pains, and sufferings emerge. Our emotions are a form of radiant energy. The astral body and its emotional nature are common among all animals. Indeed the lower aspects of our emotional body link us with animal kingdom.

Emotions affect the body through the nerves, endocrine, muscular and immune systems. As every teenager quickly learns, you can't experience an emotion without an instantaneous granular reaction. Each emotion appears in the field as a charged constellation of energy. Depending on its nature and quality the emotion can emerge within the field like a flower opening to the sun or like an explosion that showers the field with ecstatic or destabilizing energy. If the emotion is joy, the field opens and expands, sending energy radiating throughout the entire electrical and physical body. Immediately the body experiences a flood of lifeforce. Every pore seems to open to the sun. The light within your expanding, brightening and opening up to an infinite energy that surrounds you and is channelled through your energetic field. At this juncture of your life, you are more alive than ever because you are experiencing love—the universal love for you. That love, is energy i.e. always present, but changes in the field—caused by beliefs, perceptions, attitudes and most of all fears—cause the field to shut down or be injured. But when the moment of joy arrives, you open and experience the light that is all around you and the part of you that opens especifically is your heart or in other words your heart chakra. A whirling flow of energy you experience over your heart at this opening. It is filled with the light of love which in turn floods your field and your physical body.

The healing that can take place in that moment can be miraculous. Depending upon how much lifeforce is penetrating your field and physical body, that love can overcome barriers or form of stagnation that is currently causing your physical symptoms of disease, love, joy, hope and feeling of well-being. All of these are generators of energy within you that cause the field to expand and open and result in similar openings within the physical body.

You have experienced the electrical quality of emotion, hundreds or even thousands of times. Think back to your first date, the first time you touched the hand of a boy or girl whom you have liked. Suddenly you felt something tangible, an electric or altogether wonderful sensation passed through your body. Now think back to your first kiss. Need I say more?

On the other hand, if the emotions are of the opposite effect it will take place on small to moderate degrees of anger or conflict causing the energy within the field to become erratic. It is an irritating energy that causes similar nervous, muscular and hormonal irritations in your body. Too much of anger, fear or hatred spoil the field causing rifts and holes in the walls between the layers and great storms of energy within the field that wound even further. When any angry patient arrives, the field feels to me as if it is hard and pushing outward as if she or he is pushing people away.

Changes within the field cause immediate change in the human body. For example, when light reaction occurs, then fear stimulates the adrenal glands to secrete adrenaline, which in turn becomes epinephrine, dopamine and norepinephrine chemicals that trigger an incredible array of thoughts and physical reactions, among which are increased heart rate and respiration, blood glucose, and muscular activity. Fear depresses the immune response and increases heart rate and respiration and causes heightened muscular activities. If your fear becomes chronic, cholesterol levels are elevated significantly, hormones — especially catecholamines become heightened and imbalanced, respiration becomes shallow and tense and muscles remain tense and sometimes go into spasm.

Conversely, positive emotions — such as love, hope, joy and feeling of well-being and security, all these strengthen immune response and make the physical body better able to fight off disease. In this case, the emotions are smooth flowing, what most people do not realise that these changes — both positive and negative — originate in electromagnetic field that surrounds and permeates the body, and that many come from the astral layer of the field.

Emotions, of course are directly linked to our thoughts which exist in the next level up within the energetic field. Even unconscious emotions — those emotions whose sources still lie unrecognised in the unconscious — create thoughts of which we are conscious. For example, we may be angry with someone and have long internal monologues with ourselves, yet never realise the deeper reasons for our anger. Perhaps we are really angry with ourselves or with some persons in question remind us of. Indeed it is not until the emotions and thinking work harmony i.e. until our emotions are allowed to emerge and our thoughts are made free to investigate the sources of these emotions that we understand our emotional world.

The loss of energy that occurs, whenever we experience guilt, shame and unresolved anger is referred to as leak in the field. The boundary that maintains the integrity of the field is torn. Through that tear, energy leaks and is lost. We experience guilt as a loss of integrity, personal protection and a blurring of our own boundaries. We are no longer capable of protecting ourselves from another person's judgment of us. It is as if we have absorbed another person's assessment and made it our own. The boundary that supports our sense of self is injured allowing energy to be lost. We experience a palpable diminution of the lifeforce with all its familiar and well-known weakness, fatigue, self condemnation, loss of direction and a weakened sense of self. For a healer, the emotional layer of the field is an essential part of the healing process because most illnesses are very often rooted here.

After healing touch session is complete, a meditation or guided energy can help the person repattern the emotional plane, which will help close wounds arid establish new and healthier habits.

Other studies that have examined the influence of prayers have shown similar results, like healing touch prayer has been shown to affect the health of plants, fungi and bacteria. Research has demonstrated that people . can use prayers effectively to inhibit the growth of fungi even at a distance of 20 kilometres. The power of prayers demonstrate the importance of your intention while you perform healing touch, Reiki. In short, send all those you work with your love and make your healing touch sessions an act of prayer.

MENTAL BODY: THE THIRD LAYER

The third layer of the field is responsible for intellectual functions, our conscious and unconscious mind and many memories. This conscious mind, of course, refers to those aspects of ourselves and our environment of which we are aware. By unconscious I mean your personal unconscious—those thoughts, memories and dreams that have been repressed or forgotten but that exists just beneath the surface of our consciousness. The mental body coordinates physiological activity including conscious and autonomic functions. It gives you the ability to say, drive your car many kilometres while you think of everything but driving and yet arrive safely.

Among the important contents of the mental body especially from a healing point of view, are the unexamined ideas, beliefs, judgments and concepts that give rise to our behaviour and can inhibit our growth. Beliefs, judgments and attitudes that no longer serve our current state of maturity and development, exist as blockages to circulation of energy within the field when they stand rigidly in the way of new information, first in sights and larger belief systems. Like boulders in a stream or knots of tension in the muscles they block circulation of energy within the field preventing renewal and new understanding of life. Even worse, these unexamined judgments and beliefs feed the conscious mind and cause behaviours that are inappropriate to our current situation. They prevent us from seeing situation in a fresh, new light. Racism and sexism and various beliefs of superiority or inferiority are all examples of blockages in the mental plane. Beliefs that you are weak or talentless or always wrong or always right are also your unexamined judgments that impede health and development. The instance "I can do that" is an unchallenged belief that becomes energetic pattern in the field. These patterns present the circulation of energy within the field which limits our freedom and our creativity and affects our health.

As a practitioner of healing touch you will release these blockages from your client's fields. When that occurs, you will frequently hear people start talking about their frustrations, their projections or their unexamined beliefs from a whole new perspective. Some will have revelations on how they have limited themselves. Others will simply feel tremendous relief or a new sense of personal power and identity.

Once when some of the long standing beliefs are released, creativity emerges with great relief and flexibility. The person feels empowered simply because he or she has been devoid of beliefs that have prevented him or her from viewing the vast array of possibilities and opportunities — implicit with the situation.

PARA-CONSCIOUSNESS : THE FOURTH LAYER

The fourth layer contains all the extraordinary abilities, such as intuition, extra-sensory perception, image projection and spiritual sight. In addition to these abilities is one's capacity for compensation. It is observed that one person with intuition has the ability to join with another person to feel his life condition, to know his pain and suffering. Out of such intuition comes compassion for another human being.

Intuition is the ability to learn the experience of the true connection that exists among all people and indeed with a great spirit. When we experience that unity we open ourselves to the information that is passing constantly through the cosmos in the form of energy. On a one-to-one level you can experience connectedness simply by listening and feeling another person's lifeforce, various forms of oriental diagnosis and teaching methods of developing intuition by allowing the client's energy to contact your own field. In this way you can understand the person in a deepened intimate way. (Method and exercise for doing this as well as the ways to release any of your client's energies that you might have picked up has been explained separately step by step).

We practise this awakening to connectedness whenever we perform healing touch. During a session, the practitioner channels the universal energy through himself or herself to the client. The practice is based on the fundamental unity among the cosmos, the practitioner and the other human being. By doing this you are living in the awareness of connectedness which accelerates the development of your intuition and the fourth level of the field.

Your ability to allow your intuition or the fourth layer within your field to guide you depends on how clear and unobstructed the lower layer is. By removing obstructions from these levels of our being, the fourth and the higher layers can influence the mental, emotional and etheric body. Consequently our feelings of connectedness and intuition automatically improve.

THE CAUSAL BODY : THE FIFTH LAYER

Traditional approaches to the field maintain that there is a place within all of us that we know that why we are here on the earth. This layer of the field contains the knowledge of your life purpose, your many talents and the lessons you wish to learn while you are on this earth. The causal layer contains the knowledge that awakens in you if only faintly when you encounter people with whom you have agreed to work out the specific tasks, accomplish goals and overcome barriers before you come on to the earth. On this layer of the field your soul's plan for this lifetime can be found.

Virtually all religions have taught that reincarnation or the transmigration of souls, is the foundation of the life. We live multiple lifetimes on this planet so that we can learn and evolve to higher states of being. In the process we accumulate knowledge which we use in each succeeding lifetimes to help ourselves and others. In addition we make the mistakes and incur karmic lessons or debts we wish to propitiate. All of these are done and we can develop greater and greater love, knowledge, and understand meaning of life itself in an inextinguishable source. It can't be destroyed and so continues to manifest in the forms that best replicate the consciousness associated with that particular life form. The physical body perfectly replicates the consciousness of the being within it, and serves to manifest in physical form all the abilities and lessons that each individual soul wishes to experience, express and learn. All such information about your individual lifetime, as well as all previous lifetimes is contained with the causal body, the fifth layer of the field.

It is important to recognise that you do not have to believe in reincarnation to serve as a practitioner of healing touch. On the contrary, all you have to do is to care deeply about the person you are thinking to help and to serve as an instrument for the universal love and energy that will pass through you to the person you wish to help.

THE COSMIC AND SPIRITUAL CONSCIOUSNESS: THE SIXTH AND SEVENTH LAYER

The sixth and seventh layers of our being represent our most fortunate links with what each of us recognise as a great spirit of universal. creative force. Obviously all aspects of the field and the physical body are directly linked to the universal divine, but the sixth and the seventh layers actually know it and are consciously in direct contact with it. Consequently these layers offer us the experience of direct union with God. They are sometimes able to resonate within our consciousness when we are deep in prayer and meditation. It is this level of our being, that is the being experienced when a person is said to have momentary enlightenment.

About the levels of their fields much is unknown simply because they are so rare and lofty that very few people consciously experience them and then write about their experiences. What we do know is the sixth and seventh layers of the field possess a tremendous force of energy that, when it grounded in the body can create a host of psychological disorders if the person is not prepared for such an experience or if the body itself is not in sufficient health.

INTERACTION OF LAYERS WITH EACH OTHER

In order to understand better topography of field I have tried to describe the layer individually, but this separation does not reveal, how the layers interact, influence each other and function as one. While each layer of the field has its own unique function, strengths, weaknesses, abilities and talents, it must work in coordination with the entire field in order for us to express our talents and abilities and learn about life. The person who has a gift for music is using his or her entire field while playing an instrument, clearly beginning with the physical body and including the first layer (the etheric body to coordinate the voice or the muscles used to perform on an instrument), the second (placing the depth of feeling in the music), the third (providing the intellectual ability needed to learn the music and express it with nuance and precision), the fourth (experiencing music's power to unify people in harmony and sound), and fifth (music is a part of a particular person's life plan and expressing that plan provides the greatest or joys). If the musician truly reaches the great heights, he or she has the potential to express the divine sound. All the layers of these fields must work in harmony, if a person is to truly express his or her gifts.

THE CHANNEL OF SPIRIT IN YOU (The Central Tube)

After several years of experience as a practitioner of healing touch, I realised that in addition to the standard layers, there is another characteristic of field which is called the central tube. This tube or channel of energy runs down the centre of the physical- body itself (Fig. 6.) It originates at the very top of the head, where the spiritual lifeforce enters the body and runs down the centre of the body through

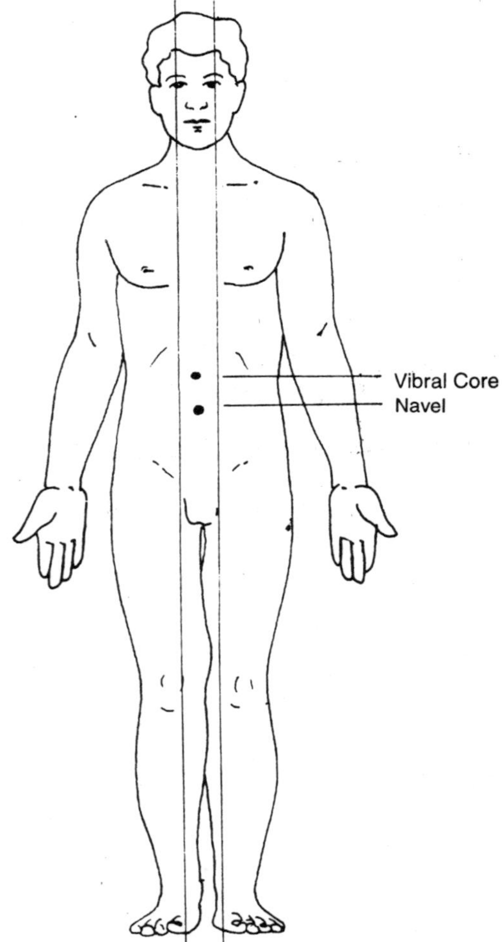

Fig. 6. The Central Tube

the neck down the centre of the digestive system to the very base of the sex organs, where the energy can pass out of body and where the earth's energy can enter into it. Along the tube are found the seven wheels of energy or chakras each of which fan out and enrich the organs in the particular area of the body. This is a kind of spiritual channel running from top to bottom.

Energy runs like a river through this tube. Blockages within the tube often appear as eddies of energy and can prevent energy from flowing clearly through this essential channel. The most frequent problems I have found among those with blockages in the tube are emotional conflicts, specifically the problems of integrating concept of the head with the emotions and instincts of the heart and lower organs. The chakras (located around the tube) represent specific aspects of our human psychology. People who have great difficulty in integrating the head, the heart and the sexual organs — their survival instincts often have blockages in the tube. Lifeforce that would otherwise flow smoothly among these three centres is blocked, causing the mind to behave as if it were separated from the emotional and sexual-survival centres. Such a person is continuously in conflict over what he or she thinks versus what he or she feels or secretly wants or is instinctively drawn to.

By eliminating these blockages we can help the person to integrate the higher and lower centres of the psyche and restore the brightness and clarity of his mind.

In the centre of the body, just below the solar plexus and just above the umbilicus is the centre of being known as the vibral core. Here our spirit and matter join and become one. This is where the vital healing energy flows from the practitioner to the client. The energy originates from the creator of the universe but flows to the practitioner, who sends it forth from the universal source to the practitioner's vibral core, then to the practitioner's hands and then to the client's vibral core where the father spirit (energy) and the mother earth (matter) mingle together to create our essential humanness. When the healer and the client work together, their energetic bodies mingle and become one. The oneness is established between their vibral cores. This vibrational union harmonises the two people and direct both of them in the healing process.

HAVE THE VISION OF DIVINE LIGHT COMING OUT OF YOUR BODY

An Important Exercise

Here is an important exercise which can be performed by you during early evening. It is best at twilight. This will help you to see the auric field around your hands.

Turn off all artificial lighting and lie on your back on the floor. Raise your hands a foot or so above your head and join your fingers in a relaxed weave. Now very gradually pull your hands apart so that your fingers gently and slowly separate as your hands move in the opposite directions. As your hands slowly separate, relax your focus gaze between your hands so that you are looking at the space between your hands and at the ceiling of your room. Slightly blur your vision. You will likely see a stream of soft light between your hands and fingers. The light will appear much like vapours that surrounds your hands and dance between your fingers. If not visible, do it again and again. Don't forget to rub your hands for nearly one minute.

THIS IS DIVINE LIGHT

MEDITATIVE ALIGNMENT EXERCISES (Attunement)

1. Sit in a chair or on a pillow on the floor with your back straight and body comfortable and relaxed. Deeply breathe and establish a deep rhythmic pattern of breathing (breathe in a regular pattern for approximately three minutes); slowly draw your attention away from your environment and focus on the in and out movement of your breath; let go off all your thoughts.

2. Bring your attention into your physical body. Take sometime to notice where you are holding your tension. Breathe deeply and evenly into the tension and visualise the tension streching out and becoming relaxed. See the area of tension becoming smooth and supple. Then say to yourself, "I have a physical body, but I am more than my physical body."

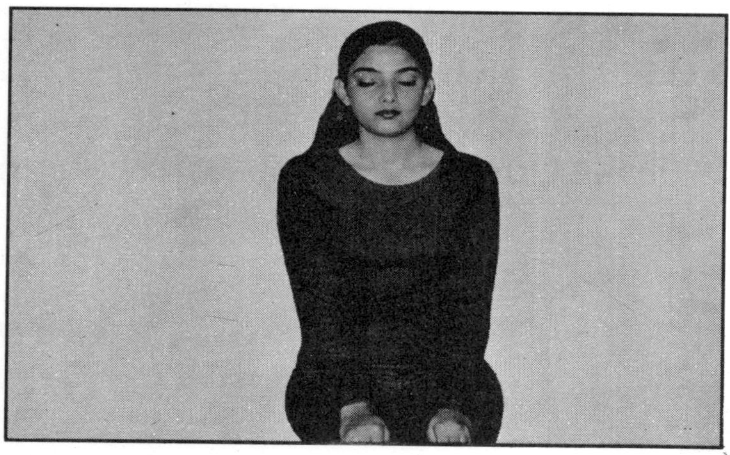

Position showing sitting in chair with back straight and body comfortable and relaxed.

3. Now bring your attention to your emotional body. Take sometime to become aware of your feelings. Take a personal inventory of what is going on within you. Notice your feelings. Do not judge them or try to change them and then breathe into those feelings and visualise yourself letting go off them. See them fading from your consciousness and say to yourself, "I have an emotional body and I am more than my emotional body."

4. Move your attention into your mental body. Take an inventory of your thoughts, notice the amount of activity going on in your mind. Breathe deeply and slowly and quieten the mind.

Release all thoughts and arrive at the place of stillness. Take a moment to experience the stillness, then say to yourself, "I have a mental body and I am more than my mental body."

5. Focus your attention at the top of your head and say to yourself, "I am the centre of pure creative awareness and higher spiritual will." I allow yourself to fully experience that statement. Feel its power and the grace that flows to you from this recognition.

6. See yourself as an energetic field, a living energy that has consciousness and love, that love flows to you from an infinite source. It can never be extinguished. You can send that energy to help others in endless ways, including helping them to heal. Say to yourself, "I am in the flow of power, I am the channel of power and that power is love" or say in high pitch voice ....

[*"I invoke the light of God within.*
I am clear and perfect channel and light is my guide."]

In the beginning, acting on this exercise may not fulfil attunement to the extreme level of energy. But, your more devotion and faith in this exercise and working for it will improve your channels day by day and you will start healing faithfully and develop the channel of flow through your body. First start healing yourself and work on your chakras and sub-chakras, to remove the existing blockages for the clear flow of divine light through your body.

The detailed position of hands to be kept to open chakra's channel has been illustrated in detail. More and more devotional practice on these chakras will bring you to be a source of divine light channel for passing to imperfect bodies to be healed of diseases.

AN EXERCISE TO FEEL THE FIELD
OF DIVINE FLOW IN YOUR BODY

1. Stand face to face with your partner at a little more than an arm's distance from each other.

2. Extend your arm directly out from your side towards your partner's shoulder but still well back from your partner keep your elbow bent slightly.

3. Cup your hand loosely and gradually bring your hand towards your partner's shoulder.

4. As your hand approaches your partner's shoulder, move your hand slowly through his or her field, slightly raising and lowering your hand a few inches. So that you can delineate the various layers and densities of field.

    Feel the field with your hand, note the changes in thickness, temperature or patterns as your hand perceives as it moves through the field.

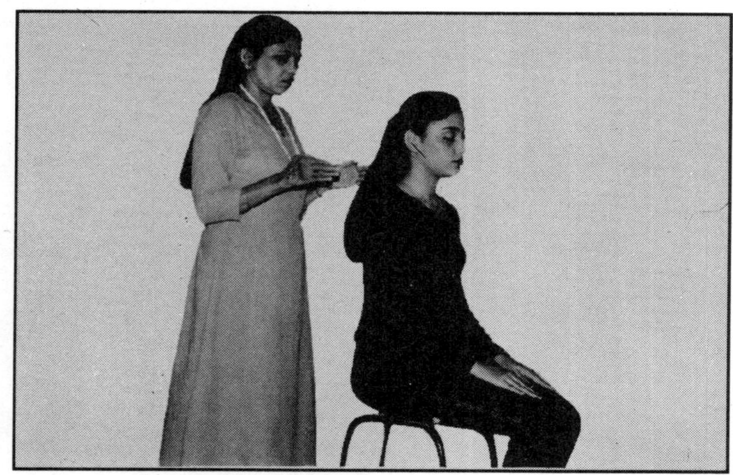

Position showing the feeling of
divine flow in the body.

10. THE CHAKRAS : YOUR SPHERES OF ENERGY

CONSCIOUSNESS AND LIFE

If we take out hand and place it gently over our heart, allowing our fingertips to touch our shirt ever so lightly and then slowly rotate hand in a clockwise direction as facing outward, we will feel comforted. If we continue to rotate our hand in that gentle, circular way, we will feel our body relax and get warmer. Gradually, we will experience a strange communication with this part of our body as if our heart area is melting in gratitude. Breathe deeply and allow that smile to warm our entire inner being. Many people who do this exercise eventually start to cry. They cry because they feel comforted, relieved and overwhelmed with gratitude as if they were being welcomed into a realm in which all their burdens could be put down, a realm in which they were embraced by an unconditional love. (Try this exercise by reversing the motion of your hand over your heart. Note the difference in feeling).

While you do this exercise, you are applying healing touch to your heart chakra, the sphere of energy that governs your heart and thymus gland and a specific realm of your consciousness. In doing this exercise you get a small glimpse of the unity of your body, mind and spirit. You also recognise that you achieve the power to gain access to your spirit and influence it in healing ways. As you progress through this book you will learn many other techniques for healing your body, mind and spirit through simple yet powerful methods of healing touch.

For the practitioner of healing touch, a knowledge of the chakras is an indispensable diagnostic tool. The chakras also are the sites on which great healing can occur. We can understand people according to their chakra imbalances, but more important, we can do so much for them by working with the chakras through healing touch. Finally the chakras demonstrate the importance of your intention, for your intention reveals the chakra from which you are expressing yourself. As we have seen, your action will have very different effects on the recipient depending on the chakras by which you are motivated. If you, as a healer, are acting from your heart chakra, you are channelling the energy that can utilize all your other abilities. The farthest energy reaches your mind and unfolds your deepest and most practical wisdom about survival. Ultimately the chakras prove what the poets have always taught: that the greatest integrating and unifying force in life is love (Fig. 7).

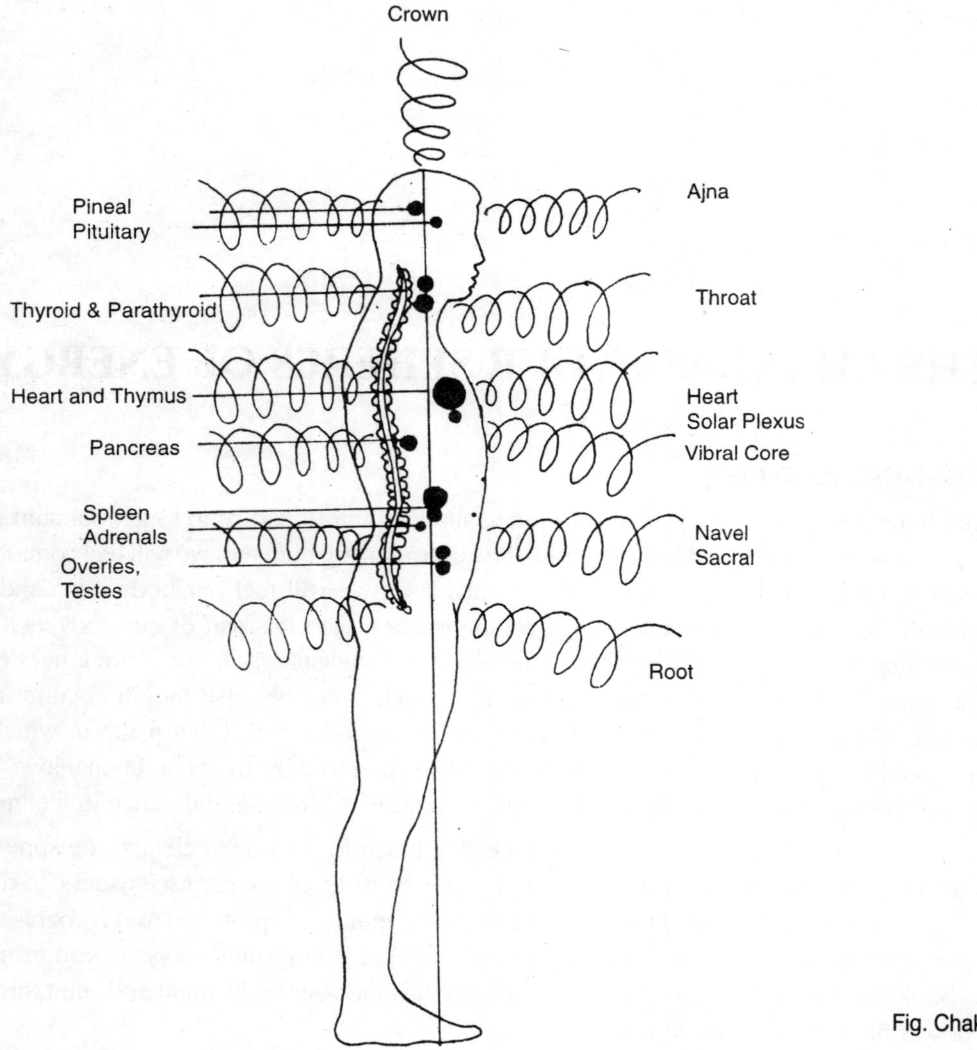

Fig. Chakra Locations

The information provided here on the chakras comes from my own experiences.

WHERE THE BODY, MIND AND SPIRIT ARE ONE

Nothing illustrates the unity of body, mind and spirit better than the chakras. Chakra is a Sanskrit word meaning **"Wheel" or "Circles of Movement."** The chakras are spirits of concentrated lifeforce — vortices of energy as they are referred to by some. They are arrayed in a straight line on the front of your body, starting at the very .base of your spine (at the perineum) and extending to the top of your head. The seven primary chakras are located as follows.

The first is found at the base of the spine, the second a few inches below the navel. The third at the solar plexus, the fourth over the heart and the fifth over the throat of the larynx, the sixth between the eye brows and the seventh just above the crown of the head. Each of the seven primary chakras radiates downward into your physical body and outward through the seven layers of your energy field. Each chakra is shaped like a cone, a spiral with its pointed end entering the body and the widening end spiraling outward into your energy field.

In addition to these primary chakras you possess smaller secondary chakras on the palm of your hands and back of your knees and the sole of your feet near the arches. There are seven smaller tertiary chakras located on your finger tips and the toe tips. You use the second and third chakras in your hands to direct energy during healing touch, and you use the second and third chakras in your feet to ground yourself while performing the practice.

As you will notice shortly, the function of each of the seven primary chakras corresponds roughly to the seven layers of the field, so that the activities of the first layer of the field (the **etheric layer**) correspond to the first chakra, the second layer of the field corresponds to the second **chakra, the third** layer with the third chakra and so on.

One of the functions of the chakras is to act as funnels for the lifeforce, each of us is **continually** bathed in an unlimited flow of **Electromagnetic Energy,** or the lifeforce that sustains **our lives. We** breathe in the lifeforce, receive it through the five senses, channel it through the field **and draw it into** us through the seven chakras.

The chakras can be understood on several levels on the gross physical level. **They channel** lifeforce to particular organs and endocrine glands. Indeed when you look **at the illustration of chakras** (see diagram) you will notice that they correspond with the most active parts of the body — the brain, eyes, speech centre, heart, middle organs, digestion, endocrine glands and sex organs. These areas obviously require a great deal of energy, but we can say the reverse as well that in their enormous activity these same areas of the body generate the most energy. These are the parts of the body that give rise to the thoughts and ideas that in turn shape our world. They recall memories that sustain relationships, they drink up light and colour, they masticate and digest food, they pump and cleanse the blood, they procreate and sustain life. In short they are the basis upon which we experience life and even participate in its creation. Little wonder, therefore that ancient sages correlated these parts of the body with special vortices of energy that could sustain such important functions.

But there is much more to these chakras than the purely physical. These seven cones also carry with them profound emotional and psychological associations, of which virtually all of us already are aware. For example, on some visceral and well established level of our knowing, each of us regards the heart as the centre of the emotions. We say about some people, "He has a lot of heart" or "She has a heart of lion" or "He is a heartless soul". To Express our deepest love we might say, "I give you my heart." Other chakra areas possess their own unique character and associations. The brain, for example, is regarded as the realm of intelligence. Objective thoughts and reasons even through the brain are directly linked to virtually every physical, psychological and emotional aspect of humanity. When trying to assess a person's character we search his eyes for insight into his soul.

In fact each chakra is the site of a specific consciousness, a realm that offers its own specific set of values. None of us has integrated all seven levels of consciousness into our being. You may be awakaned and motivated by two, three or even more chakras, but it is very rare being who is awake and functions at all seven levels of consciousness.

This brings me to an essential point. The one, two or three chakras that might be most influential in your life dictate your physical and emotional needs, your values and your spiritual awareness. The world today is being governed by the first three chakars.

The chakras, therefore represent a kind of ladder of personal, psychological and spiritual evolution. Each of us is attempting to move into next higher chakra above the ones that now directs our world view. Hence, the values and awareness are implicit in the chakra that we are striving to represent our next step in growth and development. The chakras are described in an ascending order to show how we proceed from the very rudimentary consciousness to an ever enlarging viewpoint on ourselves and life.

As we will see, moving up the chakra ladder inevitably presents the greatest challenges that life has to offer very often. One or more of the chakras blocked or partially closed mean, we are not being influenced sufficiently by the corresponding values and understanding that resides within that chakra. It will also mean that the lifeforce will be diminished in that part of the body. Yet, even when one or another chakra is closed, it still functions in some limited capacity. It is still providing nourishing lifeforce to its corresponding part of the body. If the chakra did not function on some level **we would soon be dead.** Still when chakra is working in a weakened state, the part of the body to which it corresponds is also weakened. In addition, the values and consciousness represented by that chakra do not influence us as strongly, if at all. Gradually the related organs and glands may atrophy and eventually manifest some kind of symptoms of disease. Also our lack of understanding for the part of the life represented by the chakra inevitably brings us into conflict and crisis. By understanding a person's problems and sites at which seven chakras might be fixed, the practitioner of healing touch can understand why certain physical and psychological problems manifest. The practitioner will also know which of the seven chakras the client is struggling to integrate into consciousness and therefore where the practitioner must concentrate his or her work.

As a practitioner of healing touch, you are doing more than working on physical health. You are working with the body, mind and spirit and in doing so your are treating the underlying reasons which cause sickness at the first place.

Let us turn now to an examination of the seven chakras individually and collectively to better understand their roles in our lives and in the practice of healing touch.

THE FIRST CHAKRA (The Root of Being)

Referred to in Sanskrit as the **"MULADHARA"** or the root chakra, the first wheel of energy is located at the very base of the spine and encompasses the perineum. It provides lifeforce to the Adrenal Glands which in turn produce adrenaline for instinctive and instantaneous responses to exciting events or perceived threats. This chakra provides lifeforce to the large intestine, rectum bones, legs and feet. It is also responsible for maintaining the nervous and circulatory systems. Physical symptoms that emerge when this chakra is congested, blocked or closed include constipation, haemorrhoids, obesity, sciatica pain, arthritis, knee trouble, anorexia nervosa and suicide.

The first chakra is responsible for grounding your life in physical existence. It is your instinctive centre of your energetic and spiritual root on the earth, the source of your survival instinct. It keeps you rooted in the present moment and aware of possible threats to your existence, any reaction related to your survival; including the flight or fight instinct emanates form this centre of consciousness. Conversely any self induced threat to existence, such as anorexia or an attempted suicide, is a breach of the values and consciousness inherent in this chakra.

Kundalini Yoga and Ayurvedic Medicine teach that the first chakra is responsible for maintaining our sense of smell. The human olfactory sense is quite developed though we usually don't think of ourselves as good smellers. In fact we can identify an object after smelling just nine molecules of the particular substance, which means that we can often perceive something at considerable distance from our nose.

Our faculty of smell was developed as a means of self-protection. Smell allows us to perceive whether or not something is poisonous or somehow dangerous without having to eat it, for example, or to get too close to the object in question. (Cautious children and adults invariably place unknown or foreign foods under their noses before they dare taste something that they might find revolting or dangerous). This relates directly to the chakra's overall responsibility for survival.

There is an enormous body of literature and mythology surrounding the seven chakras and much attention has been **paid to the** first chakra. Out of this mythology has come our understanding of the consciousness and values that lie within this wheel of energy.

To begin with, this chakra is associated with the earth and colour red. It is characterised by cohesiveness, inertia and a certain amount of stagnation. The first chakra makes us cautious which is a kind of inertia. It encourages us to remain focused on our number one priority, which is survival. And it prevents us from allowing too many contradictory thoughts and bits of information to enter our consciousness, which would break down the mind into fragments. This is part of its character of cohesiveness.

THE SECOND CHAKRA (Sex and Passion)

Referred to in Sanskrit as **SWADHISTHANA** or the centre, the second chakra is located a few inches below the navel in the region of the first lumbar vertebra. It provides lifeforce to the ovaries in a woman and to the testes in a man and to their related hormones. The chakra channel leads lifeforce to the male and female genitals, kidneys, bladder and circulatory system. It also serves a developing foetus with life energy. This chakra is also responsible for governing the sense of taste and deep vital breath. According to Chinese medicine the kidneys make the deep breath possible, when the kidneys are strong and vital, they draw the breath deep into the bottom of lungs. When kidneys are weak the breath is shallow and the person is timid, nervous and fearful.

Blockages, closure or any impairment of the second chakra can result in illness related to the kidneys, bladder and sex organs and the lower back. All emotional and psychological issues related to sex emanate from the second chakra including how one expresses oneself as a male or female.

The chakra's main biological functions are the maintenance of sex organs, the sex drive and the desire for the physical pleasure and all the social issues associated with entering into a sexual relationship. One can't truly experience sex alone, and consequently the second chakra leads us form the individualised state articulated by the first chakra into the search for a mate and realm of social interaction.

The second chakra is regarded as the centre of the personality. In Japan it is known as **HARA** or the centre of gravity. **HARA** is the foundation upon which one maintains physical, emotional, psychological and spiritual equilibrium. It is the centre of power and vitality. From **HARA** one maintains balance, no matter what the circumstances and therefore controls himself and his environment without lifting a finger. The second chakra is associated with the colour orange and the water elements. It is symbolised with **leviathan or sea serpent,** what the elephant is to the earth so the leviathan is to the oceans. It is the embodiment of the enormous power and mystery that lies beneath the intimidating surface of the seas. Water of course, connotes fertility, the womb and the bodily fluids that carry sperms and egg. It symbolises the unconscious mind and its infinite mysteries that lie beneath its waves. Consistent with this image is the fact that water and the serpent represent a primitive stage in the evolution of life on the planet, when living creatures inhabited the oceans exclusively.

The ocean is the mother of life on the planet, the womb from which we all emerged. Indeed, while each of us was in our mother's womb, we underwent a reptilian stage that replicated our earlier journey from the ocean water to the land.

Thus the second chakra is concerned primarily with sex and the behaviour related to having sex or entering into a relationship in which we can have sex.

THE RELATION BETWEEN FIRST AND SECOND CHAKRAS

Let us pause a minute and reflect on the first two chakras and how their value system affect our lives in very different ways. Since it is concerned with the preservation of life and of separation, the first chakra make us aware of the dangers of life and our own longing for companionship, love and sex which means it drives us to the second chakra in its truest form in pursuit of the opposite sex based on love.

Sexual love is the union of opposites, man and woman, yang and yin, heaven and earth. In all traditional, spiritual and religious practices but especially those of the east, human sexual experience is regarded as the union of divine opposites. It is seen as the way for humans to glimpse the harmony and order that occurs when two halves of the cosmic puzzle come together in love. In Yoga and tantric traditions sex permits two people to unite and thus participate in the coming together of archetypes, cosmic deities. It is one way humans can participate in the divine drama which is essential in the creation of life.

THE THIRD CHAKRA (Power, Mastery and Ego)

The Sanskrit word for the third chakra is **MANIPURA** or Gem centre. It is located at the solar plexus or the region of the eighth thoracic vertebra. The third chakra is responsible for providing lifeforce to pancreas. It also funnels electromagnetic energy to the liver, gall bladder, spleen and stomach.

The pancreas, of course is responsible for creating insulin, which makes blood sugar available to cells as fuel. The third chakra is therefore associated with metabolism and the basic work of the cells of the body. Metabolism is in fact, a tiny fire inside the cells, like tiny factories, the cells burn glucose (or blood sugar) so that they can do their work. Hence the third chakra has traditionally been associated with fire or in Ayurvedic medicine with the fire element. Blockages or closure of the third chakra results in digestive disorders, ulcers, diabetes, hypoglycemia, liver problems and disorder related to the metabolism of blood sugar and fat.

Psychologically and spiritually, the third chakra is all about your personal power and self mastery. Personal power and mastery are developed because you are required to refine yourself and mature. Hence you are advised to embrace the third chakra. In addition to fire, the third chakra is associated with the mind and the colour yellow. This chakra is represented by the ram which is the symbol of zodiac sign. Aries known for its strong will, courage, outgoing nature, leadership and indeed its stubbornness. Aries is often joined with Mars, the planet of fiery passions, war, impetuousness, emotion assertiveness, violence, courage and activity. This chakra provides you with the capacity to assert yourself and your wishes and the power to fulfil what you set out to accomplish.

Hence the atmosphere of the third chakra is all about passion, raw power and an untamed mind.

When we are deeply frustrated we often feel physical pressure or unease in the solar plexus. The third chakra is alerting us to the fact that our passions are unruly and that our personal power is being blocked or frustrated, perhaps by our own belief or by circumstances in the environment, or perhaps by both. There are two courses that can be chosen at this point, either we can self reflect, be creative and apply a new approach to the situation or we can push harder and force our will, which can lead to more frustration, anger and resentment. That is why the third chakra is often associated with violence.

RELATIONSHIP AMONG FIRST, SECOND AND THIRD CHAKRAS

Clearly, a progression of consciousness can be seen from the first, second and third chakras. Having confronted our separation and aloneness, we are driven to sexual relationship which joins us with at least one other human being and thus leads us beyond ourselves and our own priorities. The third chakra leads us back to ourselves this time focussing on self improvement and self empowerment.

In a sense the third chakra is an evolved first chakra and both the first and third chakras are interested in you, the individual. The first chakra is more concerned with your survival while the third is more concerned with a power needed to fulfil your desires. Yet these have an evolutionary step in between the first and the third chakra, a step represented by second chakra.

The second chakra leads a man and a woman into sexual relationship, which typically results in child birth. As every parent knows children force an adult back on himself, or herself, they require the parents to love and develop their talents and skills. In order to provide for their children's needs and survival, the parents are stretched by the demands of family to raise their children with love, order and understanding. They must discipline themselves and even postpone their own desires to provide for those in their care. Indeed, they must sacrifice their own needs and sometime their own lives. Women lose their lives in child birth, yet they welcome pregnancy. Fathers sacrifice the attention and maternal love of their wives so that their children can enjoy such love and attention and thereby develop fully. Fathers too give their lives for their children. Ultimately, love demands sacrifice and self development, which means that the second chakra leads inevitably into the third. In a fundamental way, awakening to the second and third chakras indeed is surrendering to them to open up the worlds above the third chakra because sex and self development involve us in complicated relationship that ultimately require love.

CRISIS OF THIRD CHAKRA

The third chakra encourages us to utilize our own power, to be responsible for our own fate. Thus it achieves self mastery. Such a consciousness leads us inevitably to one of the two crises.

The first crisis is the demagoguery, the paradox of self mastery. Indeed one of its pitfalls is that as people progress in their development an inevitable ego inflation sets in. They become more skilled, successful and also more arrogant. They can indulge in the false belief that they are masters of their own fate. This can ultimately isolate them and destroy their lives. That is only one of the dark roads that the third chakra can lead us down.

However, the second is one most of us find ourselves on the road that leads to grief, sadness and self-recrimination for not having achieved all that we wished for. Here at the third chakra, are found many of our frustrations with ourselves asking very hard and critical questions such as, why did not I do this, or become that? Why did not I make better choices along the way? These questions precipitate a life crisis, very often a mid-life crisis in which the imperatives of the third chakra—the overwhelming desire to become master of our own fate—force us to conclude that we have failed in life. We don't master ourselves so thoroughly we decide. We don't become the great persons we set out to be. Thus very often we feel bitterness and grief which becomes locked in the third chakra.

The healing of third chakra depends upon our moving upward to the fourth, which beckons us to evolve to a higher point of view, to see life in larger terms, as growth step is a particularly difficult one. Our modern culture urges all of us to be independent, self-sufficient and master of our own fate. Our culture leads us to live according to the first, second and third chakras. Our healing lies in moving upward to the fourth.

It is love that leads us to the fourth chakra.

THE FOURTH CHAKRA (Awakening to Unity)

Known traditionally by its Sanskrit name **ANAHATA meaning** "unstruck", the fourth chakra provides lifeforce to the heart. The name of heart chakra, Anahata means to emit a cosmic sound that is heard beyond the realm of five senses. It is a sound that is "unstruck" meaning it has no origin, yet it exists. Its location is the first thoracic vertebra or the area of the heart. It also provides the energy to the thymus gland, the lungs, the arms and hands. Problems related to the heart chakra manifest as symptoms in these organs and extremities, including heart disease, high blood pressure, asthma and other lung diseases.

The central ethic of the heart is love in all manifestations but most of all as compassion. Compassion means caring for others, which ieads to healing, thus the heart chakra is focused on altruism and improving the lives of one's fellow human beings. Healing begins with the heart, and healers themselves work from this chakra first if they are truly dedicated to helping others.

The heart chakra is the central conduit through which all the chakras express themselves. In this sense the heart chakra is unique but it demonstrates the universal need for love. Thus all forms of healing, all forms of expression, all ideas, all information must be expressed with love and compassion if they are to do another person any long term good. The heart chakra is therefore considered the matrix through which all the other chakras must express themselves.

When a person's consciousness progresses from the third chakra to the fourth he or she very often confronts some crisis in life. The reason is that the heart chakra, as I will explain shortly brings about the most dramatic change in consciousness.

In Ayurvedic medicine the heart chakra is associated with air element and the principle to touch. It is symbolised by the black antelope, an animal known for its speed, lightness of being and gentleness. Healing touch is done from the heart chakra.

From the heart chakra comes ability to see the unity among people, indeed, the life we all have in common. Everything that is understood in its unity and in collective terms comes from the heart chakra.

The heart chakra unites people in the mystery of love. I say it is a mystery because love has an indefinable power to unify one person with another, to unify a family, a community, to embrace humanity as a whole. As love grows, its circle widens so that the unity of life is experienced ever more deeply.

THE FIFTH CHAKRA (The World of Sound and Hearing)

The fifth chakra referred to **"VISUDDHA"** or pure is located over the throat at the third cervical vertebra which provides lifeforce to the thyroid and parathyroid glands as well as to the larynx, neck, shoulders, arms, hands and ears. It is associated with the speech centre and with hearing. Problems related to fifth chakra include disorders of thyroids and parathyroids, glands, stiff neck, hearing impairment, colds, sore throat. tonsillitis and all voice-related disorders.

The fifth chakra is the realm of communication. All forms of expression are under the influence of fifth chakra. So too is the sharing and synthesizing of ideas.

The fifth chakra is the transition into the world of ideas, symbols and communication. The first three chakras are concerned with material existence and individuality. The fourth chakra represents a transition point into the higher realms, a doorway into the world of spirit. From the fifth through the seventh chakras the level of consciousness becomes increasingly focused on the matters of spirit and immaterial existence. Consequently the consciousness in the upper three chakras becomes more and more rarefied, more subtle and spiritual in nature.

Like the first and third chakras, the fifth represents a turning inward from the more altruistic and outgoing heart centre. At the fifth chakra, the person moves into the inner world of energy, sound and light; because words and ideas illuminate the darkness that is ignorance and show us the way to resolution of conflicts and reconciliation with one another. The fifth chakra is associated with the elements which according to Ayurvedic medicine, is the vessel in which all elements mix. The colour associated with the fifth chakra is blue and its principal concerns are sound, hearing and communication. The animal that symbolizes this chakra is the moon-white elephant.

The consciousness of the lower three chakras is essentially dualistic, in that they make a clear distinction between you and me. They also tend to define people and situations as either good or bad. There is not much gray in situations, nor is there much overlap in the recognition of people's needs. Consequently there is not much understanding, but once we enter the fourth chakra, our communication through the fifth becomes increasingly universal. Our words take on greater magnitude because they unite people in understanding and in love. People are no longer seen as necessarily good or bad but as humans struggling to avoid and find happiness.

The word **VISUDDHA** or pure indicates that the ideas and values native to the fifth chakra are pure and perfect and those who reach the fifth chakra are able to express the purity and perfection of spiritual ideals.

RELATIONSHIP BETWEEN FOURTH AND FIFTH CHAKRAS

The fifth chakra represents a new level of detachment unknown to the fourth. The heart chakra is still very much attached to the material plane. In that it cares very deeply for other people and the life we all share. At the fifth chakra one understands the impermanence of material life and can see clearly where permanence and infinite truths really lie. The fifth chakra represents the kind of detachment spoken of in Buddhism in which the world is recognised as **Maya** or illusion. Hence crossing over from the fourth to the fifth chakra requires a further letting go of this impermanent world for the eternal world of spirit.

THE SIXTH CHAKRA (The World of Wisdom and Forms)

Known by its Sanskrit name **AJNA** meaning "command", the sixth chakra is located over the forehead slightly above the eyebrows between the eyes. The sixth chakra provides lifeforce to the eyes, much of the control nervous system and the brain. It also funnels energy to the pituitary and pineal glands, both endocrine organs located in the middle of the brain. These two glands work in harmony to support the individual and unified functions of the sixth and seventh chakras.

Most of the authorities say that the sixth chakra is associated with the pituitary gland, which is the master gland of the endocrine system. It controls virtually all endocrine functions and thereby influences the entire body both in its everyday operations and in the body's growth and development.

The sixth chakra is said to control various states of concentration and consciousness. This is the realm of omniscience. Whenever someone breaks through to this level of consciousness, extra-sensory perception, clairvoyance, visions, psychokinesis and other paranormal experiences occur. The sixth chakra is associated with the colour indigo. The chakra is symbolised by OM, the cosmic sound. Om represents the alpha and the omega, the beginning and the end of all things. There are no elements associated with the sixth chakra, since it is beyond the material existence. It is the world of cosmic law, harmony, perfect order and vibration. Thus the sixth chakra is the world of perfect knowing, the world of wisdom.

THE SEVENTH CHAKRA (Oneness)

The seventh or crown chakra is referred to in Sanskrit as **"SAHASRA"** meaning "thousand" or lotus of thousand petals. It is located at the back of the head slightly above the crown. Some maintain that it is actually however, above the head at this spot.

This chakra nourishes the cerebral cortex and much of the central nervous system. Its primary function is to unify understanding and integrate all ideas and states of consciousness. The crown chakra is responsible for synchronizing all the human senses and faculties and thus making the world coherent. Malfunctions that occur in the crown chakra manifest as depression, alienation and the inability to learn or comprehend ideas, situation and people.

The crown chakra is the transcendental state beyond consciousness, what the Buddhists call the Void and the Hindus call the Brahman. It is the ultimate oneness, the state beyond description.

The seventh chakra is associated with pineal gland, an endocrine organ that serves to maintain mood among other things. Indeed many believed that the pineal gland was so called third eye or the eye of intuition. Remarkably, the pineal is in fact highly sensitive to light. When deprived of light such as in winter, the pineal gland secretes abundant quantities of a hormone called Melatonin which consumes the chemical neurotransmitter Serotonin. The brain uses serotonin to help great feelings of well-being, positive thoughts and to enhance its ability to concentrate. It is also the chemical basis for deep and restful sleep.

When pineal gland is deprived of adequate sunlight it produces more melatonin, which in turn depresses serotonin levels. This results in a widely suffered disorder called seasonal affective disorder (SAD). SAD is exactly a disorder in which people feel depressed, fatigued and withdrawn. Most people who experience SAD suffer it in winter or when they are deprived of natural lighting for extensive periods. The cure is simply to increase one's exposure to sunlight or full spectrum lighting. This causes the pineal to produce less melatonin which makes serotonin levels rise and results in increased feelings of well-being, positive emotions, better sleep and the removal of depression.

The colour associated with the crown chakra is violet although many eastern Indian traditions maintain that there is no colour associated with crown chakra. The chakra represents the ocean of life to which we all return. It is the ultimate and indefinable state of love and bliss.

THE ENERGY SPIRAL (Harmonising High and Low — Heaven and Earth)

My experience has taught me that the system of Chinese acupuncture is absolutely correct in its assessment that life energy "Ki" flows in channels or what the Chinese refer to as Meridians, does more than that. Energy also flows in spirals or eddies especially in primary and secondary chakras. In addition, lifeforce weaves among the seven chakras, connecting and unifying them into a fully integrated whole.

As I have described earlier, each chakra provides a concentrated flow of lifeforce to a specific part of the body. It also represents a particular type of consciousness that must be integrated into our being. Were it not for the spiral energy, there would have been seven major sub-divisions of consciousness operations in opposite to each other, much like seven heads of state running the same country. The net effect especially on the physical and mental levels, would be chaos. Thus the spiral of energy unifies the physical, psychological and spiritual functions of the seven chakras and thus creates integration.

The spiral energy has the distinct pattern, like a single line of threat that holds seven buttons in a place on a shirt. The line itself begins at the heart chakra emanating out of the heart and turning down into the solar plexus or third chakra. There it re-enters the body and exists at back, where it loops upward and re-enters the back of the throat or throat chakra. From the fifth chakra or throat the energy moves out of the front of the body and loops downward into the second chakra located in the area of the large intestine and sex organs. From there it exits, moves upward in a semi-circle and re-enters the body at the back of the head of the sixth chakra or third eye. From the third eye the energy leaves through the front of the body and turns downward again in a large semi-circle, so that it enters the body of the root chakra or at the base of pelvis. From the pelvis the energy arcs upwards to the crown chakra located at the top of the head and within the crown chakra lies all the knowledge and life plan of the soul. Thus the movement of energy through the chakra system is 4, 3, 5, 2, 6, 1 and 7.

Traditional people believed that the soul's journey on earth is already mapped out and that knowledge of one's life plan lies within each of us. Our challenge is to know ourselves and thus truly to understand why we are here on earth.

HEADACHES (When the Cause is not just in the Head)

One of my clients, forty-five years old housewife and mother of two, suffered from regular headaches, migraines, overweight, and severe premenstrual syndrome (PMS) that included nausea and night sweats.

One of the first thing I noticed while examining her was that the energy around her second chakra located over the lower abdomen and responsible for providing lifeforce to the sex organs, kidneys, bladder, large intestine and adrenal glands felt irregular as if the chakra did not have an integrated consistency. I felt clearly that this part of her field was swollen. While other areas were weak or even withdrawn as if there was a gaping hold in the field, I continued my work on her. I kept getting the image of an open wound over the area of the second chakra which corresponded with the physical problems as she was having in her sex organs and adrenal glands. Even more telling was the fact that this part of her field seemed to me even more irregular and swollen whenever she had headaches.

From an energetic point of view, this made perfect sense, since the second and the sixth chakras are related through the spiral of energy. Clearly, the source of her headaches was the imbalance in the area of her second chakra.

I worked on her second and sixth chakras. First, I sent energy to the second chakra and then closed the wound by moving my hands in a very gentle pattern, as if I were literally bringing together tissues that had been torn apart. Then I turned my attention to the sixth chakra, which was congested and blocked. Here I drew energy away from the chakra, opened it up, and increased the circulation within this part of the field.

After a few months of treatment, the wound in the abdomen seemed to be less swollen and started to heal. At the sametime her headaches and perimenopausal symptoms had been clearly relieved.

It was not until the tenth month of treatment that she began to loose weight—now without effort. This happy circumstance coincided with what she experienced as a dramatic shift in her consciousness. She reported feeling better, was able to express her needs. She had always had great difficulty in asking for emotional or psychological support. She was a big giver, thinking as if she was loving and supportive of others and that same love and support would come back to her.

THE CHAKRAS

Chakra -1 Root Chakra

Location :	—	Base of spine, perineum
Glands :	—	Adrenals
Organs :	—	Legs, feet, bones, large intestine
Function:	—	Survival, grounding, life promoting vital physical energy
Malfunctions:	—	Constipation, haemorrhoids, obesity, sciatica arthritis, knee trouble, anorexia nervosa

Chakra -2 Splenic or Sacral

Location :	—	Two to three fingers below navel lower abdomen, first lumbar vertebra
Glands :	—	Ovaries, testicles
Organs:	—	Uterus, genitals, kidney, bladder, circulatory system
Functions :	—	Assimilation, life promoting emotions, sexuality, desire and pleasure
Malfunctions.:	—	Kidney/bladder trouble, female and male organic and emotional-sexual problems, lower back problems

Chakra-3 Solar Plexus

Location :	—	Eighth thoracic vertebra, just blow notch where ribs come together to form Xyphoid process to navel
Glands :	—	Pancreas, adrenals
Functions :	—	Will power, personal power, taking in of energy from outside of self, growth, healing
Malfunctions :	—	Digestive trouble, ulcers, diabetes hypoglycemia, liver disorder, fat metabolism

Chakra -4 Heart

Location :	—	First thoracic vertebra, heart
Gland :	—	Thymus
Organs:	—	Heart, lungs, arms, hands
Functions:	—	Self love, love toward others, taking in life nourishment in general, mental energy consciousness, healing
Malfunctions :	—	Heart disease (including high blood pressure) asthma and lung diseases

Chakra-5 Throat

Location :	—	Third cervical vertebra
Glands :	—	Thyroid and parathyroid
Organs:	—	Neck, shoulders, arms, hands, ears
Function :	—	Communication expressive energy volition, will (discernment and power of choosing) synthesizing of symbols into ideals
Malfunction :	—	Thyroid problems, hearing problems stiff neck, colds, sore throats

Chakra-6 Brow or Ajna

Location :	—	First cervical vertebra in back (space between and slightly above eyes on forehead)
Gland :	—	Pituitary (working in harmony with pineal)
Organ:	—	Eyes
Functions :	—	Seeing, intuition, synthesizing
Malfunctions :	—	Headache, vision problems, nightmares,

Chakra – 7 Crown

Location :	—	Top of head and slightly back where soft spot of baby's head is located
Gland :	—	Pineal (working in harmony with pituitary)
Organs :	—	Cerebral cortex, central nervous system
Functions :	—	Integration and understanding
Malfunctions :	—	Depression, alienation, inability to learn or comprehend

As known of anatomy and physiology of the chakras, their relationship to the physical body is also essential in the practice of healing touch. The chakras offer the healer a set of portals into the body, mind and spirit of the person on whom we are working. These portals are the concentration of life energy. Within the chakras are the roots of many old wounds, blockages and patterns that must be released if healing is to occur. Thus the chakras offer the healer not only insights into the person's past but great opportunity to assist the person's rebirth.

EXERCISE — THE CHAKRA SPIRAL (Refer the Chakra diagram)

1. Envision a beam of rainbow light coming out of your heart in an arc and entering your solar plexus.

2. See the light passing through the solar plexus out of the back, curve upward and enter the body at the back of the throat.

3. See it passing through the throat and move downward into the second or sacral chakra.

4. Envision the light passing through the body of the second chakra, exit the back and turn upward and re-enter the body at the back of the head at the third eye or sixth chakra.

5. Through the front of the third eye see the beam of light move downward and enter the body at first or root chakra.

6. Visualise the light passing through the root chakra, exiting the back, arching upward and re-entering the body at the crown chakra.

7. From the crown chakra see the light moving down through the centre of the body to the bottom of the feet.

8. Once the arc touches the bottom of the feet, envision your entire field being lit up by the rainbow light so that the field is radiant with colour and light.

9. From the feet send an arc of light to the earth.

10. From the earth, see the light re-enter your body in the feet and turn upward, exiting the crown chakra and returning to the source of light and life.

11. Feel the rainbow light fill up every cell, tissue and organ of your body with radiant light, each organ absorbs the colour of energy that it needs for health and vitality.

12. When you feel full of light and life, open your eyes and let your light shine. If you become fatigued or imbalanced at anytime of the day you need only breathe in this radiant light to be restored.

If you tape these meditations with your own voice and play the tape to guide you through these meditations, your healing will be more profound.

Fig. 8. Rainbow Transfer Disk

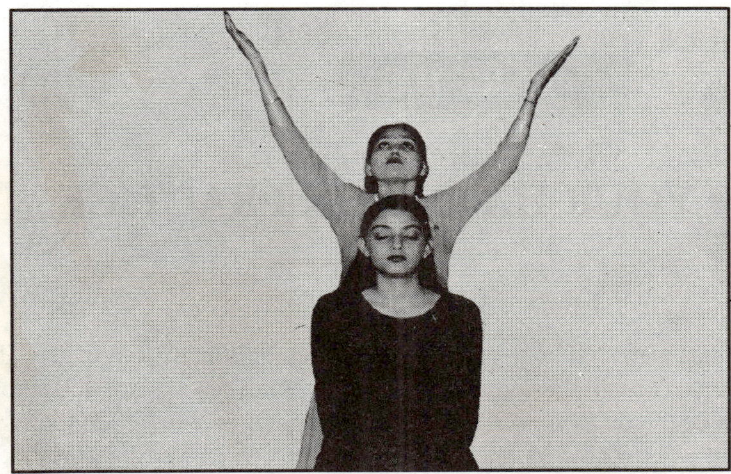

a

Position a, b showing the
positions of rainbow light
bringing on the body

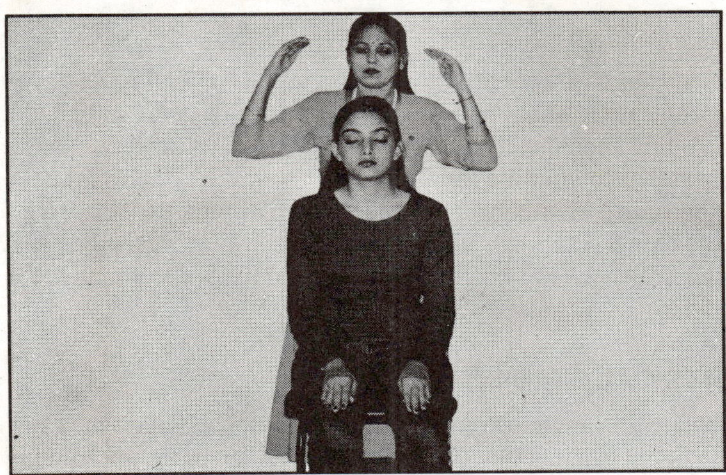

b

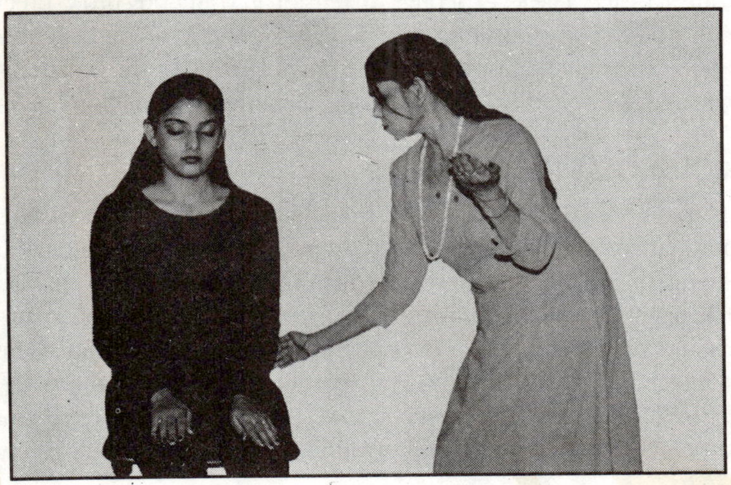

Position showing treatment on
back of Hara Chakra

PART II

11. KEEP YOUR HANDS ON PRACTICE

CENTRING YOURSELF

Centring yourself in essence, means to shift your consciousness from instability of everyday life to the quiet colour of your own spiritual core. In the centre of your inner being lies a peace and stability that can't be shaken by events outside of you as your consciousness becomes ever more founded upon this inner spiritual base, where you will become more emotionally stable and powerful in balanced ways.

THE VITAL CENTRE

To centre yourself, by contrast, means to anchor your awareness in the spiritual roots of your life. To be centred in your spiritual roots means to shift your consciousness from daily life tumult to the centre of your soul, the place within you that continually draws life energy from its universal source. Here at your vital centre is the place from which your life truly springs.

Life itself is energy and the source of energy is the one, the great spirit, the Tao. To attune your consciousness to the centre of being is to align yourself with the will of the universe and to be nourished by its never ending flow of life energy. (I will offer several methods of meditations to help you achieve a centred state shortly).

MENTAL PEACE AND PHYSICAL STABILITY

The effects of such a shift in awareness are transformative in every respect. Rather than being tossed around by the external travails of ephemeral world, you are now grounded in the unchanging world of universal lifeforce. Hence you are at peace. The level of physical tension in your body drops precipitously. Scientific research has shown that people in meditation exhibit high degrees of alertness, concentration and synchronicity between the left and right hemispheres of the brain. Heart rate and breathing patterns slow, blood pressure stabilises, and skin conductivity decreases, a sign that circulation has improved.

CULTURAL AND RELIGIOUS TRADITIONS

Various cultures and religious traditions have developed for reaching understandings of what it truly means to be centred. The entire Japanese culture is founded upon the ethic that all behaviour should flow from the vital centre of being, or what the Japanese called HARA. Perhaps for this reason, centring makes you acutely aware of yourself as a whole human being — that is you become aware of your physical body, your emotions and your spiritual consciousness as an integrated totality. Centring is a meditative act and an act of integration and harmony. Perhaps because centre is the place of such "infinite mysteries", we recognise that, from here, all that is sacred springs into the material world. Thus to centre oneself means to approach the sacred or divine within.

Centring therefore is a meditative act that transforms you physically, psychologically and spiritually. The practitioner of healing touch begins a session by centring himself / herself. In this way he/she places himself/herself in right relationship with the universal energy and thus attains the right stand point for participating in the flow of that energy.

THE INSTRUMENT OF DIVINE SOURCE

This is the mental framework that the practitioner of healing touch attempts to achieve. When you are centred you have no judgements about the person you are working with nor any attachment to the outcome. You are not the source of healing. You are not in control of what takes place. The energy flows from the divine source through you and to the recipient of healing touch. You as a practitioner of healing touch, submit yourself as an instrument to that divine source, whatever be the outcome for the client in between the Creator of the universe and the recipient. In a way, you as the practitioner are a witness to the outcome.

ATTITUDES AND DEVOTIONS

Thus the most important attitudes that the practitioner must maintain towards a client as well as towards himself or herself are compassion, love, honesty (especially within himself/herself) and humility. This is how the practitioner of healing touch confronts the sacred drama, that he or she is witnessing and assisting.

This also implies as to why it is so important to begin every session of healing touch by centring yourself. By centring yourself in your own spiritual roots, you are not so easily distracted by anyone's emotions or desires or even by the explicit needs of the client. Rather you are respectful to the client and his or her relationship with the Creator. Once you are centred, you come into communion with the source of the energy that truly heals. Whatever that energy then desires to happen, will happen effortlessly.

GROUNDING IS THE CLEAREST CHANNEL (Of your being present)

DEALING WITH THE POWERS

Once you have centred yourself, of course, you must firmly maintain your centre through the course of your healing touch session. To do that you must sustain your concentration and be fully present with your client. You can't suddenly drift off in your mind and begin to think about the many demands in your own life. Such wandering of thoughts will affect the flow of energy that is travelling through you to your client, and thus make the session less effective. Also the more you wander, the more you diminish the sense of sacred. The client's sacred awareness is the part of what allows him or her to accept the life energy that is being offered. The best way for you to sincerely invoke the sacred is through your own centredness and concentration.

Most forms of the ceremony ring false and ultimately cast you in the wrong light. You are a professional practitioner who must maintain his or her professional standpoint. You are dealing with powers far beyond your comprehension and therefore must be respectful to the true source of healing energy which you transmit.

As I pointed out earlier the best and perhaps the only way to strike the right balance between your earthly role and your heavenly ideals is to remain centred and focused. In the centre all paradoxes are reconciled and the sense of the sacred is invoked without your doing anything. In order to keep myself focused and centred I do a visualisation before the session and recite a prayer during the process. Therefore before you conduct your healing touch session do the following:—

First place your feet apart firmly on the floor. Feel the energy in your legs and feet anchored itself on the floor. Visualise it going deeply into the earth so that the earth holds you in its embrace. Feel yourself being supported by the earth and nourished by the energy that flows upward from the great Mother. At the same time, feel the upper levels of your own energy reach up into the heavens, just as the limbs of a tree reach into the sky. Feel the love of the heaven showering down on the limbs of your field and surround and envelop you. See the love and energy come up from the earth and mingle with that of the heavens. Visualise that energy channelling itself into your entire body and down into your arms and hands, see it flowing from your hands. You now have the healing energy to channel to your client.

Before I turn to my client, however I recite a prayer; over and over again throughout the healing session to remain focused on the work. I share this prayer for adopting it yourself. The prayer is as follows:—

"Father, Mother, God, I place myself and this patient in your Holy light for the highest good of all. I ask that you work through me to bring healing to this patient. I ask that thy well be done, and I am grateful for this healing."

Finally as you do your energy work on your client, visualise the darkness, boulders and blockages that are being released from your client's field as being absorbed into the light and love of the heavens or earth. The earth takes these energetic blockage stones and old patterns and dissolves them into the soil, transforming them into elements that support life and renew growth.

Be sure to do the egg meditation, given in the book, before you begin to work with your client. This will protect you from the energetic imbalances and illness which your client may be suffering from.

KNOW HOW YOU SHOULD FEEL BEFORE YOU PROCEED (The Self-feelings)

Your centring and grounding meditation will put you in touch with your emotions and physical body. You will know how you feel and if you allow your emotions to fully surface, you will know why you have such feelings. Do not resist or repress such emotions, or the event that surrounds them, but rather embrace and honour these feelings. No matter what surface, whether it is anger, shame or humiliation or conflict, try to examine the feelings and have compassion for yourself. Such emotions and the events that triggered them — are part of what it means to be human. With continued meditation, you will be able to integrate these and other feelings. You will be able to see the courage you had to have to go through such events. In time, you will be able to honour yourself in ways that perhaps you can't do now. You will also become more proficient at opening your heart and entering into a consciousness of non-judgement and acceptance.

However, if you cannot reconcile these emotions in the moment or create peace within yourself, you are better off avoiding the day's healing touch sessions. Powerful emotions especially anger or hatred are inappropriate to a healing touch session. There is a good chance that you will transmit such vibrations to your client or you may not be able to maintain your concentration and groundedness to protect yourself from your client's energy or illness. You are better avoiding the whole interaction and postponing it to another day. In the meantime, work on yourself. The greatest demands made on a practitioner of healing touch are those the practitioner makes of himself or herself. He or she must be attached to the outcome. The practitioner must become more centred in the spiritual roots of his or her being and thus clearer about who, he or she is and what the client is and who the healer is.

BEING CENTRED MEANS RESPECTING YOUR LIMITS
(Restoring the Health and Happiness)

As a practitioner of healing touch, you are performing an invaluable service to your client, to the healing arts and to the world at large. You are providing your client with an enormous boost of healing energy — the energy that is essential for the client's restoration and recovery. By offering this service you are giving people a new tool to restore health and happiness as well as new approach to understanding, health, illness and indeed the life itself. Finally you are serving as an instrument of love and healing, something in very short supply in our world today.

PROMOTING THE LIFEFORCE

Yet despite this incredibly important role, many practitioners of healing touch nevertheless feel they must be more and in the process make the mistake of overstepping their own boundries and the clients'. You must always keep in mind the scope of your practice in order to be effective in your job as a healer. Always remember that your central function is to serve as a conduit for healing energy. You promote the flow of the lifeforce in other people, whatever your client does with that energy is between him or her and God. The person already knows, what he or she needs to be healed though this knowledge may not be conscious.

Nevertheless, you must release the client into the hands of the universal healer in order to do the most good. You are not responsible for the client's recovery any more than you are responsible for the client's disharmony or disease. You are assisting the client in her or his journey through life and specifically, in her or his attempts to get well. You are the helper—the server, the practitioner of a powerful healing tool. You do not have to diagnose or provide insight into the person's past disharmonies. You do not have to be a psychotherapist or a medical doctor or a nurse; these are not your professions.

JUDGEMENT WITH REAL EXPERIENCE

People will want you to be more at times. Indeed you will be tempted to be more in part, because the practice requires so much faith, especially in the beginning when you lack experience and have not seen the incredible effects you can have on people just by doing this seemingly simple job. This lack of experience may tempt you to fill the knowledge gap with promises or speculations. Resist these temptations with all your strength. Indeed become both a practitioner and an investigator of this practice. See for yourself what it can do. Fill up your life and practice with real experience. Come to know exactly how the practice affects other people, how it changes lives and restores health. When you do this, your words will be based on what is true and real, rather than on what you think and have read. The practice works but you must experience it working before you know in your heart that it works. Let yourself have that experience.

Follow these three rules and you will be safe in all situations.

THE THREE RULES

1. Be honest with yourself, when you don't know something, admit it to yourself. Embracing your humanness is one of the most wonderful and trasformative experiences you will ever have. The more you can do this simple act the more you stand in the light of truth. The greater your own transformation, the more powerful you become.

2. Be honest with your client, don't be trapped into inflating your role or your knowledge or your ego, even if it means making the client uncomfortable temporarily. People naturally want reassurance and you will want to give it but sometimes that mutual desire can lure you into implying things or promising things that you can't be certain of. It is better to say, "I don't know" than to offer people promises that later may turn out to be false or illusory. You are centered and powerful, whenever you speak, speak the truth, even if the truth is merely admitting your limitations.

3. Respect yourself—you are taking up a role that, in other culture and traditions was among the most revered and honoured functions in human society. Today all practitioners of the holistic healing are pioneers, offering people powerful tools for establishing health. We are bringing back to the modern world the keys to health that temporarily have been forgotten. Slowly but inexorably holistic healing is being restored to the place that was once the natural place for herbalists, acupuncturists, practitioners of Chinese medicine, Ayurveda, bodyworkers and practitioners of healing touch. As long as you are clear about your practice and what you do, you are performing an essential service that is not being duplicated by any other profession. You belong to the healing art and you do not have to be any more than what you are. As you gain experience in this practice, you will learn firsthand that this is quite enough.

MEDITATION FOR CENTRING
MEDITATION—I

Sit in a chair with your back straight and your feet flat on the floor, hands resting on your knees. Relax. Take in a deep breath and begin an easy exhale making an *aaahh* sound with your voice box . After a few seconds (two or three) suspend the noise and exhale without closing the throat. The throat should feel open as it did when you made the *aaahh* sound. After a few seconds let the breath exhale. Repeat this two times. You should notice by the third time that you are able to hold your breath longer than earlier. When you open your eyes, the room should appear brighter, you are centred and probably in an alpha brain wave state.

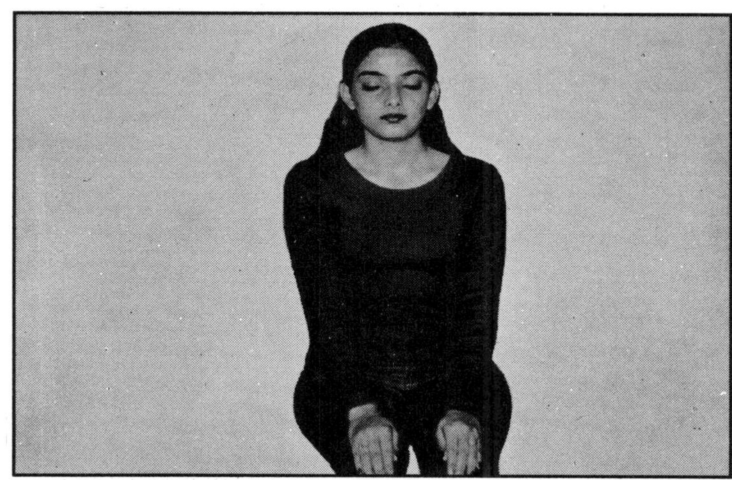

Position showing sitting in a chair with back straight and feet flat, resting hands on knees.

MEDITATION-2 (The Egg Meditation)

1. Sit on a comfortable chair with your feet flat on the floor and hands on your knees.
2. Take a few deep even breaths and then begin to breathe rhythmically, concentrate on your breath, watch the breath.
3. Meanwhile, let go all thoughts, if any thought enters your mind. Watch it float into and out of your consciousness. Feel your consciousness enter more deeply into your body.

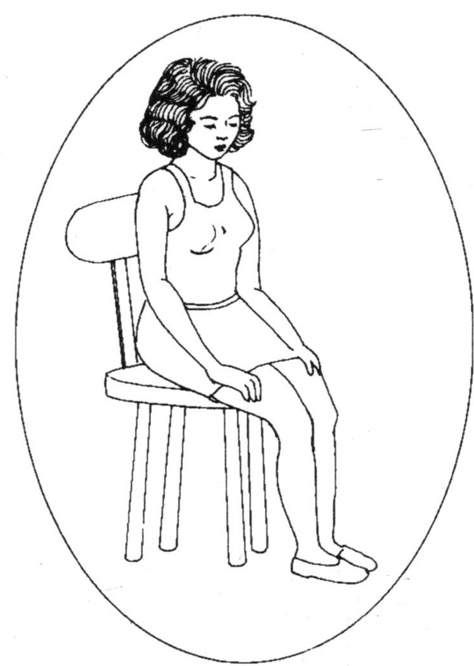

Fig. 9 Egg Meditation.

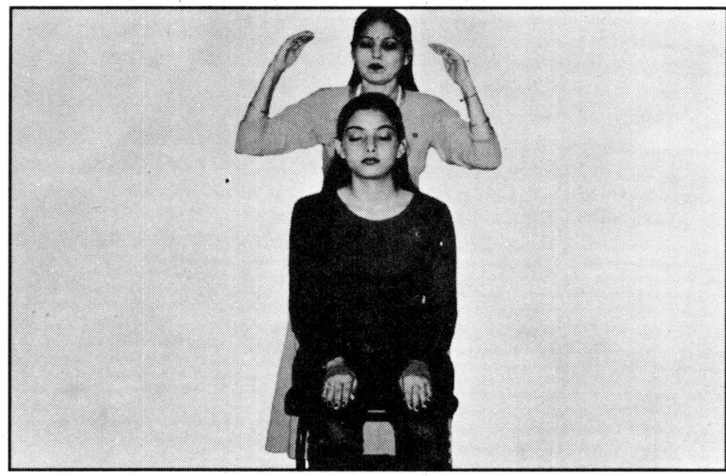

Sitting comfortable with feet flat on floor and hands on knees.

4.   Picture yourself enclosed in an egg shaped bubble that surrounds you at a distance of about an arm's length. Feel the outer edge as kind of a strong, semi-permeable membrane, something like a plexiglass shield that allows only positive, loving energy to escape your inner being and the bubble. The bubble only allows such loving supportive and positive energy to enter the bubble and embrace you as well.
5.   Balance the front and back of bubble or egg so that the energy feels equal on all sides. This balances the output of energy between the front and back chakras.
6.   Maintain a steady, slow, rhythmic breath noting any places in your body where you are holding tension. Breathe into that tension and release it.
7.   Notice your posture, maintain your centredness and an erect posture with your breath.
8.   See the protective energetic shield as a force of invulnerable love. It is designed to protect you while it allows you to help others.

PRESERVING THE INTEGRITY

This meditation is not designed to place boundaries between you and your client or between you and the world. Rather it is designed to maintain the integrity of your own energetic field to close any leaks and to allow you to focus the healing energy that you are channelling in your work. The egg meditation is designed to create a powerful sphere around you so that you will be protected from your client's energetic imbalances, disharmonies, and any illness the client may be suffering from. This bubble is composed of your loving energy and thus vibrates at the rate that is not conductive to your client disharmony or imbalance. Anything your clients shed or release during the session therefore, will not be able to attach itself to you.

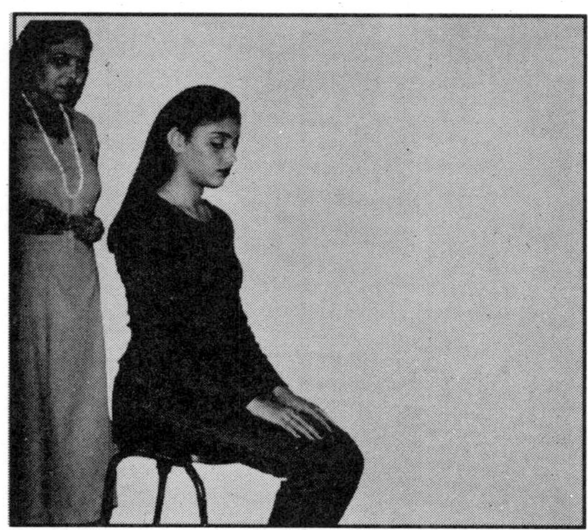

Sitting peacefully in chair wih back straight and feet flat on floor.

MEDITATION-3

In his Book *"Awaken Healing Energy Through The Tao"*, Korean healer and teacher Mantah Chia provides a meditation which teaches us to circulate the "KI" throughout the body. This meditation will help each of us as a practitioner to restore our own health and maintain balance and harmony. Once again the responsibility of the practitioner — especially one who works with transmission of energy — is to keep his or her own field clean and health strong.

PRACTISING THE STEPS

Sit in a quite peaceful room on a comfortable chair, with your back straight and your feet flat on the floor. Rub your hands, feet, arms and legs with your hands. Rotate your neck, place both your hands on lower abdomen with your right hand on top of your left. Your eyes can be open or closed, though closing them will make it easier to visualise during the meditation. Then perform the following steps:—

1. Look down into your body and smile down the front line of the upper part of your body, smile into your eyes, smile to your face, neck, throat, heart, blood and circulatory system, lungs, kidneys, adrenals, liver, pancreas and spleen.

2. Now smile down to the midline of your digestive tract, smile to oesophagus and stomach, swallow your saliva and let it carry the smile down into those organs. Smile down into your small intestine, down into your large intestine, rectum and anus. Continue to swallow saliva and visualise it. Carry your smile downward through your entire digestive tract.

3. Focus on the back of your body, send your smile down the spine vertebra by vertebra.

4. Release your jaws and touch the tongue to the palate.

5. Complete the meditation by collecting the energy of the navel. Spiral the energy inside the navel one and half inches deep.

   Women should spiral the energy thirty six times counter clockwise and 24 times clockwise.

   Men should spiral the energy in the opposite direction 36 times clockwise and 24 times counter clockwise.

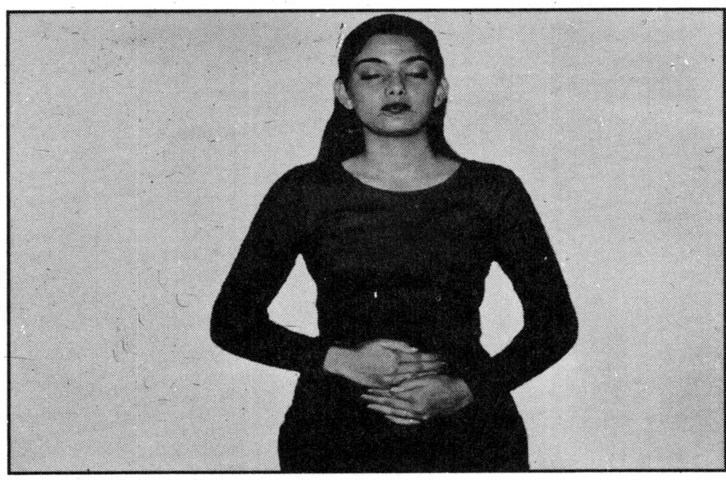

Sitting peacefully in chair with back straight and feet flat on floor

This inner smile will have profound changes on your life if done every day, as it begins to repattern the energy flow through your entire body.

The following meditation is designed to help you to centre and clear your own energy.

MEDITATION-4
(Centring and Clearing)

1   Take some deep breaths, relaxing your mind, letting go of all thoughts and words. Feel the relaxed rhythm of your breath.

2   Picture a small globe of light that is your soul about six-inches above the head. Above that, picture a larger globe of light that is the sun or the source of all living things (light of love).

3   Slowly visualise a beam of light full of all colours of rainbow from the source through your soul into your crown. Feel the crown chakra take the colour that it needs to expand this area. Release what is no longer useful into the light of love.

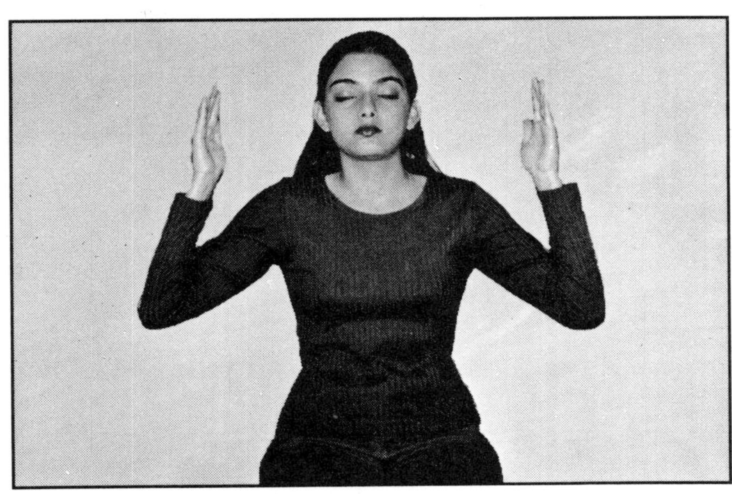

Showing the position of divine light (rainbow) moving down to the human body.

4   Drop the rainbow light into the brow of the third eye, feel the colour that is needed, expand from the rainbow and be released into the chakra. Feel the area expand and release what is no longer needed into the light of love.

5   Let the rainbow light descend into the throat chakra filling it with light, expanding and releasing.

6   Fill the heart space, expanding and releasing.

7   Visualise the light moving into the solar plexus expanding and releasing.

8   Next, visualise the energy moving down into the sacral chakra expanding and releasing.

9   Now fill the root chakra with this light, expanding and releasing.

10   Split the light, seeing it travel down both legs exiting through the arches in the feet going deeply into the earth.

11   Feel the rainbow colours fill you. Feel the peace and balance. Feel the connection with the source as you ground to the earth.

12   When you are ready and it feels right, open your eyes and let your light shine.

All of these techniques will centre you in your spiritual roots. They will also help to balance your energetic field, will open the tube down the centre of the field to allow the free flow of energy through the body and ultimately will help to heal you.

Now let us turn our attention to yet another layer for helping others — specifically using the hands to heal.

12. ENERGY FIELD

ASSESSMENT

Whenever I begin to work at any person, I always spend sometime, trying to understand the client's/patient's specific issues. I always begin with asking the client/patient to fill out an intake questionnaire that describes his or her current symptoms and conditions. The questionnaire requests information on current health complaints, i.e. if any herbs or medication being taken and the main reasons for seeing me and the person is not seeing or consulting a physician or some other health professionals at the time he or she comes to me. Healing touch is meant to complement the work of a physician, not to compete with him. **This is especially important if the person is suffering from a serious illness**.

Once the questionnaire is filled up, I always discuss any health, psychological or interpersonal disharmonies he or she may be experiencing as part of an initial interview. I want to get to know the person, and I will be working within such an intimate and important way. The discussion can involve any aspect of a person's life that is a source of stress, disharmony ranging from a personal health issue to a material or financial problem. In addition to getting to know the person, I also try to figure out where in the field the person's problems may be rooted. As I listen to and observe him or her, I try to discern with chakras or the area within the field which may be involved in the person's disharmony and where I should begin working.

PROBING THE ENERGY FIELD

Once I have some insight into the problem, I assess the energy field. I do all this for my client, even those whom I have been seeing regularly for some time. I begin by having the person sit on a stool, so that all sides of the field and body are exposed. (This will allow you to move your hands through the front and back of the person's field). Also I ask my client to take off his or her shoes before I start the session. This helps to determine whether or not the energy is flowing from the feet. When I assess that part of the field, I stand behind the seated person, centre myself and as I do, I stand with my left hand raised above my head with the palm of my hand facing the sky. My right arm is down at my side, slightly away from my body with my palm facing downward towards the earth. Now I start receiving the lifeforce from the two poles of life, so to speak heaven and earth. While in this position I pray to my God.

When I feel myself deeply centred, I bring my hands together and feel the spongy ball soft, fluffy and resilient — between my hands. It is about the size of a basketball, perhaps a little smaller. I feel the ball in front of me at the level of my vibral core (Fig. 10.) I then move the ball in my hands towards the person's vibral core at his back. After visualising the connection of my vibral core to the patient through the energy ball, I then move to my patient's right side and place my hands about a foot above his head. I dissolve the energy ball into his field

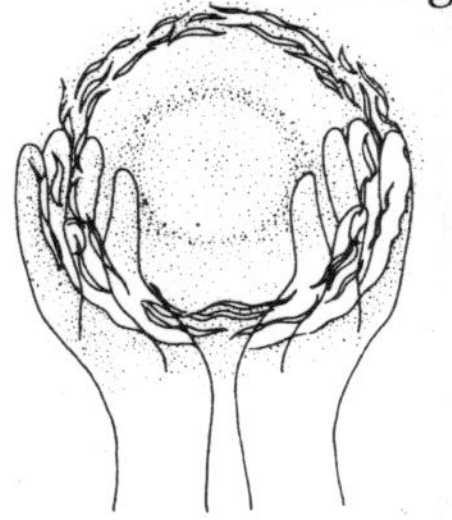

Fig. 10
The Spongy energy Ball

and visualise it enriching his field with lifeforce slowly. I allow my hands to come apart and simultaneously move down the front and back of the patient's field all the time while assessing his energy (Fig. 11). My hands are anywhere from six to eighteen inches from the person's body. Meanwhile, I am always reciting my prayer to remain centred and empty of distracting thoughts.

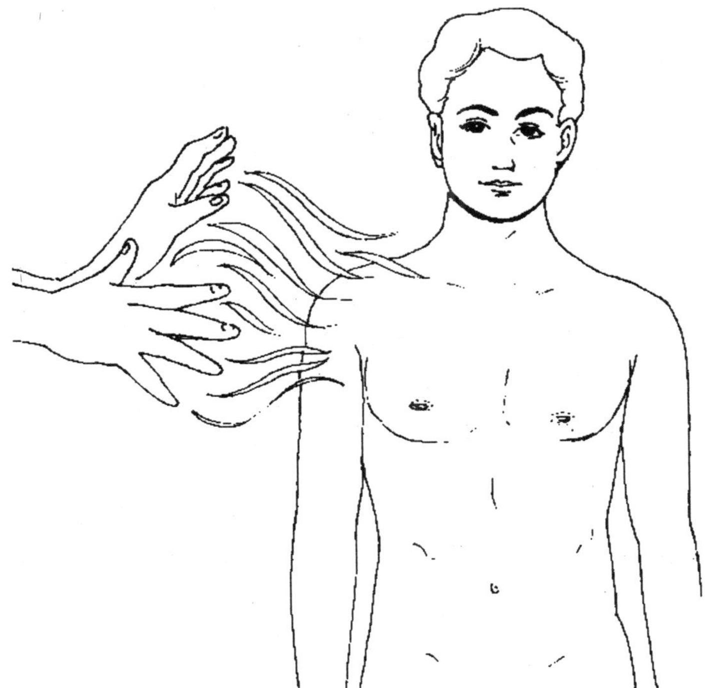

Fig. 11 Transferring of Energy to shoulder from Energy Ball.

WATCHING AND LISTENING BY TOUCH
(The Technique of Assessment)

I assess the field with my hands, but in effect I am touching the field with my entire being. I am so attuned to the energy that I am feeling it with a type of perception that is the synthesis of all my physical perceptions and yet is beyond my physical perceptions. It is as if my physical perceptions and those of my higherself all combine to form a singular intelligence, a unified perception that goes just beyond my everyday senses. Thus as I touch the field, I am listening to it with my hands, I am seeing with my fingers, I am sensing something that might be thought of as smell or taste but goes beyond these as well.

As I conduct my assesment I move my hands downward from the top of the client's head and down the front and back of the body. I run my hands gently over the field in the area of the heart (right hand) and the back of the lung (left hand) over the stomach and kidneys over the lower intestinal tract and to the spine over the front and back of the legs and to the feet. Meanwhile I note any imbalance or deviation from that resilient ball of "cotton candy". I feel how resilient and closed the field feels in most places if there is an egg-shaped energy with a specific boundary area. As I move my hands farther along the periphery of the field, I may begin to perceive aberrations.

TEMPERATURE AND DENSITY CHANGES
(Understanding the Conditions)

The sensation of different places of body is very subtle and resilience changes in temperature are also common, some places may feel cool, some places in the field are warm and occasionally I encounter significant heat. In general you typically do not feel a change in temperature when going over the client's field. However, whenever you do notice a decline in temperature — a relatively cool or cold spot, it can often mean a decrease in energy and may appear over places where there is little lifeforce. Those energy dips may indicate that the particular part of the body was wounded long ago, causing a diminished flow of blood, lymph and lifeforce to that area, thus creating the conditions for disharmony of some kind. The person may not experience the underlying conditions until the disharmony reaches to an acute phase. But long before the physical body experiences the disorder the underlying energetic causes of disharmony would already present.

EXAMPLES OF THE PHENOMENON

Lower back injuries are good examples of this phenomenon. It is quite common for people to experience a low back injury simply by bending down and picking up a newspaper. Hardly a strenuous task. In fact, the condition for injury were there within the back muscles and vertebrae for a long time, sometimes for more than a decade.

These extremes create an acute imbalance in the muscles of the back, manifesting an excessive contraction among certain muscles and excessive weakness in others. Actually the spinal vertebrae are kept in alignment by muscle tension that is essentially equal on the left and right sides of the spine.

However, muscles on one side usually become too contracted and loose their flexibility. They can no longer expand and contract within their normal ranges. Other muscles become excessively weak and thus can no longer support the vertebrae or other muscles, meaning that one side of the back muscles is pulling harder than the other side. Eventually the smallest action — such as picking up a newspaper can cause the contracted muscle to go into spasm and in the process pull the vertebrae to one side of the back, on the other side the weak muscles give way, allowing the spine to curve unnaturally in the direction of concentrated muscle. This causes the spine to force the vertebrae to pinch nerves and is perceived as an acute injury. Once it reaches the acute phase the area becomes inflamed and hot. **Heat is often a sign of increased circulation, inflammation and sometimes fever**.

BINDING BLOCKAGES (Removing the Barriers)

To understand the nature of energetic blockages you must recognise that energy is constantly moving through the field in great channels like a rushing river. As long as the energy is circulating through the field and physical body, there is an abundance of lifeforce flowing to organs, tissues and cells and thus there is health and harmony within the entire system. Disharmony arises when the energy is blocked, your job as a practitioner of healing touch is to remove those blockages and to send additional lifeforce to areas that have been deprived of energy.

Deficiencies in the field can be perceived as the absence of energy and sometimes as a hole or what I refer to as a leak. Holes or leaks arise not just from blockages elsewhere in the field but also from traumas experienced early in life that inflicted wounds on the energetic body.

HOLES IN THE FIELD (The Negative Patterns)

Holes or leaks are energetic patterns within the field that allow energy to escape causing the person to experience a sudden change in emotions, (usally bringing on negative emotions), a loss of energy and a loss of his or her personal integrity. A common symptom of a leak is a negative emotional pattern that is consistent but usually irrational. Leaks trigger feelings of guilt, shame, anger, low self-esteem and personal failure.

EMOTIONAL PATTERNS IN CHILDHOOD

Leaks in the field and their corresponding emotional patterns are established in childhood when parents or guardians teach children how to react to difficult situations that may involve personal responsibility. They are also caused by physical or psychological abuse. Such abuse injures the field, literally causing a tear or rip or hole. We must remember that vebral or physical abuse is an energetic and vibrational act as well as a physical act.

A parent need not strike a child to make the child feel injured. The injury can be accomplished just as effectively and sometimes even more permanently — with a word or a set of words, especially if those words are shouted in anger or rage. Sometimes that is the very reason, the words are said in the first place, though few people would admit it that, they are meant to wound. Effect of such verbal or vibrational attacks on the field are analogous to striking your arm with your fist. If you strike your arm for a certain amount of time, you will cause the capillaries to be broken and your arm will turn black and blue.

If you persist you will eventually break the skin and if you persist still longer you will break the bone. Energetic attacks on one's field are done with the emotional vibration and the intent is embedded in words and attitudes. This vibration causes an actual wound in the field, just as striking your arm causes a physical wound in your flesh. An emotional or psychological wound will leak life energy from the child — and later the adult's field until it is healed.

To some extent a hole in the field is always leaking a relatively small amount of energy even in those situations, when the person is not made to feel inferior or shameful; leaks will continually drain energy and that is why the person who has such leaks will continually drain energy. The person who has such leaks closed even for a short period of time, experiences a sudden increase in energy and overall vitality. Therefore, say that closing leaks is one of the most important functions in the healing touch process.

GUILT (The Wound that Stays Alive)

Guilt and shame are the most common emotions to surface whenever leaks in the field are exposed. Guilt makes you feel that you should have done something that you did not, or that you should not have done something that you did. The implicit belief that gives rise to guilt is that you could have been more than you were, which is a delusion. You can't be more than you are at any given moment. Each situation arises and you meet it with physical, psychological and spiritual resources available in that moment. You can be nothing more nor anything less.

Guilt is a wound in the field that leaks energy. Certain energetic patterns in the field and in the person's behaviour and or thinking, may, keep that wound from healing. As a consequence, each time one meets a situation that resembles the one that caused the original wound, and the same feelings occur.

Guilt and shame in a subtle, yet powerful way cause all of us to loose our sense of integrity, self protection and centredness. Whoever the person is, who has made you feel guilty has managed to open one of these leaky places. Once that happens, you give yourself over to the person's judgement of you, as if he or she had greater hold on truth. Your own personal integrity has broken down, you feel weaker, more assured, energetically ill defined, as if you no longer have a clear sense as to who you are, where from you begin and where you end up. This loss of clarity is due to the breakdown of your own energetic boundary—a boundary that protects you, identifies you, encloses you within it and gives you a feeling of integrity, wholeness and strength.

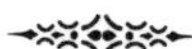

13. CLUES TO GUIDE THE COURSE OF HEALING

TRACING OUT THE IMBALANCES

Once an imbalance is located in the field, no matter of what type it is, I note that area, its nearest chakra and its correspondence to the body. I always look for clues that will reveal the source or sources of the imbalance. If the imbalance is over the heart area, for example, I note the possibility of a disharmony in the heart chakra, the possibility of an emotional issue and perhaps some form of heart disease. If it is over the lower abdomen, I always wonder about the health of the large intestines or sex organs. If it is over the solar plexus, I always wonder about the liver (particularly if the imbalance is on the right side of the body) or the spleen/pancreas, (if it is over the left side of the body) or the stomach, (if it is directly in the centre).

An imbalance over the solar plexus or just below it might also suggest that the stomach and small intestines are in distress. Also keep in mind the spiral energy, which reveals how the energy moves through and nourishes the chakras, i.e. from fourth chakra to the third, then fifth to the second, sixth chakra to the first and then to the seventh chakra. Headaches may be caused by a first or second chakra imbalance (a sixth chakra disorder).

Sore throats (a fifth chakra disorder) may be caused by a third or second chakra imblance. Whenever I encounter a known symptom, I look for the corresponding chakra imbalance. I also examine the chakras directly above and below the disorder. Our looking for any evidence of excessive or deficient energy may cause imbalance in its neighbouring chakra. This is particularly true if the condition is chronic and standard medical treatment fails to cure it.

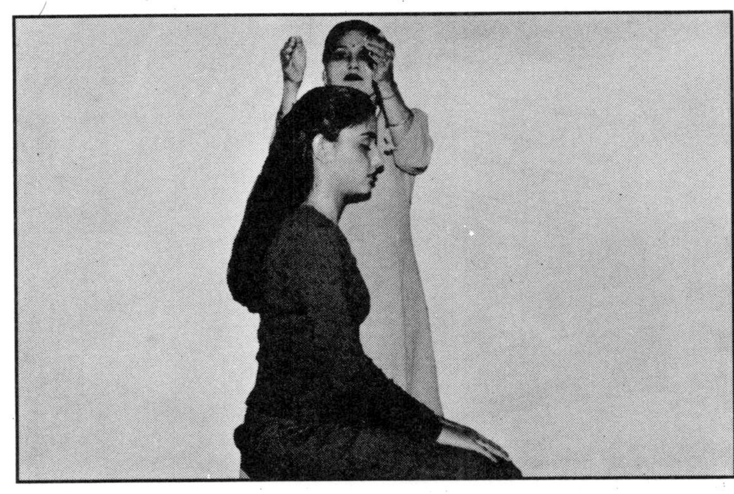

Position showing the bringing of the universal lifeforce to the patient's body.

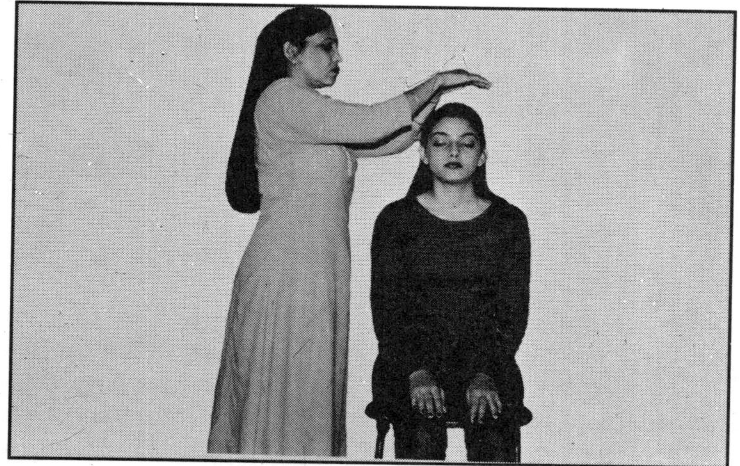

Position showing working of the universal lifeforce on crown chakra.

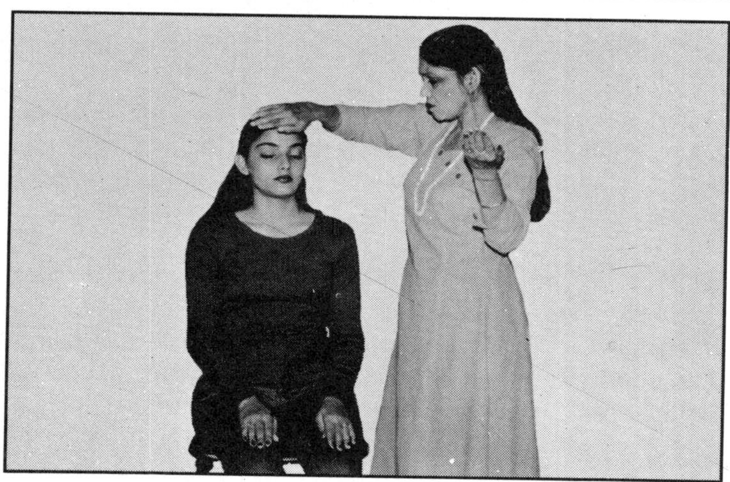

Position showing working of the universal lifeforce on brow chakra.

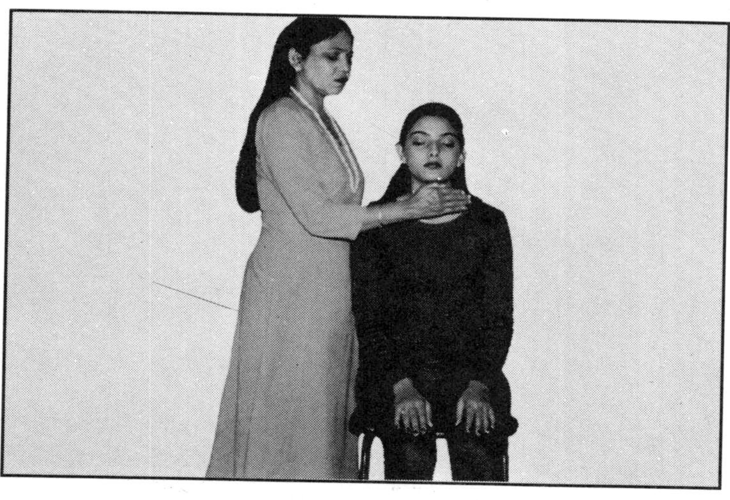

Position showing working of the universal lifeforce on throat chakra.

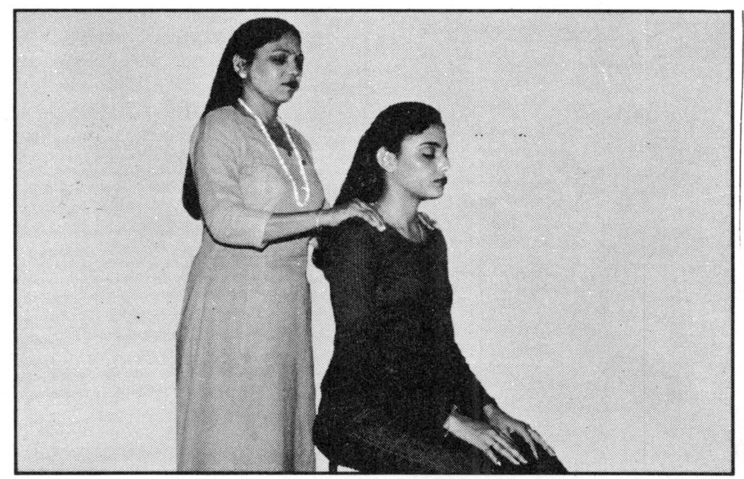

Position showing working of the universal lifeforce on shoulder of the patient.

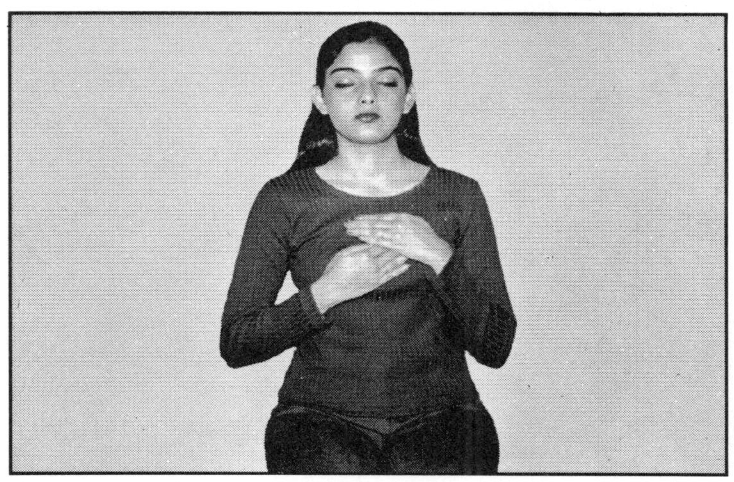

Position showing the working of the universal lifeforce on heart chakra.

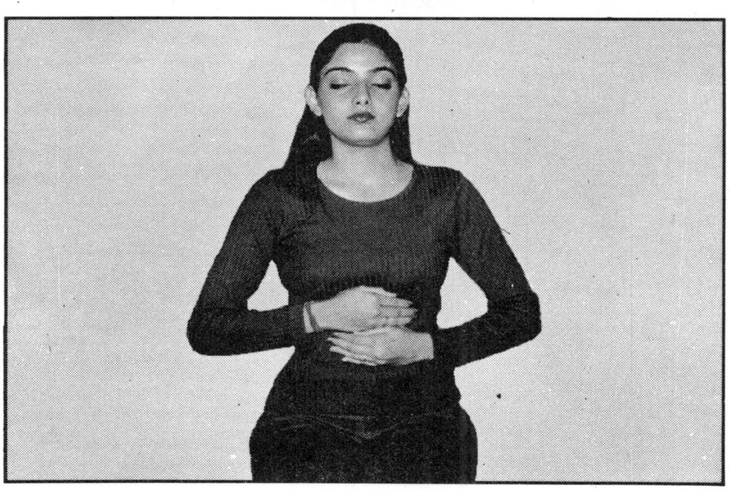

Position showing the working of the universal lifeforce on solar plexus.

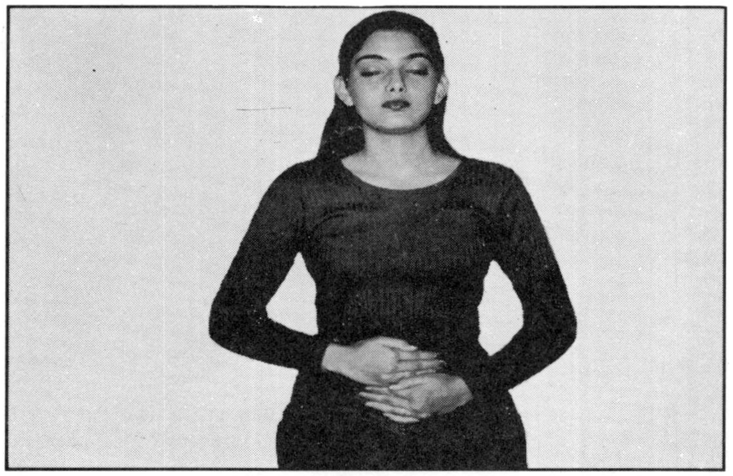

Position showing working of the universal lifeforce on hara chakra.

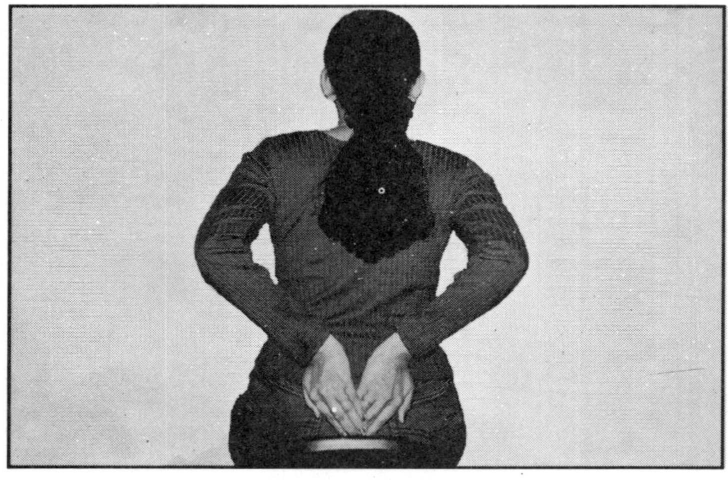

Position showing working of the universal lifeforce on root chakra.

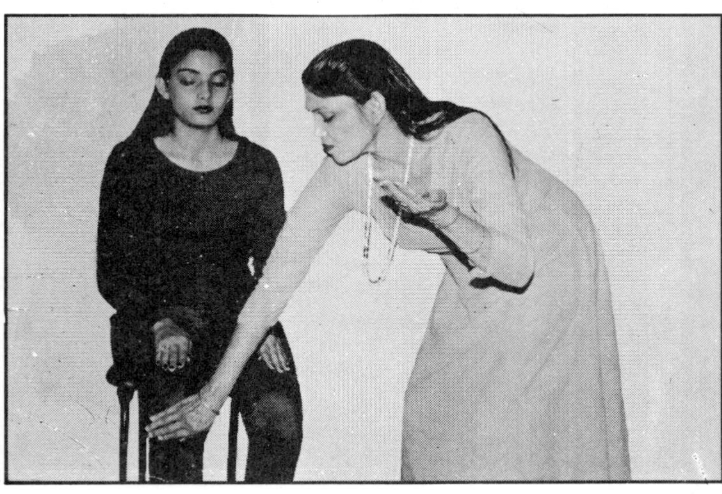

Position showing working of the universal lifeforce on knee chakra (Left).

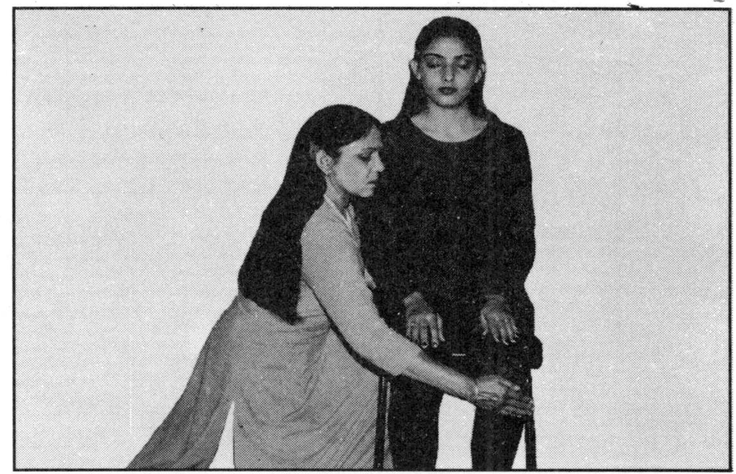

Position showing working of the universal lifeforce on knee charka (right).

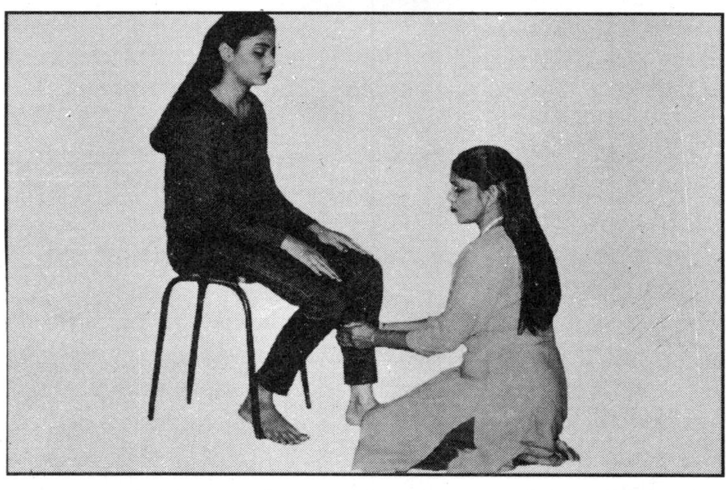

Position showing working of the universal lifeforce on calves.

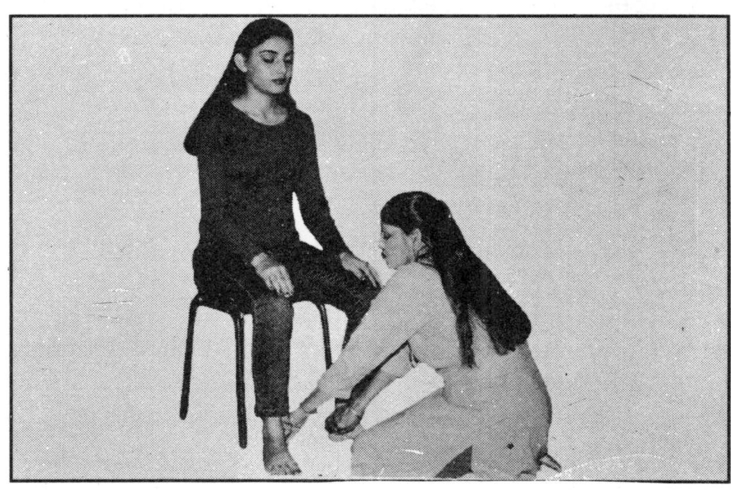

Position showing working of the universal lifeforce on foot chakra.

GROUNDING THE PATIENT
(Opening the Feet)

At the conclusion of assessment process comes a step what I call it as "Opening the Feet", or allowing the energy that is flowing down through the body to exit the feet and unify with the earth. This step provides a deep sense of physical, psychological and spiritual stability to the person on whom you are working. It also allows the energy that is backed up and blocked in the upper part of the body to be released. This step alone often harmonises the entire field and can relieve many painful symptoms in the upper body, especially headaches because it draws the energy down from the upper parts of the body field into the lower parts.

THE TECHNIQUE

Once I have reached the bottoms of the legs in my assessment, I gently massage the muscles and tendons behind the knees, especially the points directly in the centre behind the knees — the site of secondary chakras, you will recall, I massage the site in a slow and consistent fashion. This is the first and sometimes the only time I touch the physical body. After a few minutes of gently massaging the back of the knee, I gradually move down to calf and on to the achilles tendon and then to the bottom of the foot of the same leg massaging deeply, gently and rhythmically. (It is to be worked on each leg and foot individually).

While doing this work I consciously try to pull the energy down from upper part of the body into the lower legs and feet. This massage and pulling of energy centres the person, balances the energy throughout the body and stabilizes the patient's field.

I then attempt to "open the feet" by holding the secondary chakras at the arches of the feet . This will allow the energy that I have brought down into the feet to flow out and make its natural link with the earth thus giving the person a sense of being "grounded" or physically and psychologically stable.

After I have held one foot for a time and feel with my entire being the flow of energy leaving the foot, I perform the same exercise on the other foot and once again ask the recipient to visualise the energy penetrating deeply into the feet from the rest of the body on the inhalation and out of the feet on the exhalation.

When I am sure that energy is flowing through the feet, I resume the first position with my hands over the recipient's head. I then slowly but steadily run my hands over the recipient's field once again to determine how the energy has changed. Each time a healing touch practitioner passes his or her hands through a recipient's field, so as to keep it steady.

In the meanwhile, I forget myself entirely in the process. I am thinking of nothing but my prayer that allows me to be empty. It gives my mind something to be occupied with, while my higher self directs my actions. Now I am ready to work on the field.

ASSOCIATIVE IDEAS
(Ancient Therapies)

The practice of any traditional healing therapy inevitably leads you into an exploration of other ancient practices, which you will find to share many underlying themes. Healing touch is consistent and even shares many of the same principles of other ancient therapies especially of Chinese medicine.

ASSOCIATION OF ORGANS AND EMOTIONS

After more and more years of practice I have found that the Chinese were right in their association of organs and emotions. The more imbalanced the lever is, for example, the more a person is prone to anger. The more imbalanced the heart is, the less joy and laughter the person experiences. My experiences have given me additional insight into the link between the organs and emotion.

The practitioner of healing touch is always trying to restore balance to the body, mind and spirit. If you keep these guidelines in your mind as you are doing your assessment, you will be able to know, where the blockages in the field lie, even if you can't feel the energy as yet.

Below is a list of organs and their associated psychological conditions.

Organ	Personality characteristics when organ is balanced	Emotions and Psychology when significantly imbalanced
LIVER	Strong ability to express strong will; good appearance.	Anger, frustrations, weak will, inability to express oneself, overtly timid.
SPLEEN	Good self-esteem, centred personality, lack of worry, compassion and understanding.	Worry, anxiety, nervousness.
STOMACH	Strong appetite for life, good ability to enjoy a wide variety of food and types of experiences.	Nervous, poor appetite for life, very picky about food, people and types of experiences he or she can tolerate.
HEART	Can give and feel love, can identify with others, can feel connected to others.	Walls self off from love and affection, feels isolated and tends to sustain isolation. May be given to hysteria, depression, low self-esteem.
PANCREAS	Good sense of boundaries.	Suffers from chronic guilt.
GALL BLADDER	Decisive, good digestion.	Indecisive, poor digestion
SMALL INTESTINE	Can determine what is good in experience and what should be discarded.	Has trouble in finding the good in people, situations and one's own experiences in life.
SKIN	Good sense of boundaries, positive sense of self, good self-esteem, good elimination from kidneys and large intestine.	Weak sense of boundaries, poor self-esteem and sense of self, poor elimination from kidneys and large intestine.

Contd.

Organ	Personality characteristics when organ is balanced	Emotions and Psychology when significantly imbalanced
LARGE INTESTINE	Able to go off the past, not over - burdened with sadness or grief.	Constipation, holding on to old memories, sadness, and grief, unable to let go of old hurts, trouble in letting go of the past, diarrhoea, unable to get most out of experience, let go too easily of people and relationships.
THYROID	Good self expression.	Hypothyroid: low energy and generally weak self expression. Hyperthyroid : racing, unable to deeply appreciate the moment or one's own contributions to an endeavour.
SEX ORGANS	Good expression of one's own unique self and creativity.	Holding back one's expression and creativity.
KIDNEYS	Confident and generally secure personality.	Suffers from deep-rooted fears.
LUNGS	Good energy and vitality, strong ability to take in and enjoy life.	Repressed emotions, low energy (oxygen is the basis of energy), low self-esteem, strong sense of one's own weeknesses or frailty.

IN SEARCH OF BALANCE
(Relationship — Body, Mind and Spirit)

The body, mind and spirit are always searching for balance in all ways, especially energetically. Whenever you see excessive strength, you will also discover weakness nearby. Once you discover the imbalance, you will have to move the energy from the area of excess to the places where it is deficient.

The practitioner of healing touch is always trying to restore balance to the body, mind and spirit. If you keep these guidelines in your mind as you are doing your assessment, you will be able to know, where the blockages in the field lie, even if you canät feel the energy as yet.

THREE POINT MEDITATION
(The Concept of a Whole Unit)

As you recall we have mentioned that it is the whole field that becomes charged with energy from the universal source before the energy works. The healer works as a whole unit, the hands can merely direct and be specific with energy.

The first part of the following exercise teaches you to use your own field to reach out and scan the other person and the second part teaches you to send healing energy through your field to the other person.

This exercise can be done with two or more people. If there are more than two people, pick the person who is going to be scanned and have him or her sit in the middle with the rest of the group forming a circle around him or her. (Fig. 12.)

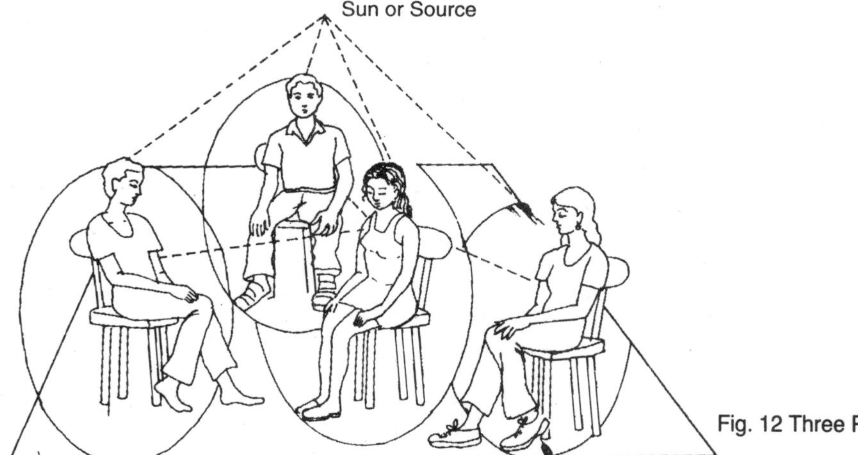

Fig. 12 Three Point Meditation

1. Start this exercise by using the meditative clearing exercise, choosing one person to guide the imagery. Picture the sun or source over the centre of the whole group (not over each one individually). Do this for about five minutes.
   The person who has been chosen to guide this meditation will now guide the rest through the imagery.

   - Person in the centre should focus on what he needs to heal within any part of the body, emotion or mind, while also keeping himself centred in his egg meditation.

   - The rest of the group should be centred in their individual energy eggs and begin to move their energy from the front of their egg to gently make contact with the person in the centre of the circle in a natural energy made. Stay here for about five minutes and just feel or get a sense of what is going on with this person. Note any images you have, any physical sensation, any thoughts etc.

   - After five minutes gently withdraw your energy. Open your eyes and have each person in the group share with the person in the centre what each received. The person in the centre should also share what he received. Remember that you have been in the centre person's sacred space. Not only is this information confidential within the group but you have been privy to secrets within the person and you should be gentle with how you share the thoughts. Remember that the purpose of healing touch is "To help and to heal" from a non- judgemental place.

Chat for a short time, although some association may have no relevance at the time. That happens.

2.   In the same circle, centre yourselves again by breathing. The person in the centre should open himself to receive healing energies. The group should bring the healing energy from the source through each to the centre person through each individual field.

Continue this for about five minutes. Your energy is in the "gentle push" stage. At the end of five minutes consciously feel your energy go into neutral and withdraw your energy from the centre person's sacred space.

Each one takes a turn being in the middle, each being supportive of the other. It is important to remember that when you are in another's sacred space, you know everything about that person. It may not be conscious in you but on some level there is a great awareness. You must remember not only to be non-judgemental but also to honour this space as you would your own.

SERVING OTHERS (The Sacred Space)

After the assessment of patient's physical and energetic bodies, I start to work on the field usally at a distance of about eighteen inches, a distance that is traditionally known as sacred space. Within this area, a person's sensitivity and self protectiveness are more acute, and consequently you do not want to violate this space, especially during the first few treatments, because you may not yet have established a bond of trust. Even whenever I work on people, I am very familiar with, I still try to remain beyond the eighteen inch boundary during our first two sessions together.

The obvious contradiction to this is my touching of the secondary chakras at the back of the knees and my massaging the back of the legs, tendons in the calves and the bottoms of the feet. This work which I call opening the feet is so important to balancing a person's energy that there simply is no way around it. Nevertheless, I approach the body and these secondary chakras with great respect and appreciation for this person and his willingness to allow me to work with him.

Generally in most cases opening of feet is performed at the conclusion of the assessment. Once that is done, I start at the top of the field and move downward to the feet. I am aware of the energy flowing to me from the cosmos, above and the earth below. I feel the energy passing from my field to my body, up from my heart and down to my hands. My hands are flowing with healing energy as passing them over the patient's field.

INSTRUMENT FOR THE UNIVERSAL LIFEFORCE

It is first and most important part of the work that I should be only an instrument for the universal lifeforce, that energy is flowing through me and into the person I am working with. It's that simple. Thus, the very basis of the patient requires very little from me, because the lifeforce flowing from the universal healer is doing the healing. I am attempting to direct and facilitate that flow of energy from an infinite source to the person in need of assistance. As I always tell my students that once a practitioner reorganises and achieves this stand point, she/he is in a position to help a person. His/her ego is out of way and can't be an obstruction to the process. This is what I mean when I always advise them, "Less is more".

As I send lifeforce to the field of the patient, I am particularly conscious of the places in the field that I had perceived to be imbalanced, while doing my assessment or where a symptom may be manifesting. Of course, I do not have to perceive blockages or holes in the field to recognise and treat a broken arm or a physical wound or some form of disorder. I can treat the imbalance by sending life energy to that part of the body. That is beauty of healing touch. At bottom, I am sending love, healing energy. The body and the great spirit together know better than I what to do with that energy.

REMOVING BLOCKAGES (Boulders and Stones)

In general, all symptoms arise out of balance, either there is too much energy in the area or too little. As a general rule, you are trying to move the excess energy into the places where there is deficiency. Once I discover the imbalance in the energy field, I always focus on it and attempt to restore circulation of the lifeforce to that area. If the area is blocked or stagnant, I try to remove gently the obstruction, often perceived as a large stone from that part of the field. These boulders are perceived as large, dense clumps of energy.

I have found that before you try to remove the blockages from the field, it is helpful to ask the person with whom you are working to visualise the energy flowing freely within his body without obstruction, especially the energy that flows up and down the central tube.

ENCOURAGING FREE FLOW OF ENERGY WITHIN THE PATIENT (Experiencing the Energy)

Before describing about the excessive or diminished energy in the patient of different fields, it is very necessary to know certain processes as explained hereafter. First of all what we should do is to perform the exercise for **experiencing the energy.**

This exercise will give you the experience of feeling the energy in your hands. It is a good exercise to perform before you work on someone's field.

Exercises

1. Hold your palms face up with arms slightly extended from your body.

2. Rapidly open and close both palms thirty to forty times.

3. Bring your slightly cupped hands, slowly towards each other in front of you, noting the "spongy" ball of energy between your hands, when they are about four inches apart.

   Now our basic approach is to meet with problem of pulling the energy out where it is blocked and excessive and push the energy into the places where it is deficient. So you help yourself, get a feeling for working on pulling and pushing the energy experience the different sensations of healing touch/Reiki, the universal lifeforce. Try the following exercises.

a. First sit opposite to each other (patient and healer) in a straight backed chair with your feet flat on the floor and your knees almost touching those of your patient. Take a minute or two to breathe deeply and centre yourselves.

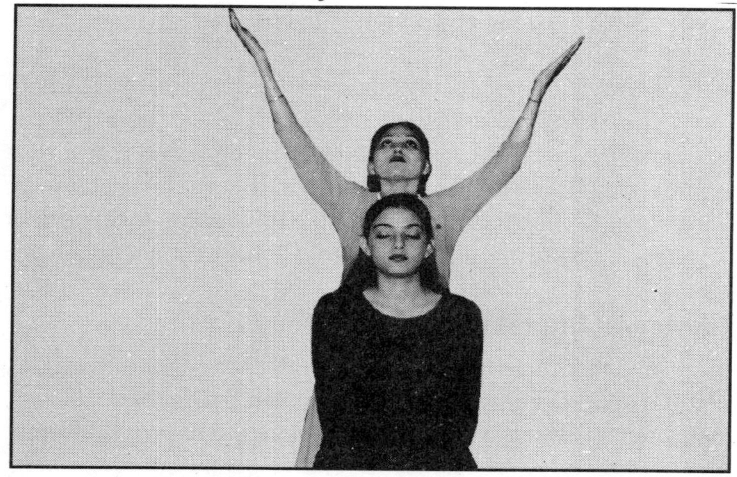

Showing the position of bringing
Rainbow light on the patient's body

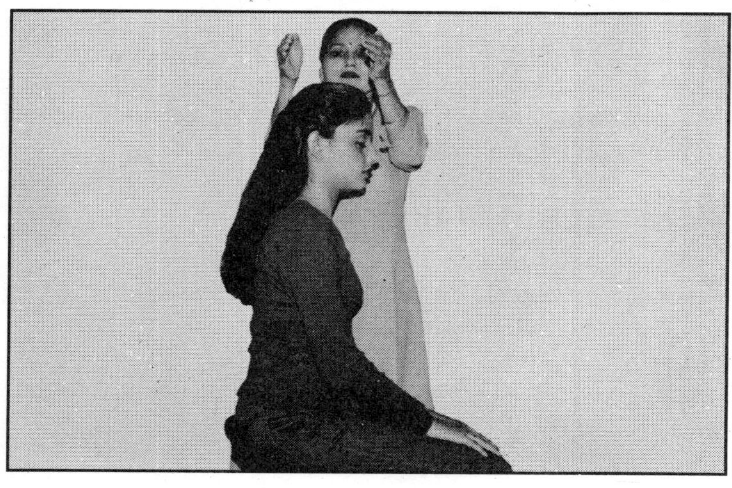

Showing the position of bringing
Rainbow light on the patient's body

b.   Now rest your arms and hands on your thighs with your left palm facing upward and your right palm facing downward. Have your patient place her/his right palm on top of your left palm and his/her left palm under your right palm. (For this exercise you may actually touch each other's palms).

Before you begin sending or receiving energy you and your partner should try to determine, how the energy is flowing between both of you. Does it go out of your left hand and into your partner's right? Does the energy pass from your partner's right hand to your left? How does the energy that you receive from your partner affect your body? How does it travel through your body, that is, does it enter your right hand, for example, travel up the arm through the shoulders and out of the left hand? Try to feel the movement of energy before you try to affect the energy. Don't worry if you can't feel the flow of energy. Most important, don't think you should just feel. It takes time and practice to become sensitive to the movements of this energy.

SENDING OR PUSHING OF ENERGY
(Boosting the Life Energy)

Once you have tried to establish the direction of the energy, see if you can direct it with your hands and mind, decide with which hand you are going to push the energy to the patient out of the left or right. Now use the exhalation of your breath to send the energy from the palm that you have choosen to send with. As you exhale, visualise the energy going out of your palm and into the opposite hand of your partner. The person who is receiving energy should stay in neutral mode and be senstive to the energy. Visualise the line of flow, that is to see how the energy travels through your partner, such as from her/his arms, across his/her shoulders, and/or down his/her other arm returning to the hand opposite your own. Feel your other hand receiving the energy. Ask your partner whether or not he/she can feel the energy flow. Take turn pushing with other hand. Also take turns receiving and sending the energy.

In general sending energy to your client will raise or boost the life-energy you send to places those are weak or deficient of "KI" or lifeforce.

PULLING THE ENERGY FROM PARTNER
(Determining the Energy Flow)

The next energy flow to learn is pulling the energy. Pulling the energy will diminish the lifeforce in that area. You do this in places, where the energy is excessive. Repeat the previous exercise, but instead of pushing the energy with the exhalation, visualise pulling the energy out of your partner's hand as you inhale. Try to determine how the energy is flowing within yourself and your partner. Where is the energy coming from that you are pulling from your partner? It is coming from shoulder, back and neck. Ask your partner if he or she has any physical sensations while you are pulling the energy.

STOPPING THE ENERGY FLOW
(Mastering the Way)

Finally let us try to stop the energy from flowing between you and your partner. Visualise the energy remaining at the state of rest between you and your partner. Both of you are only one who are closed to each other. Shut off. Determine how this feels and compare it to the previous exercise.

These exercises will help you learn how to master the ways in which you can direct energy through your hands. You can practise sending and receiving energy all the day. Whenever you shake a person's hand, send your energy or receive his/her. When you touch another person on the shoulder or the arm, try to sense the person's energy or send some of your own. In short try to expand the sense of touch. It is actually a lot easier than you think. Try not to make practice excessively intellectual or difficult. All you need to do is experience and practise it.

KEEP THE TREATMENTS SHORT
(The General Rules)

Generally, the healing touch/Reiki/universal energy sessions are short, anywhere from five to thirty minutes, depending on the age of the person and his/her health. The general rules are as following:—
(a)   The younger the patient the shorter the treatment time.
(b)   More severe the disharmony of the person, the shorter the treatment.

For example, for treatment of infants upto 1 year of age usally takes 30 seconds. For the child of this age you would do gentle healing touch over the area of disharmony or over the general body, especially in the case of premature babies or infants who are struggling with some types of systemic problems.

At the age group between one to five years usually children are treated for one minute (depending upon the situation how long the child will sit still)

Very ill patients (especially those who are bedridden) are treated for not less than five minutes but not more than seven minutes. You can apply the treatment daily.

THOSE WHO SUFFER FROM ACUTE ILLNESS — LESS IS MORE

The general rule is that "Less is more" meaning that few minutes of healing touch will promote healing without overwhelming the body (such as first stage of cold). If you work on a person with a cold or flue too long, you may trigger even stronger symptoms and more sufferings than would otherwise have occured. Cold is actually the body's attempt to eliminate accumulated wastes and toxins especially those that have been taken in from the environment which can be found in the air water and food. Gradually these waste products accumulate in the fluid between tissue cells, tension in muscles, fascia and other tissues prevent the waste from moving into the lymph. Tension also prevents the lymphs from moving the waste out of the tissues and into the liver for elimination. Hence waste accumulates. This toxic environment in the tissues provides the right conditions for virus and bacteria to flourish and to set on a cold.

CLOSING OF HOLES (The Important Task)

It is a vitally important task for the practitioner of healing touch to close the holes or leaks in the field. This will allow the person to experience, even for a short time his/her true wholeness and integrity. Such an experience triggers the healing process. Once the patient glimpses his best-self, he/she unconsciously and consciously begins to move out of blockages and stagnation. The more you work on a person, the more you can "repattern" the field to close the leaks permanently or teach the person to close the leaks whenever he or she feels vulnerable.

LEAKS AND HOLES—TYPICAL OCCURRENCE

Typical leaks or holes occur near the areas of the field that are loaded with energy, often stuck or blocked from flowing into the hole. The field will try to heal itself of leaks but blockages may prevent the lifeforce from flowing smoothly to the hole or leak. Leaks are often near those chakras that are related to the various kinds of issues the person may be experiencing. (Those issues may well have been discussed during your intake interview or as a part of healing session). If it's an issue veering around money for example, then perhaps the hole is located near first chakra — responsible for survival issues, the third chakra — responsible for the will and drive or the fifth chakra— responsible for self expression.

If issue involves relationship with the opposite sex then perhaps it involves the second chakra — responsible for sexuality or the third chakra — responsible for will and self empowerment or the fourth chakra responsible for ability to experience love.

If the issue involves the discovery of the person's specific work then perhaps it involves the **Second Chakra** responsible for discerning what it is the person truly loves or **Fifth Chakra** responsible for self expression or the **Sixth Chakra** — responsible for one's deep understanding of self.

HARMONISING THE FIELD

If any person comes to you complaining of a specific health issue, search the field around the nearest related chakra. If you do not feel a leak or hole reassess the field and open the feet. You may need to spend five minutes of the treatment holding the feet and encouraging the person to breathe deeply down into the feet. (Very often people who are difficult to assess are shallow breathers and consequently suffer from stagnant life energy. These imbalances can very often be relieved by asking the person to spend five minutes breathing deeply while you are opening the secondary chakras in their feet). Be patient with your assessment. It may take several sessions before you understand the person's energetic imbalances. Meanwhile you are harmonising the field through your healing touch and by opening the chakra in the feet.

CHANNELLING THE EXTRA LIFEFORCE

To close the holes and leaks, I always run my hands along boundaries of the field that are healthy and strong and draw the excess energy to hole or leak. I try to channel additional lifeforce to the hole, filling it with energy and then close over the wounded area by smoothing my hands over the leak. I give the leak a kind of maternal love, flowing within that love is the healing energy, that is flowing through me to the client. I always visualise the healing energy flowing into the leak, filling it and healing the wound. I see the wound closing and the integrity of the field being reestablished. I work to balance the energy so that it flows smoothly throughout the region where there was formely a wound. Once again, the field is closed, strong, resilient and whole.

This process of closing a leak or hole usually takes several sessions, simply because wounds are chronics and the field is patterned to maintain that wound.

When holes or leaks in the field are closed even temporarily, the person feels the experiences of wholeness. His/her field is now intact and energy that was leaking is now flowing within him/her. This experience may give him/her a sudden burst of energy or may make him/her feel tired as areas of his/her body is experiencing energy for the first time in many years.

But more important is, body, mind, and spirit feel contained within one's own boundaries and identity. The effect is profound but it reminds one on all levels of what it feels like to be whole. It is a glimpse of all that one is and can be. The full self healing of those holes takes place long after the session is over. The person's own field will heal itself. The closing of holes by the practitioner awakens the healing forces within the field and directs them to those places within the field that must be restored to integrity.

COMPLAINTS OF PAIN

If someone tells you that she or he is experiencing a mild ache or pain after treatment and for the pain is acute or lingers for more than two hours, ask the person to consult his/her physician. In general you can't cause any serious side effect—including pain by administering healing touch. On the other hand, the infusion of lifeforce can create temporary discomfort especially in the person who has suffered long term blockages and stagnations.

The most common pain that may result after the healing touch session occurs after you have cleared an area of obstructions and old energetic patterns begin to break down. Once these blockages are removed, energy, blood and lymph flow in greater abundance into areas that were previously blocked and deficient of all three elixirs of life. When blood, lymph and KI starts to move into the parts of the field and physical body that were stagnant or blocked, the tissues can be highly sensitive and therefore might experience temporary discomfort or mild pain.

Whenever client expresses or experiences the pain but especially if that pain emerges after a treatment then first open the feet, place your hands over the site of the pain and send that place soothing and comforting healing energy, visualise the tissues opening as if they were just now arising after a long sleep, and accepting the increased circulation. Once you have done this, move one hand over the nearest chakras opening and place the other hand over the back where the chakras exist.

Now create a new energy ball between your hands, see the energy ball fill-up the entire area with soft healing energy and light. See the tissues becoming supple and relaxed. Finally make sure the energy is flowing freely from the bottoms of the feet. Then balance the healing chakra and close it. When this step is completed, ask the client to lie down for ten minutes. The energy that has been channelled to the client will build on itself over the next twentyfour hours boosting the immune and healing forces and harmonising imbalances.

TAKING AWAY ENERGETIC WASTE OUT OF THE CHANNEL (The Process)

Very often when I work with people, I finish my treatment by clearing the central tube. I do this type of treatment only after I have established a strong bond of trust because it requires the practitioner to touch the client's head, shoulders, and back. I have found that clearing of tube is highly effective at eliminating old emotional wounds, memories and attachments to old relationships which limits the person's outlook and growth, even when the person does not realise that he still holds on to such memories or relationships. It is also a powerful way to raise the lifeforce. Keep in mind that clearing the tube is usally done at the end of the treatment. That means by the time you clear the tube you have centred and completed your assessment and finished your energy work. Here are the steps that you can use to clear your patient's central tube:

(a)   Move to the back of your patient and gently place your hands on the back of his neck with your thumbs gently pressing the muscles on each side of the vertebrae at the base of head. Massage these points ever gently so that the muscles relax.

(b)   Slowly move your thumbs down the left and right sides of each vertebra, pausing at each vertebra to massage the muscles on each side of the spine. Do not stop until you reach the base of the spine.

(c)   Your intention in this first phase of the clearing is to loosen the muscles and gain the body's trust. The client may well trust you intellectually, but you must now convince his body that it can release its armour and allow you to probe its soft and vulnerable interior. Massage gently and firmly. You want your client to feel good, to relax and to put down his armours so that you can go deeper with each step of clearing.

(d)   Repeat the procedure again, moving from top of the spine to its base with the same loving healing hands.

(e)   Do the procedure a third time. As you move down the spine this time, go a little deeper, try to wake up the spinal nerves so that energy is released into the system.

(f)   Start again from the top vertebra only this time, move your own lifeforce beyond your hands, so that your "etheric hands" move deeply into the client's inner field and directly into the central tube running through the centre of the body. Your energetic hands are now deep within the tube and you can sense where the blockages in the tube are located. Loosen merely the blockages that you sense and then keep moving downward through the tube. Allow yourself to perceive any information in your client's field which may be communicating to you about these blockages. But more important stay focused on your work, stay centred and keep reciting your prayer. That is the tool you use to keep yourself centred.

(g)   When you reach the base of the spine, keep your thumbs at the base and rest your thumbs on each side of buttocks, between your hands create an energy ball, visualise the energy forming and becoming stronger and more vital at the base of the client's spine. You are not strengthening the client's "Ki" or lifeforce. Take a few minutes and allow the energy ball to grow and become strong.

(h)   When you feel that ball is strong enough and of very good quality "KI" slowly begin to move your thumbs up on either side of vertebrae while visualising the energy gently moving with your hands. As the energy moves upward it serves as a vacuum cleaner, gathering all the old blockages and debris from the tube.

(i)   As you reach the back of client's heart chakra, pause and ask the client to take a deep breath with his inhalation continue moving up the spine to the base of the head. Try to visualise and feel the ball growing ever more powerful as you move up the spine.

(j)   At the base of the neck, gently place your hands and palms on either side of the client's head. Ask him to exhale and also visualise all the release out of the top of his head, which he no longer needs. At the same time gently squeeze his head between your hands and pull the ball of energy and debris that it holds out at the top of his central tube at the top of his head.

(k)   As you raise your hands high above your client's head, release the debris into the light of love to be transformed by the Great Healer.

      If the client feels congestion in his neck repeat the process from step (f) to end.

Many people describe the feeling upon being released from central tube debris as an "energy rush". Others feel lighter and still others feel tired and they need rest for a while.

TREATMENT PLAN (Initial Interview)

A good treatment plan always begins with a good initial interview. Healer should take a complete history of the client as well as complaints. An extended family history should be obtained, along with information on any medicines, herbs or vitamins or dietary supplements which the patient is currently taking. It is also imperative that the healer should have a working knowledge of the disease or disharmony the patient wants to work on. Once you have established what the client sees as a problem, a case plan can be developed to guide both you and the patient through the treatment.

There is a five step process that takes into consideration the patient's medical diagnosis and leads the healer to develop a plan of action to enhance the healing of the patient. The steps are as following:—

1.   ASSESSMENT:- This includes all information obtained in the initial interview.

2.   ANALYSIS: This includes analysis of patient's problem.

3.   PLAN: In healing touch, the plan is the energy work based on prioritizing the problems and established patient-centred goals, along with the specific intervention and rationale. This also includes the networking and list of other professionals involved on the care team. The plan of energy work remains the same. What changes each week are the symptoms the patient arrives with and the changes that have occurred in the field as a result of the past week's work. Part of the plan is to talk with the patient and help him recognise the changes and evaluate the effect of the work having on him or her.

4.   IMPLEMENTATION : This is putting the case plan, into action to fulfil the patient's centred goals.

5.   EVALUATION :- This includes determining the value and results of the treatment plan and evaluating the patient's progress. The evaluation comes from the patient, the family and other health care professionals involved (physiotherapist, psychotherapist, massage therapist and any other practitioner if treated for), and most important from the healer observing the patient's response to the therapeutic touch process.

Whenever a patient comes to you for healing touch, it is very important that he/she has a recent physical examination report by a doctor and you must be aware of any physical problem or limitation the patient may have.

14. CONCLUSION

WORKING WITH REIKI

As briefed in its history chapter, Reiki (pronounced Ray-Key), is an art of laying on hands, a healing technique and it is thousands of years old. It is presumed to have originated as a Tibetan Buddhist practice that was rediscovered in late 18th century by Dr. Mikao Usui. It is a very simple yet powerful technique and can be learned by anyone.

REI—MEANS SPIRITUAL WISDOM

As per Mrs. Takata, the world "Rei" means universal and this definition is accepted by most of her followers. However Mrs. Takata also indicated that this interpretation is a very general one. The Kanji ideograms have seven different levels of meaning. They vary from the mundane to the highly esoteric, so while it is true that REI can be interpreted as universal, meaning that it is present everywhere. Research into the esoteric meaning of Japanese Kanji character for REI has given a much deeper understanding of this ideogram. The word Rei as it is used in REIKI is more accurately interpreted to mean Supernatural Knowledge or spiritual consciousness. This is the wisdom that comes from God or the higher self. This is the God-consciousness which is all knowing. It understands each person completely. It knows the causes of all problems and difficulties and knows what to do to heal them.

KI—THE LIFEFORCE

Ki—means the same as CHI - in Chinese and Prana in Sanskrit. It has also been called odic-force, orgone and bio-plasma. It has been given many other names by various cultures that have been aware of it.

KI—is the lifeforce. It is also called the Universal Energy. This is non-physical energy that animates all living things. As long as something is alive, it has lifeforce circulating through it and surrounding it and when it dies the lifeforce departs. If your lifeforce is low or if there is any restriction in its flow, you will be more vulnerable to illness. When it is high and flowing freely, you are less likely to get sick. Lifeforce plays an important role in every thing we do. It animates the body and is also the primary energy of our emotions, thoughts and spiritual life.

The Chinese place great importance on the lifeforce or what they call CHI. They have studied it for thousands of years and have discovered that there are many different kinds of CHI. The Yellow Emperor's "Classic of Internal Medicine" which is over 4000 years old lists thirty two types of CHI.

KI is used by martial artists in their physical training and mental development. It is used in meditative breathing exercises called PRANAYAMA and by the shamans of all cultures for divination, psychic awareness, manifestation and healing. KI is present all around us and can be accumulated and guided by the mind.

SPIRITUALLY – GUIDED LIFEFORCE ENERGY

It is the God-consciousness called REI that guides the lifeforce or Ki in the practice of healing. Therefore, REIKI can be defined as the spiritually guided lifeforce energy. This is a meaningful interpretation of the word Reiki. It more closely describes the experience most people have of it. Also Reiki guides itself with its own wisdom and is unresponsive to the direction of the practitioner.

DO ALL HEALERS USE REIKI?

All healers use lifeforce or KI, BUT NOT ALL USE REIKI. Reiki is a special kind of lifeforce that can only be channelled by someone who has been attuned to it. It is possible that some people are born with Reiki or have acquired it some other way. Most healers who have not received the Reiki attunement from Reiki masters are not using Reiki but uses another kind of lifeforce. People who do the healing work consistently report an increase of at least fifty percent in the strength of their own healing energies after completing the training.

ATTUNEMENT

Reiki is not taught in the way other healing techniques are taught. It is transferred to the student by the Reiki master during an attunement process. This process opens the crown, heart and palm chakras and creates a special link between the student and the Reiki channel.

The Reiki attunement is a powerful spiritual experience. The attunement energies are channelled into the student through the master. The process is guided by the Rei or God-consciousness and makes adjustments in the process depending on the need of individual student. The attunement is also attended by Reiki Guides and other spiritual people who help to implement the process. Many reports are in existence having mystical experiences involving personal massages, healings, visions and past life experiences.

The attunement can also increase psychic sensitivity. Some students report experiences involving opening of the third eye, increased intuitive awareness, and other psychic abilities after receiving a Reiki attunement. Once you have received the attunement, you will have Reiki for the remaining years of your life. It does not wear off and you can never loose it. Experiments have found that additional attunements of same level can add to the value of that level and these benefits include refinement of the Reiki energy in channelling increased strength of energy, healing of personal problems, clarity of mind, increased psychic sensitivity and a raised level of consciousness.

The Reiki attunement can start a cleaning process that affects the physical body as well as the mind and emotions. Toxin that have been stored in the body may be released along with feelings and thought patterns that are no longer useful. Therefore, a process of purification prior to the attunement is recommended to improve the benefit one receives.

REIKI NEVER CAUSES HARM

Because it is guided by God-consciousness, it can never do any harm to human mind and physical body. It always knows, what a person needs and will adjust itself to create the effect that is appropriate for him. One never need worry about whether to give Reiki or not. It is always helpful.

In addition, the practitioner does not direct the healing and does not decide where to work on or what to heal. The practitioner is not in danger of taking on the karma of the client because the practitioner is not doing the healing. It is much easier for the ego to stay out of the way and allow the presence of God to clearly shine through your whole.

REIKI ENERGY IS NEVER DEPLETED

Because it is a channelled healing, the Reiki practitioner's energies are never depleted. In fact, the Reiki consciousness considers both the practitioner and client to be in need of healing, so both get treated. Because of this giving a treatment always increases one's energy and leaves one surrounded with loving feelings of well-being.

BIPOLAR NATURE OF REIKI

Clairvoyant observation has indicated that Reiki is bipolar in nature. It is made up of both male and female healing energies. The male part comes from above. It is associated with the crown and higher chakras and is called Shiva in Tile Tantra system. The female part comes from below, is associated with the root chakra and is called Shakti in tantra system. These two energies communicate with each other and decide how much of each polarity is in need so that when the energies leave the hands, they have the proper combination of male and female healing energies for the person being treated. It is interesting to note that when more than one person is treating on a client, the Reiki communicates with all the practitioners involved in, giving someone more of the male energy to channel and others more of the female energy, so that the proper mix is maintained for the client.

HOW TO TREAT

- First of all treat yourself. You are REIKI and can be in as perfect of health as your ego will allow yourself to express.

- Secondly, treat all your surrounding persons especially family members. Normally the family unit would have provided you with many benefits so that transmitting the health of Reiki to them is an excellent way to complete the exchange.

- Thirdly, it is important for a healer to stress upon the questions being asked by the healee because Reiki is a system based on intent. The prospective client should express his intent for health requesting the treatment.

- Naturally, if a person is in coma, any child or someone from his family can ask for healing. It is very much appropriate to give Reiki.

- By keeping in your mind, "you are free to accept or reject a healing at your will", if you feel yourself disturbed mentally.

- Be cautious in treating an accident victim you don't know. In such cases it is legally advisable not to say anything about your healing ability.

- Simply attempt to administer Reiki in an inconspicuous manner which fortunately is very easy with Reiki.

- Speaking of infants, don't think babies or even foetuses are too young to receive treatments.

- Persons hospitalized or under conventional medical care can also be treated with Reiki.

- If the patient takes medication, instruct him to regularly consult with his physician, because the Reiki rebalances his body, the prescribed dosage might have to be lessened to avoid overdoses.

- **It is important to remember that you should never feel forced or obligated to heal someone or feel guilty for not taking the time to heal wherever and whenever requested.**
- **The big bonus with Reiki is that whenever you are treating someone else you are also receiving a healing at the same time.**
- **One is never tired nor depleted after giving a treatment, since one is using universal life energy for it.**

SOME BASIC POINTS TO TREAT THE PATIENT

- Create an environment as quite comfortable and soothing as possible for treatment.
- In your house choose a room or small area to be regularly used for client treatment. This REIKI space will become familiar (and thus psychologically comfortable) for clients who require successive treatments and also becomes charged with the nature of Reiki itself, thereby facilitating the healing experience.
- Wear comfortable clothing that won't interfere with the treatment positions.
- **For Female Patients:** remove glasses, jacket, shoes belt (if any), scarves, jewellery around the neck, no girdles or tight pantyhose.
- **For Male Patients:** remove glasses, vest, jacket, tie, belt shoes and also empty the pockets.
- No terribly snug pants in male/female case.
- REIKI finish does require direct physical contact with the skin.
- Have the client lie down if possible, so gravity can aid in pulling Reiki into his body.
- Make sure that the client's feet are not crossed. This tends to the short circuit of the energy flow.
- Remember that the comfort of yourself and the client is the most important thing in Reiki during a treatment.
- Tell the client that he may feel worse after the first or second treatment either due to severe imbalance in an organ (or the body generally) or because you may stop treatment just as the illness has been brought back from the chronic stage to its acute stage before eventual release. If this happens a minimum three, preferably four consecutive daily treatments will be required, unless healing takes place after the first or second treatment.
- Keep your fingers together otherwise energy will be scattered with spending 3 to 5 minutes on each position.
- A cold spot indicates a disfunctioning or impaired circulation. Hold that area until it is warmed up.
- Reiki is pulled through the body at a rate corresponding to the need of the client.
- Reiki Finish :- When the patient has accepted all the Reiki needed at one session, conclude his/her treatment with the Reiki finish. It is like icing on a cake.

On completion of the treatment of the front body, draw anticlockwise energy spiral with the index and middle fingers (together) on the patient beginning from shoulders down to arms and to the finger tips and from shoulders to the tips of toes.

TRADITIONAL REIKI POSITIONS FOR SELF AND OTHERS' TREATMENT

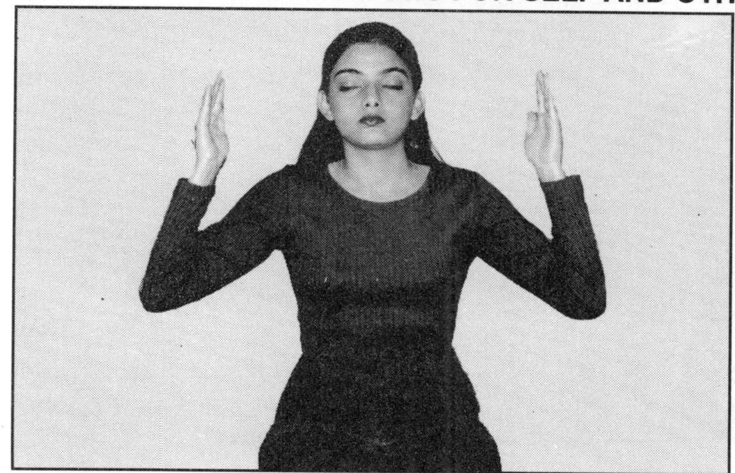

Position showing receiving of the universal lifeforce in the body.

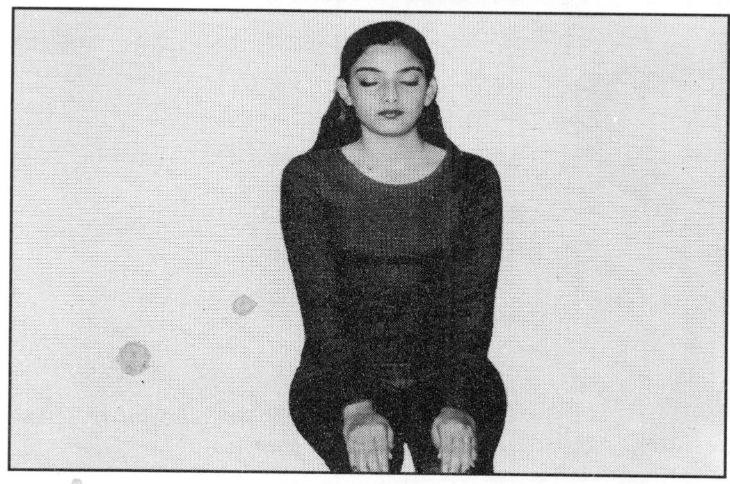

Position showing sitting back straight in chair meditating deep breath and watching internal body.

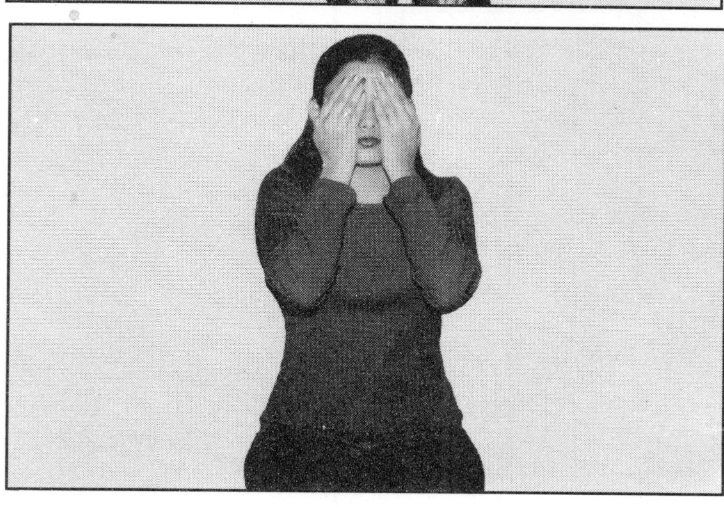

Position showing giving treatment for eyes.

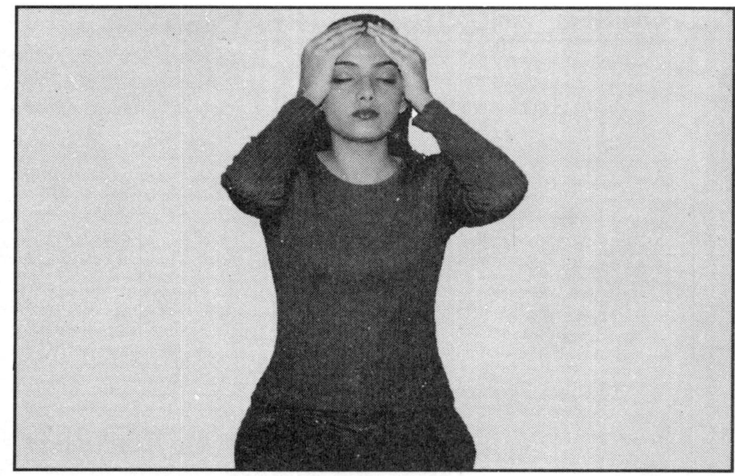

Position showing giving treatment for pituitaries by keeping the hands on the temples.

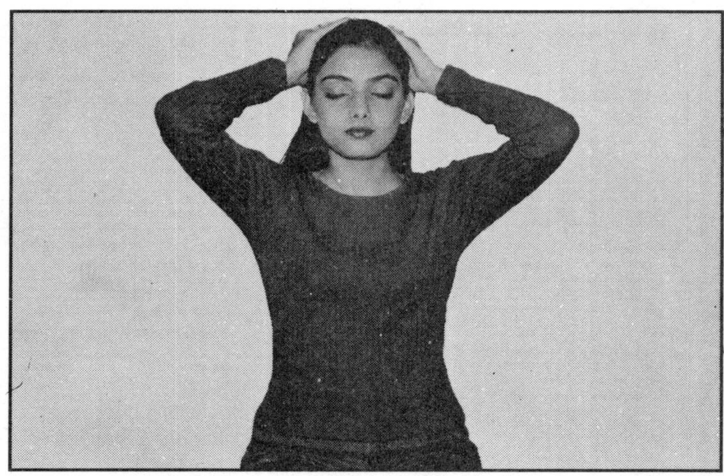

Postion showing treatment on the crown chakra.

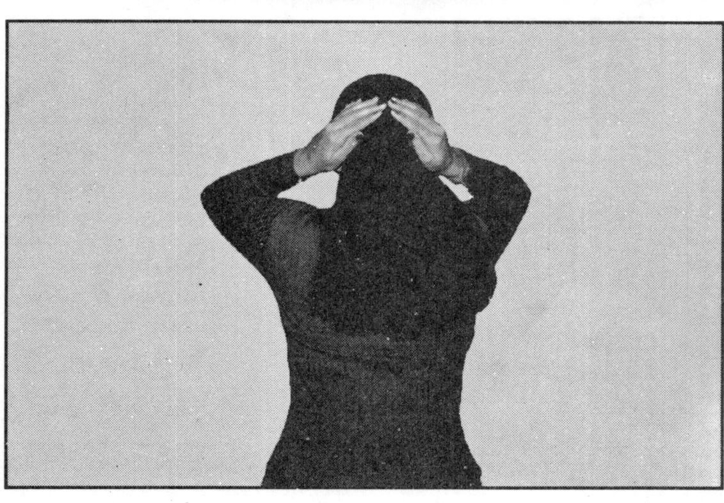

Position showing treatment on the crown chakra.

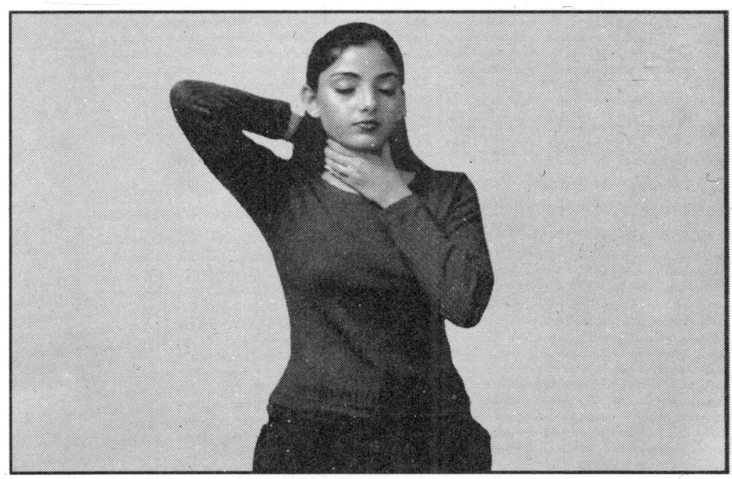

Position showing treatment on the throat charka.

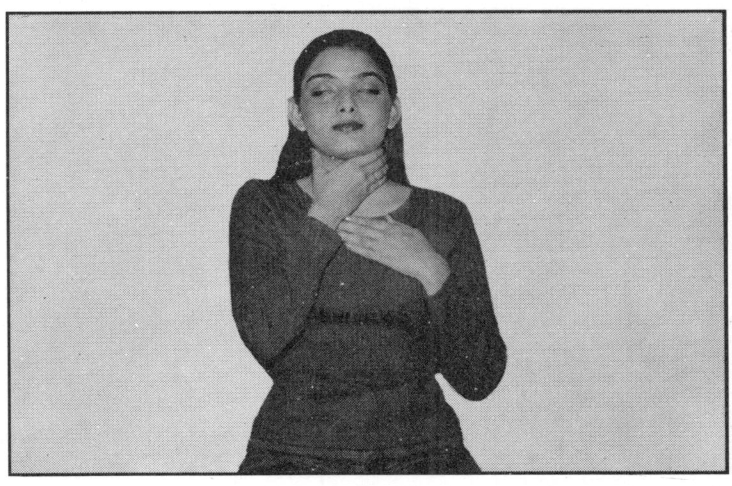

Position showing treatment on the thyroid and thymus glands.

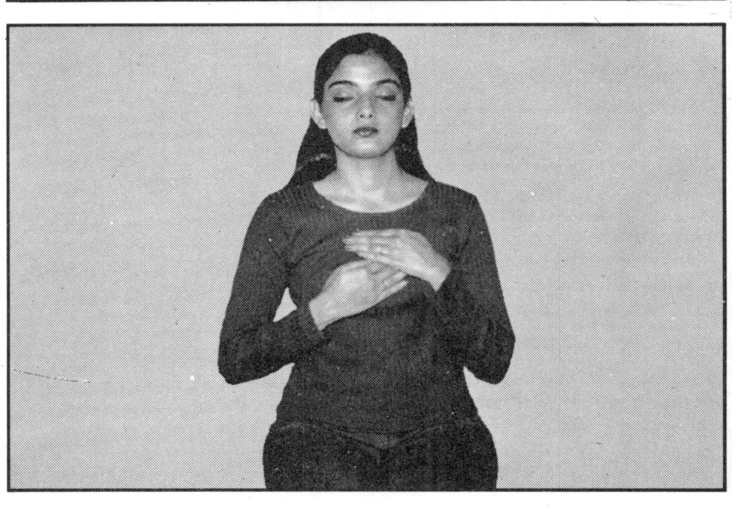

Position showing treatment on the heart chakra.

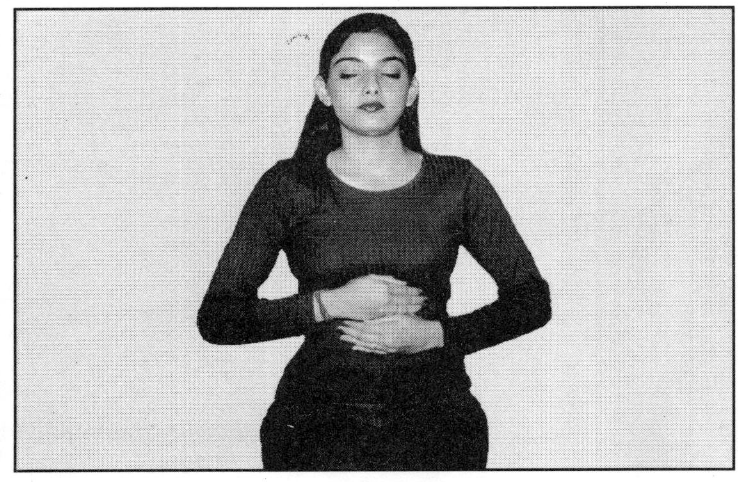

Position showing treatment on the solar plexus.

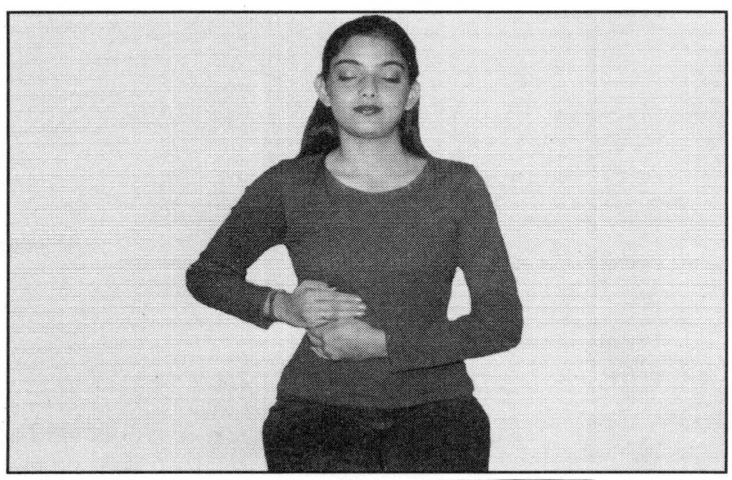

Position showing treatment on the liver.

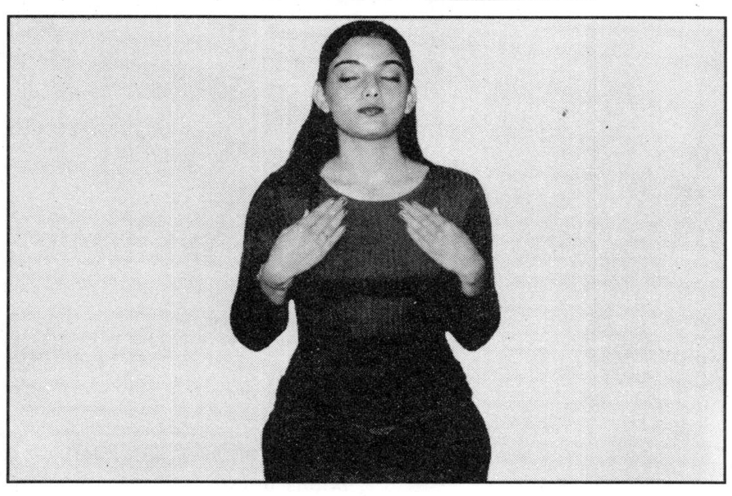

Position showing treatment on the lungs.

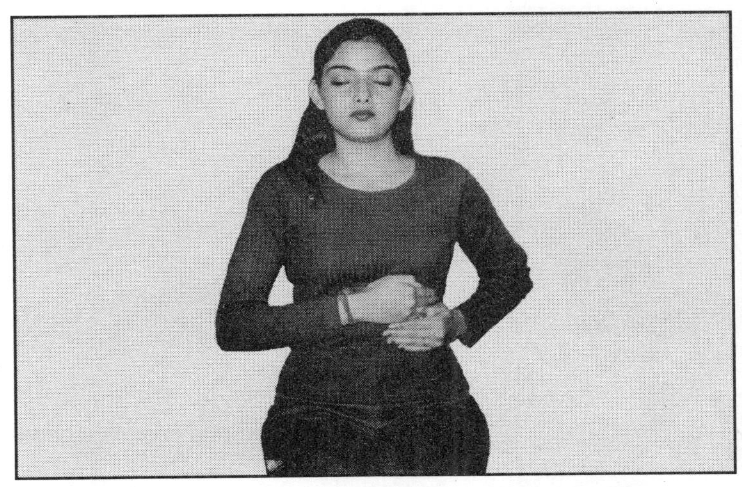

*Position showing treatment on
the spleen and pancreas.*

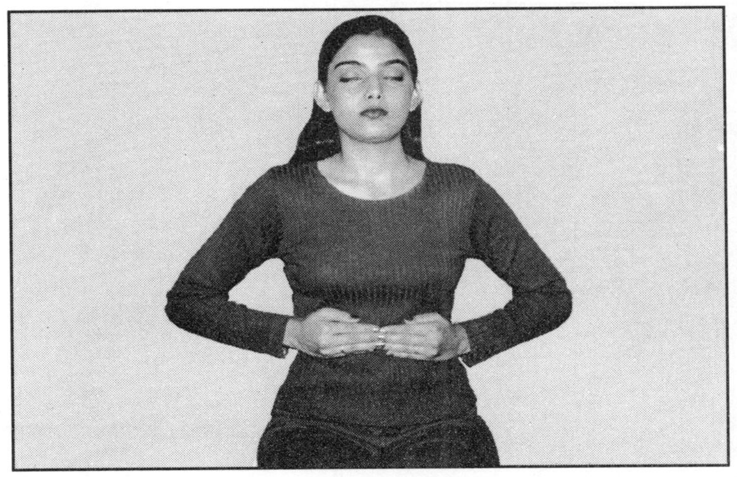

*Position showing treatment on solar
plexus.*

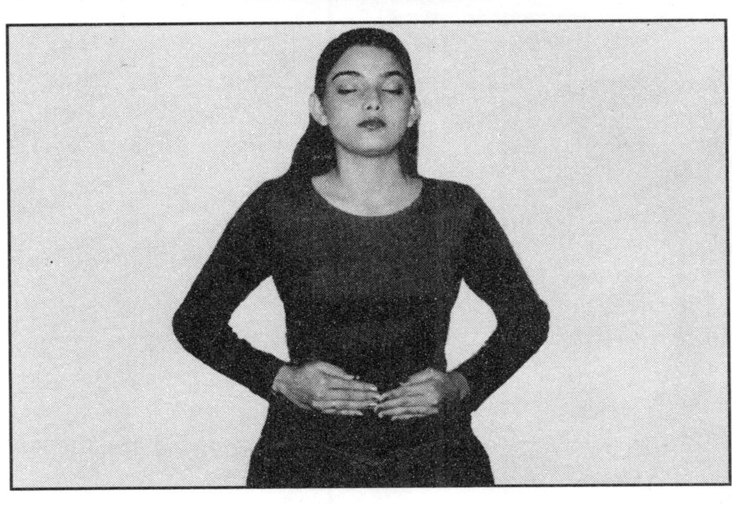

*Position showing treatment on
hara chakra.*

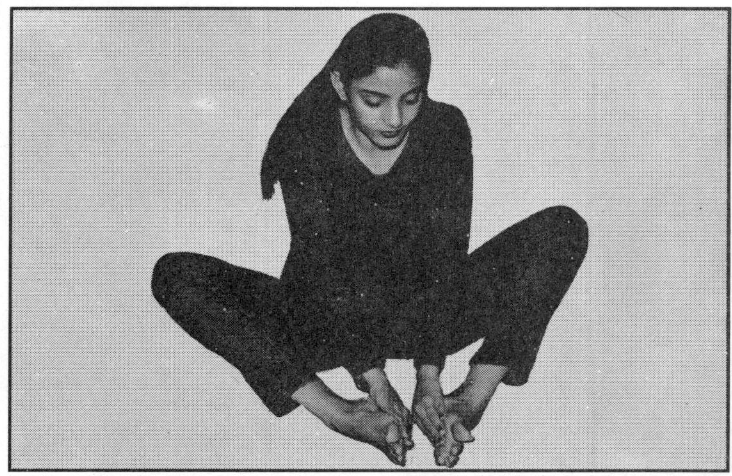

Position showing treatment on the foot chakra

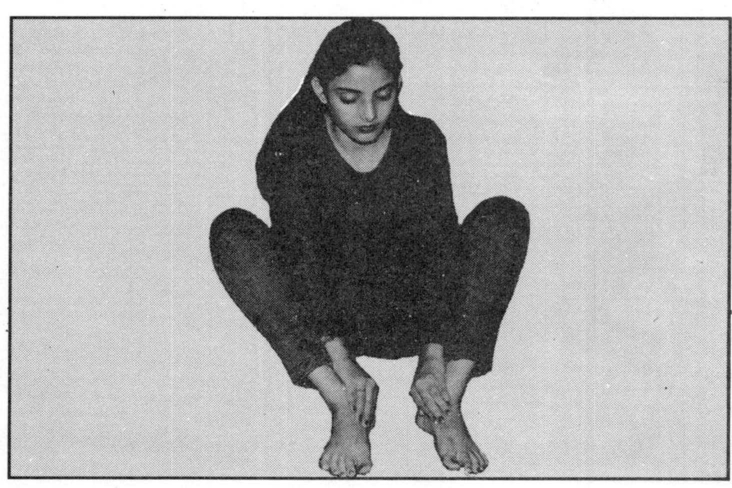

Position showing treatment on the ankle chakra.

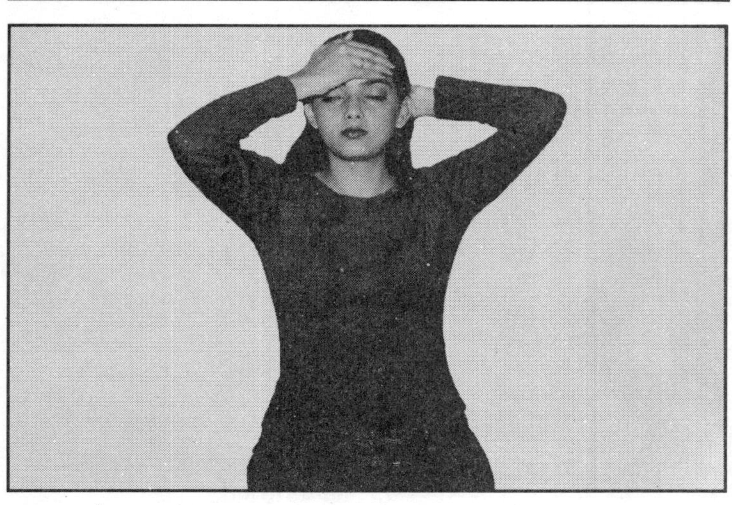

Position showing treatment on the brow chakra.

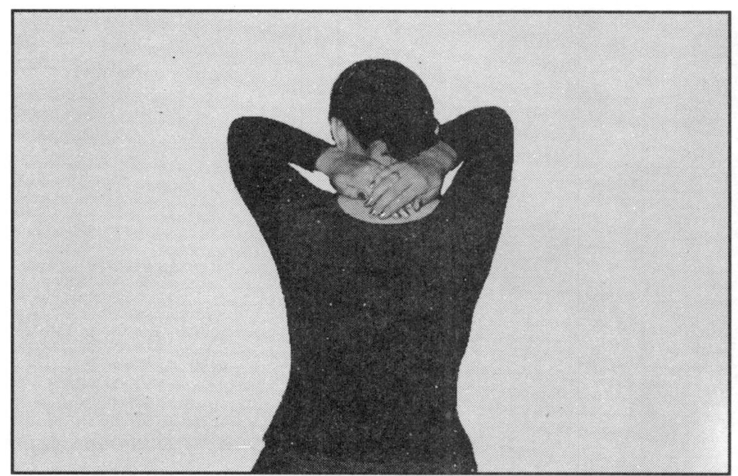

Position showing treatment on the back of thyroid.

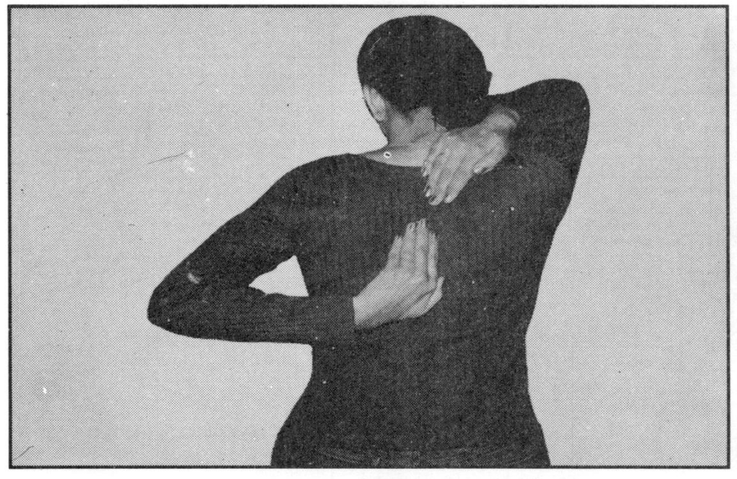

Position showing treatment on the back of heart chakra.

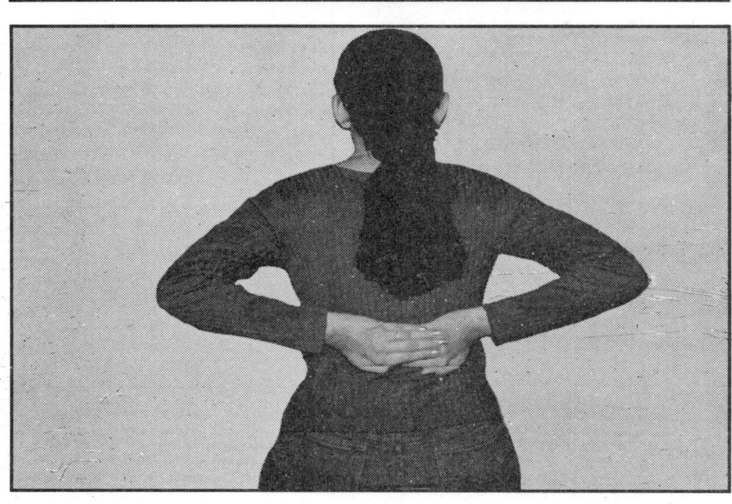

Position showing treatment on back of solar plexus.

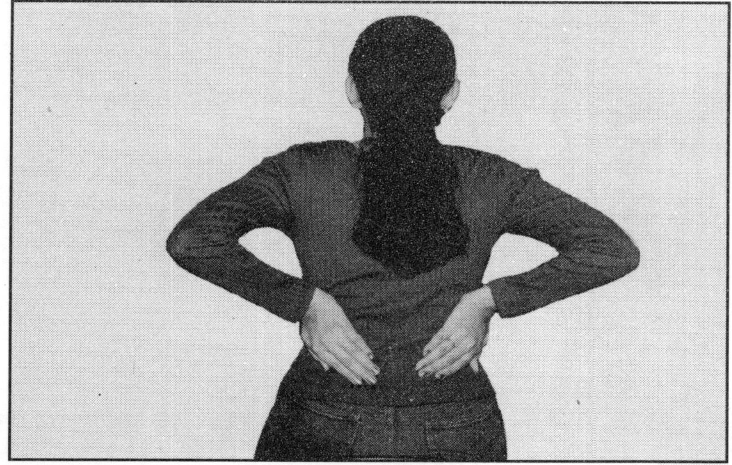

Position showing treatment on the kidneys.

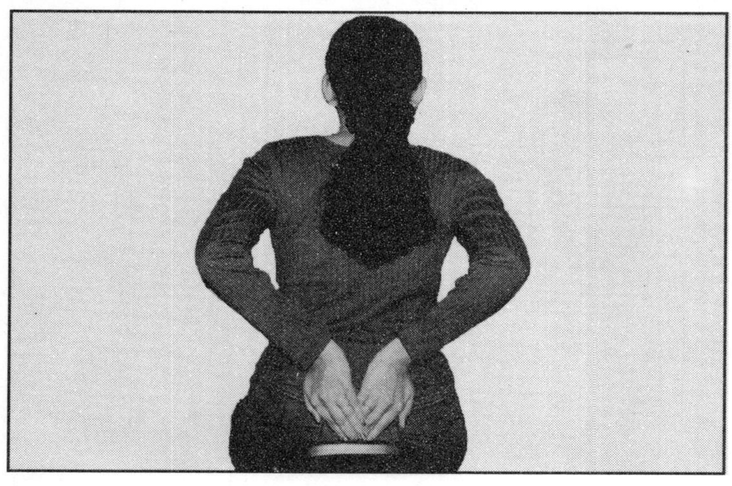

Position showing treatment on back of hara chakra.

SELF TREATMENT SHORT PROCESS.
(When Time is Less).

If you have used 3 to 5 minutes for each position, the session would have lasted between 45 minutes to an hour. If you can spare more time, it is preferred that you should do the whole body first and then spend time for your specific problem. If you do not have enough time, then go straight to the specific problem area. Reiki directs itself and will often flow to places beyond where your hands are placed.

The healer who will accept nothing is "egotistical". They are putting themselves in a position where they would not allow a person to pay off his human obligations. They are keeping that person indebted, not only in this life time but also into eternity.

Always remember, the two must complete itself. If everything comes in and does not go out, you will become like the dead sea and die. If everything goes out, you will dry up and become like the mud bed. If there is a balanced in and out flow, you are like a beautiful lake — everything in and around it grows and blossoms.

Energy work treatment with the patient in the sitting position and balancing of the chakras with the patient in lying down position.

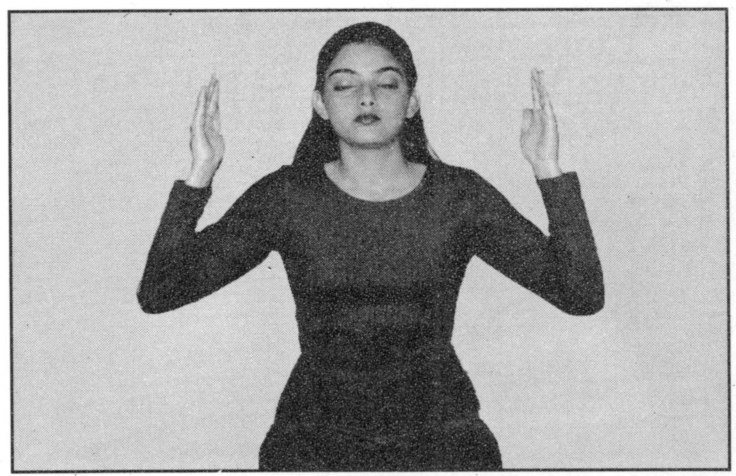

Receiving the Universal lifeforce.

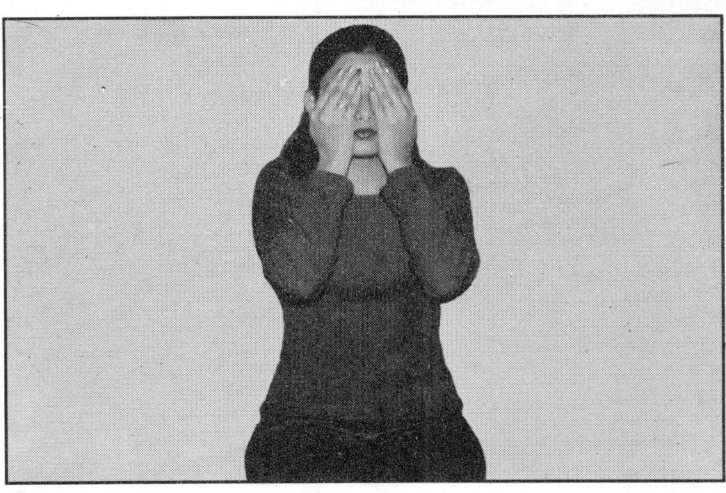

Place hands over the face with the fingers at the top of the forehead and palm over the eyes.

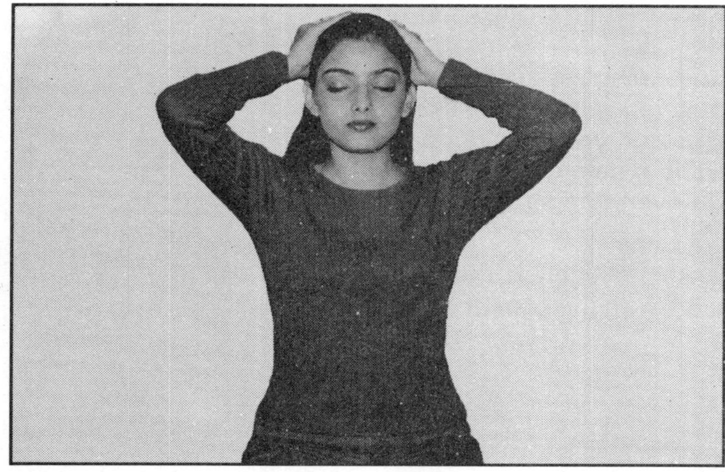

Place hands on top of head touching the crown with middle fingers touching.

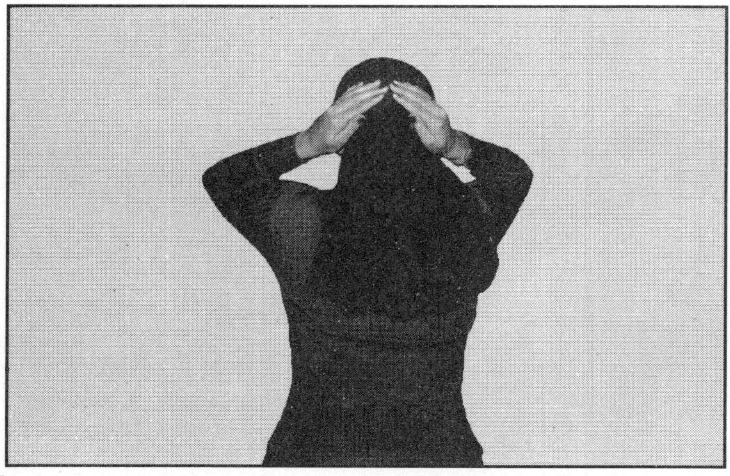

Place hands on back of your head.

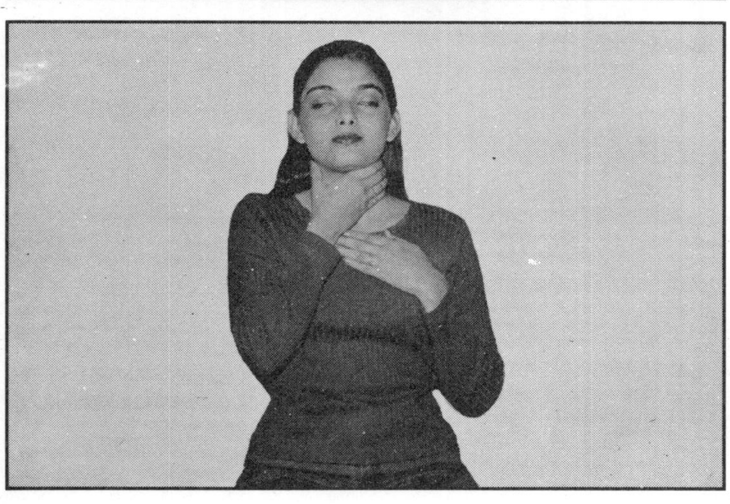

Place right hand over the throat and left hand over the heart.

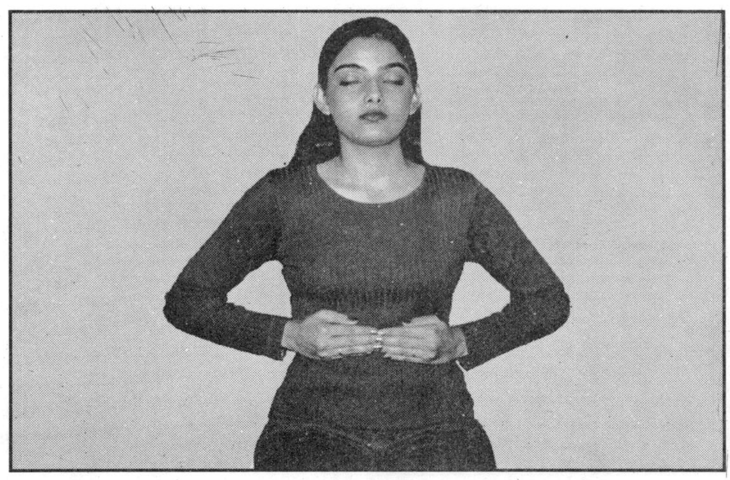

Place both hands with middle fingers touching just below breast line.

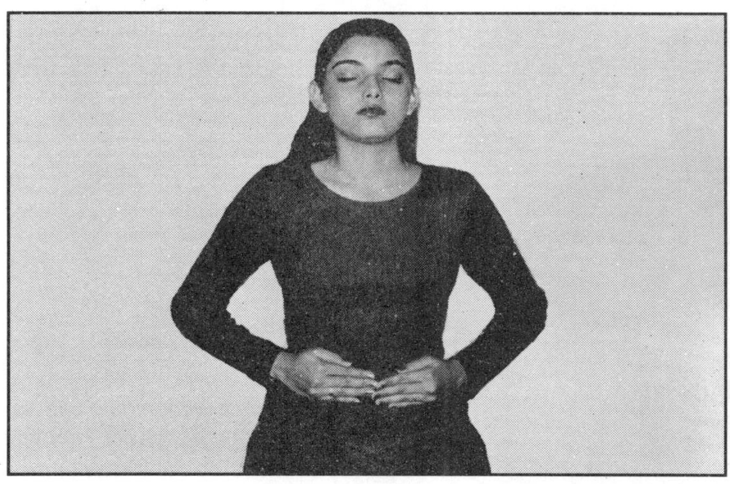

Move hands one hand-width down placing them over the stomach with middle fingers touching navel area.

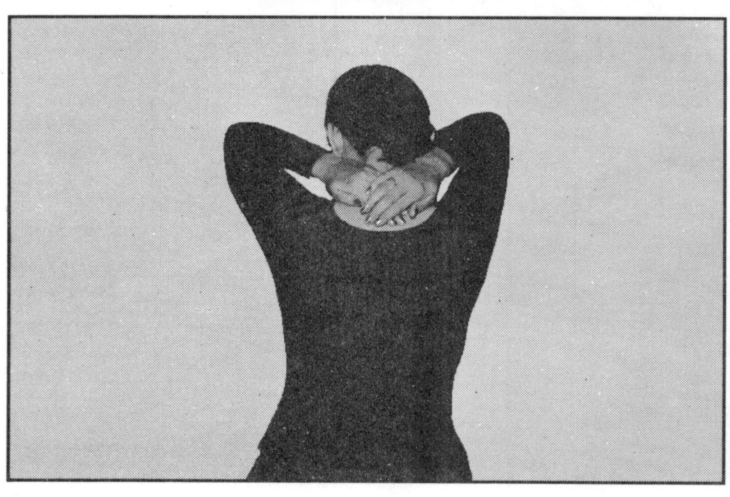

Place hands on the shoulder muscles with middle fingers touching the spine.

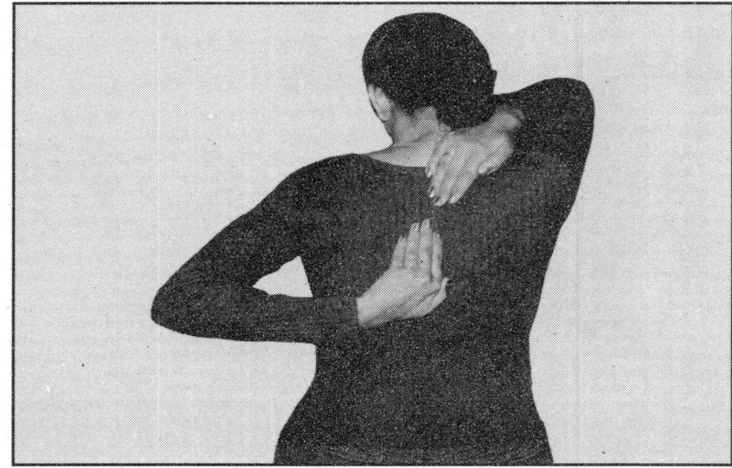

Reach round and behind back with left hand and place right hand on the shoulder blade.

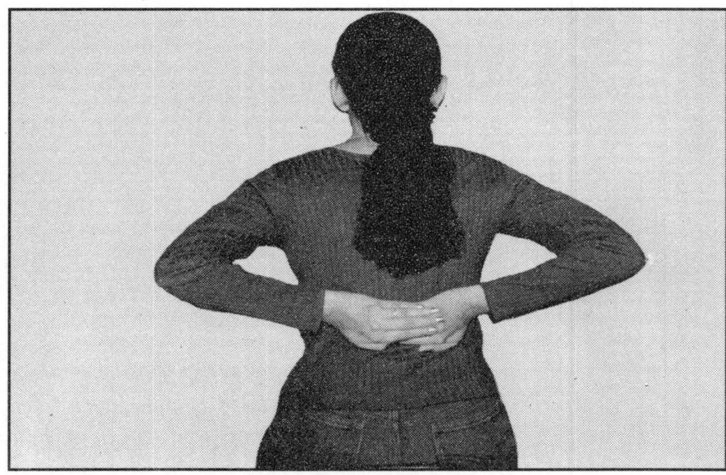

Place hands with middle fingers touching one hand width above the kidneys.

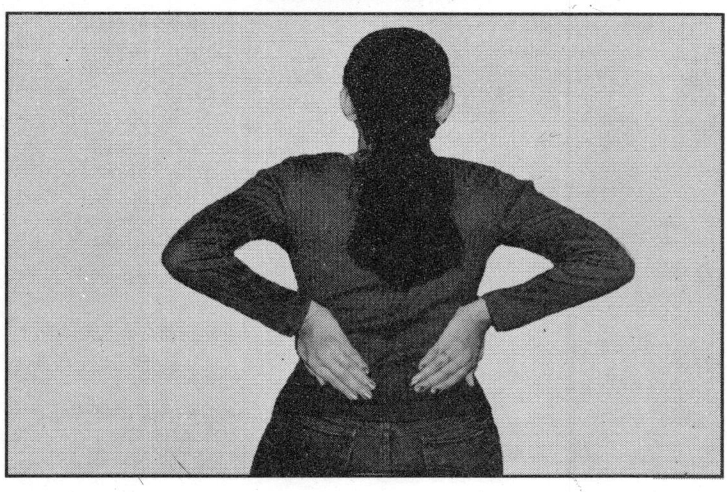

Place hands above waist line on the kidneys.

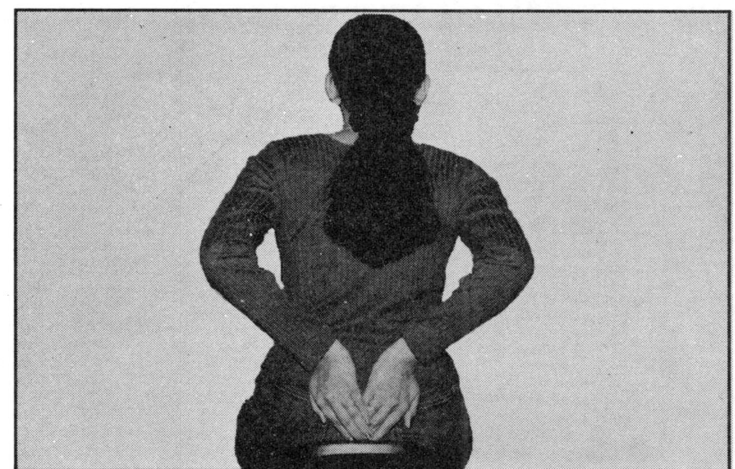

Place hands on the lower back with finger tips pointing downward and touching the tip of the tail bone (Coccyx).

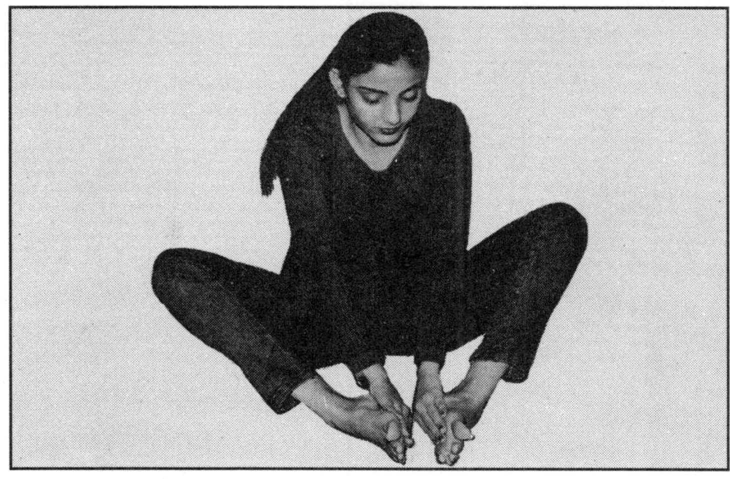

Place hands at your feet soles and ankles, fingers combined and cup shaped.

ENERGY WORK TREATMENT WITH PATIENT

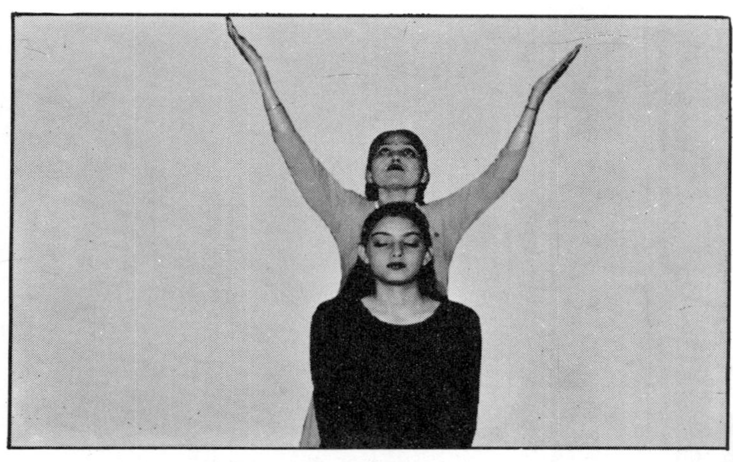

Step - 1
Practitioner opening Rainbow disc and pulling energy down to herself.

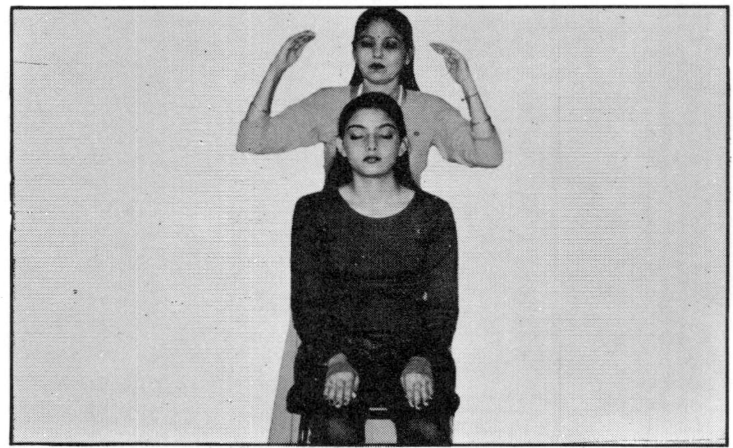

Step - 2

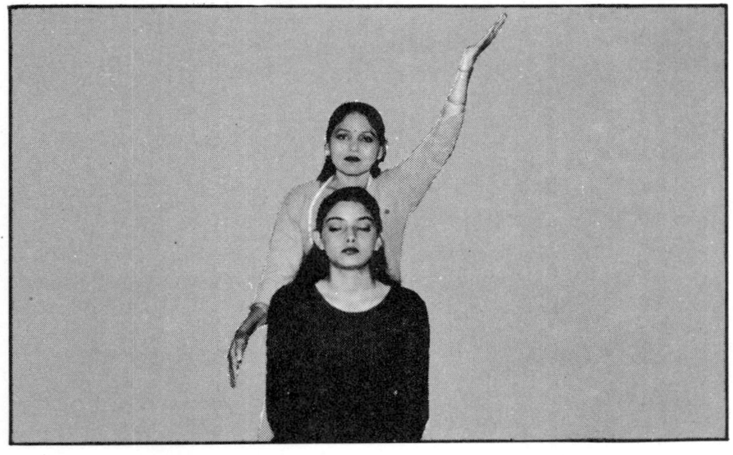

Step - 3

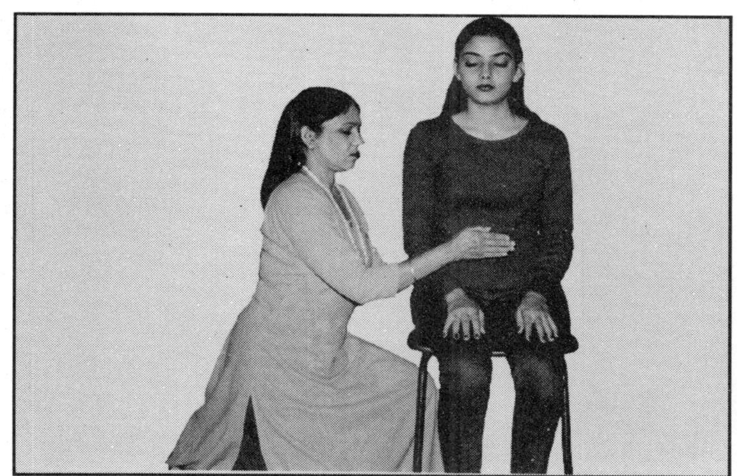

Step - 4

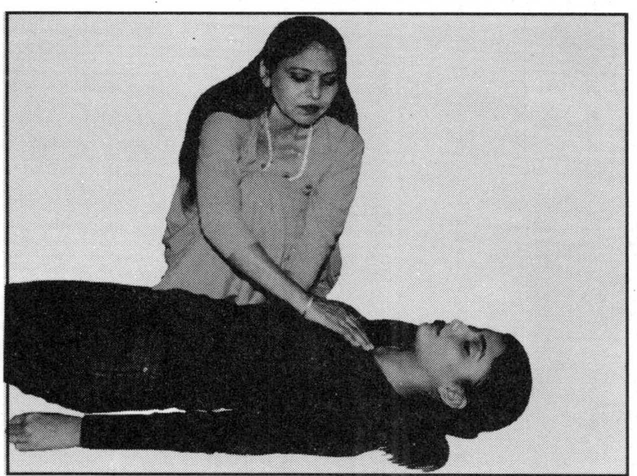

Step - 5

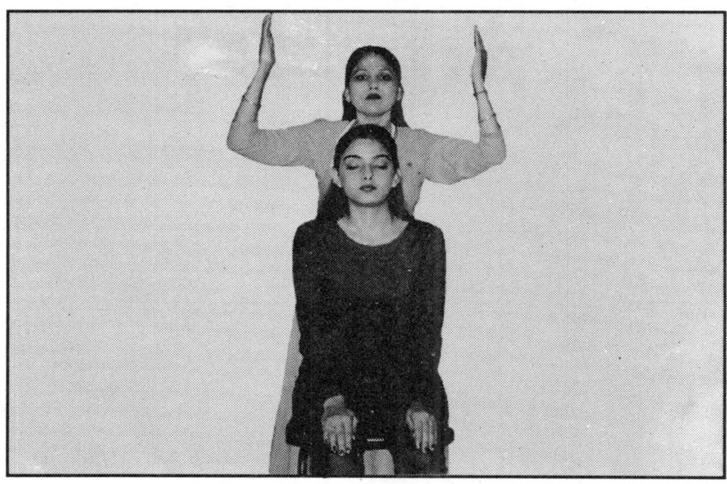

Step - 6
*Practitioner opening rainbow-disc
and pulling down energy for the
patient*

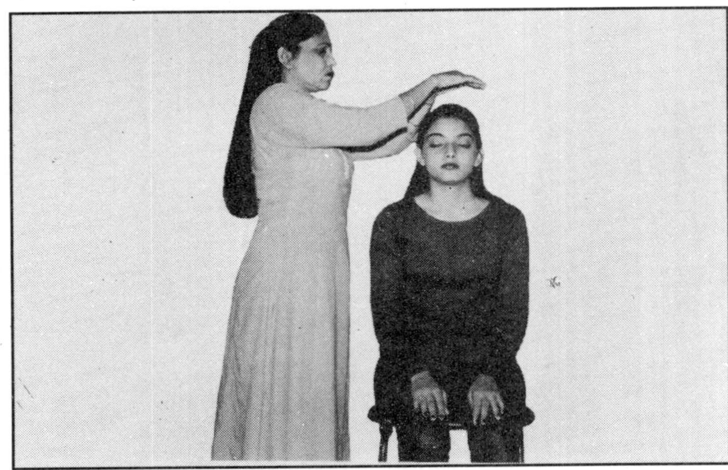

Step - 7
Practitioner performing initial assessment.

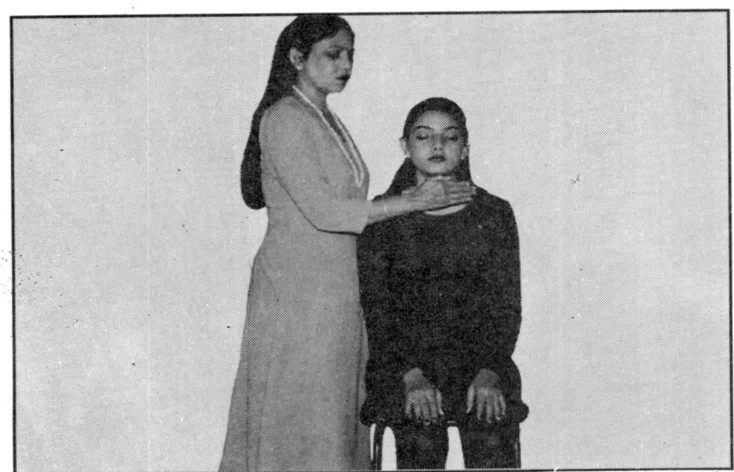

Step - 8

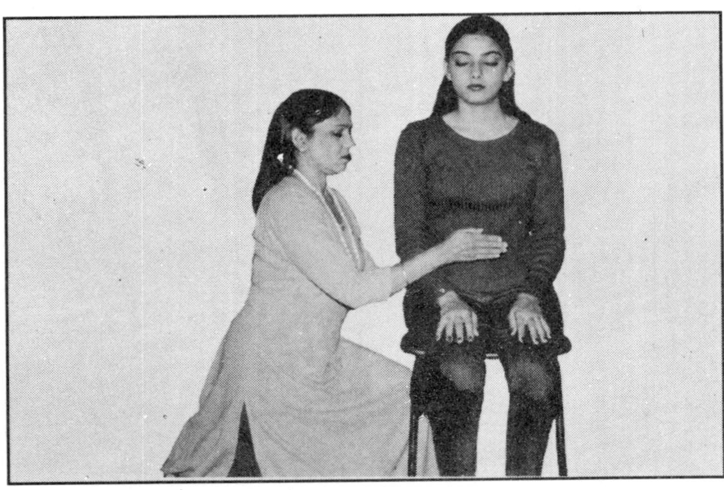

Step - 9

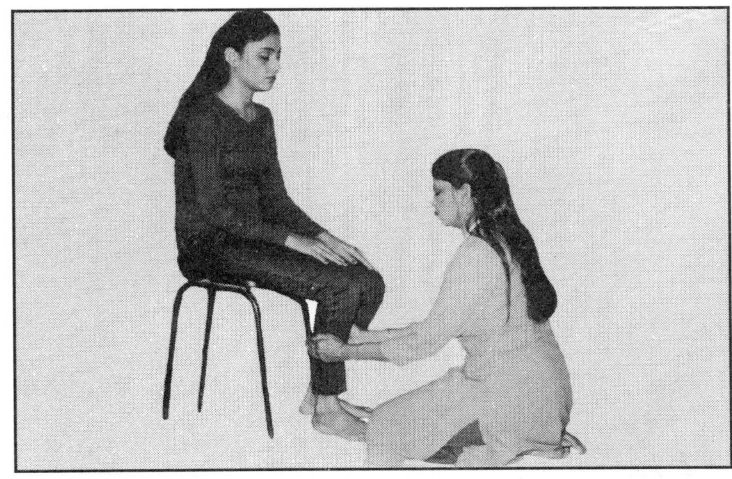

Step - 10

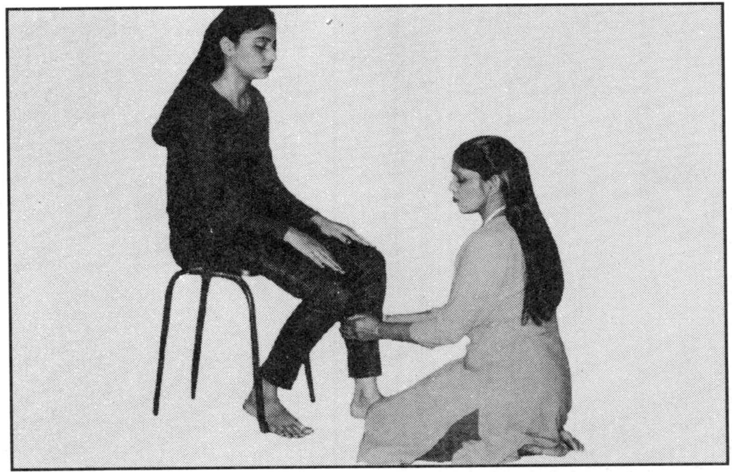

Step - 11

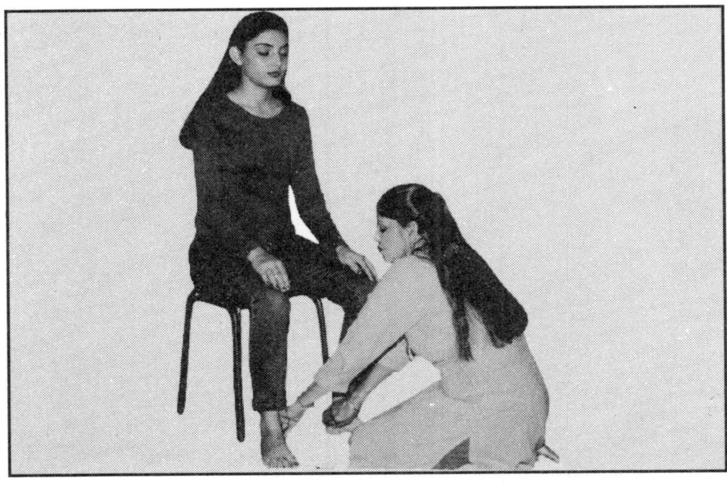

Step - 12
Practitioner opening the patient's
feet and balancing the energy flow.

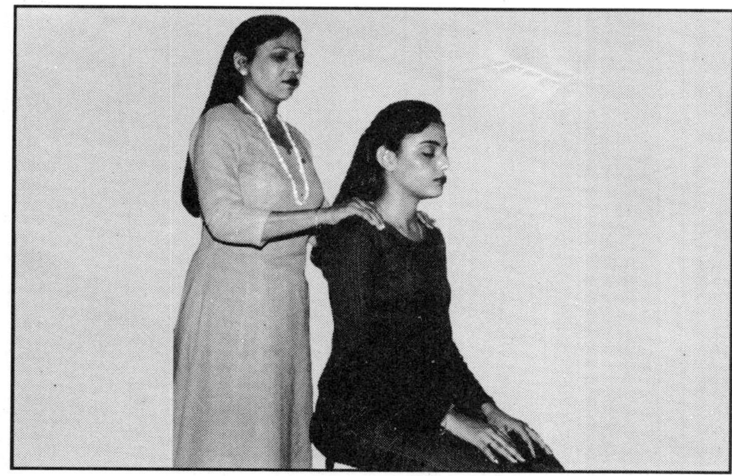

Step - 13
Practitioner opening the shoulders and directing energy flow down each arm (same procedure as opening of feet)

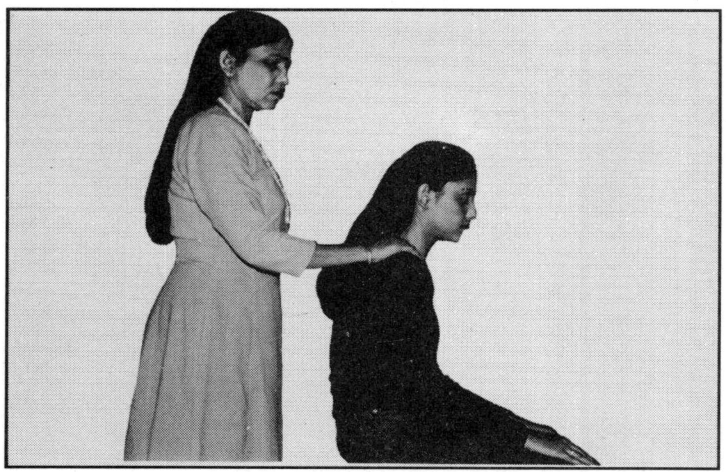

Step - 14

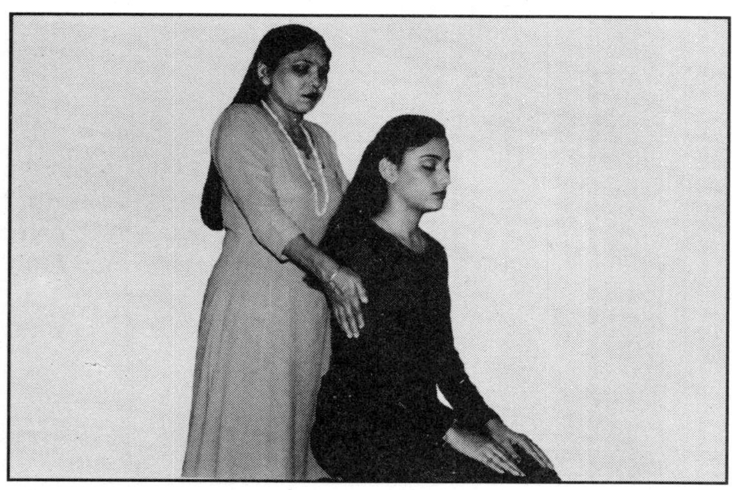

Step - 15

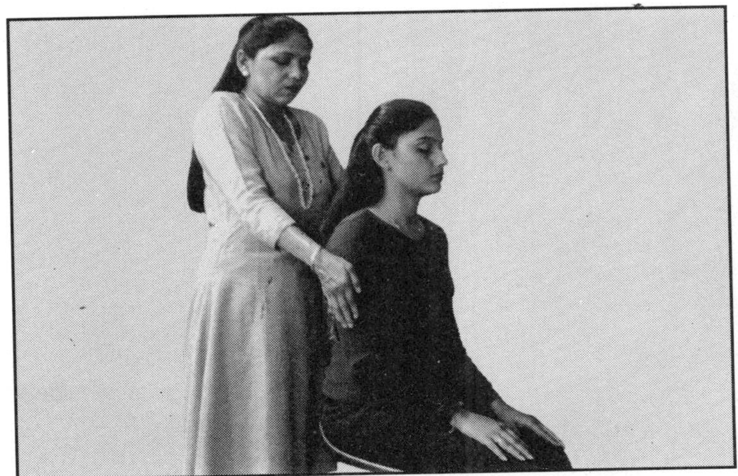

Step - 16

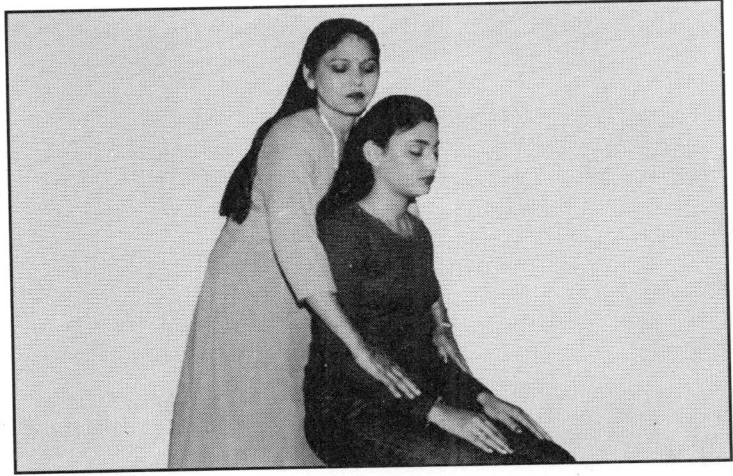

Step - 17

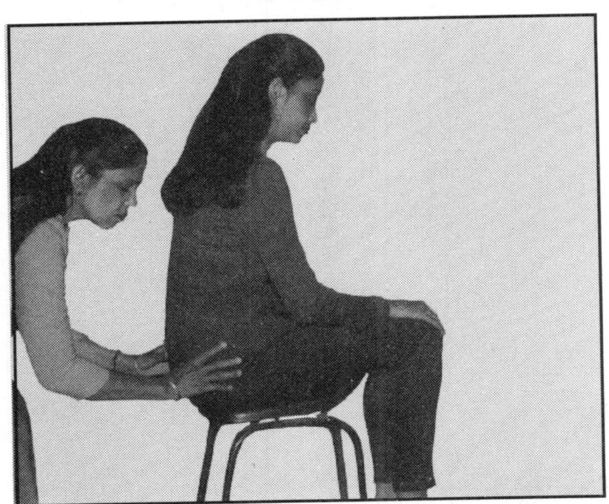

At this point in the Treatment, the practitioner needs to perform another, which can be done by repeating step 7 to 11.

Step - 18
Practitioner gently moving down the patient's spine

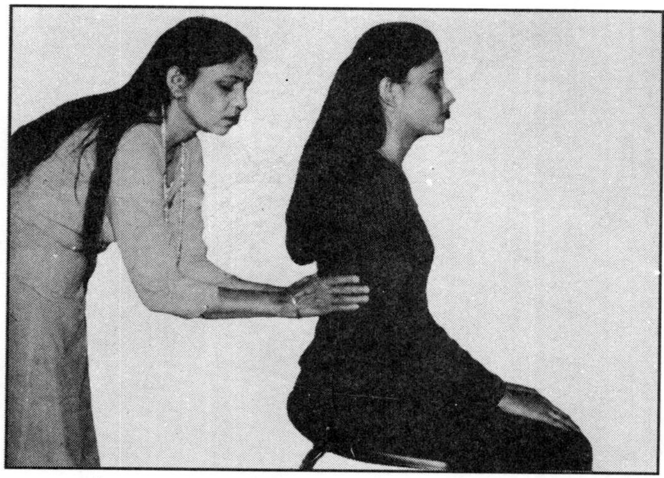

Step - 19
Practitioner building the Energy ball to raise the life force.

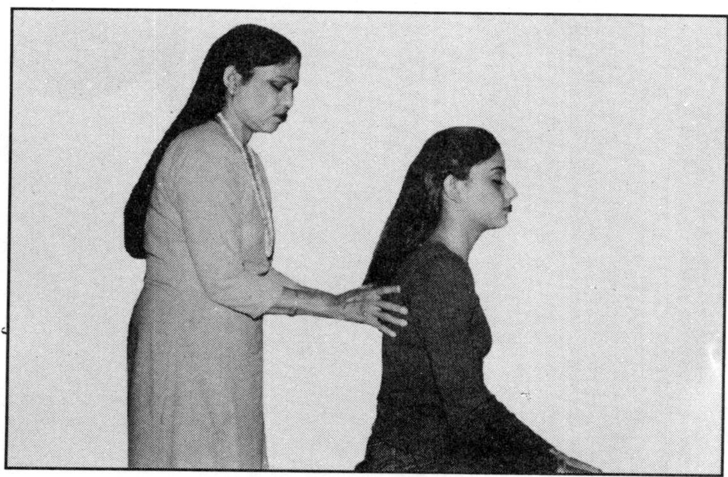

Step - 20
Practitioner slowly moving up the patient's spine while visualizing the energy ball

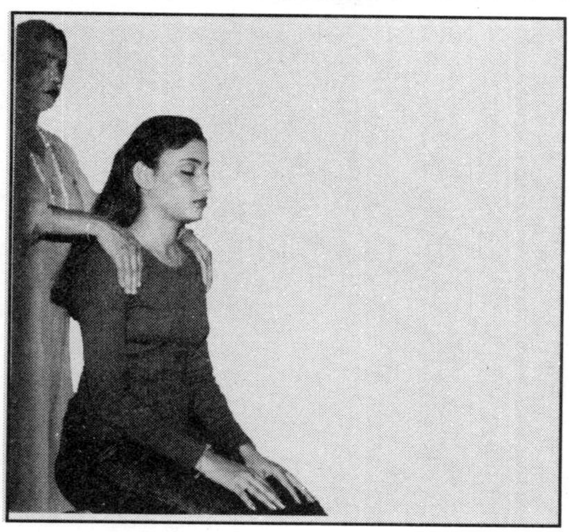

Step - 21

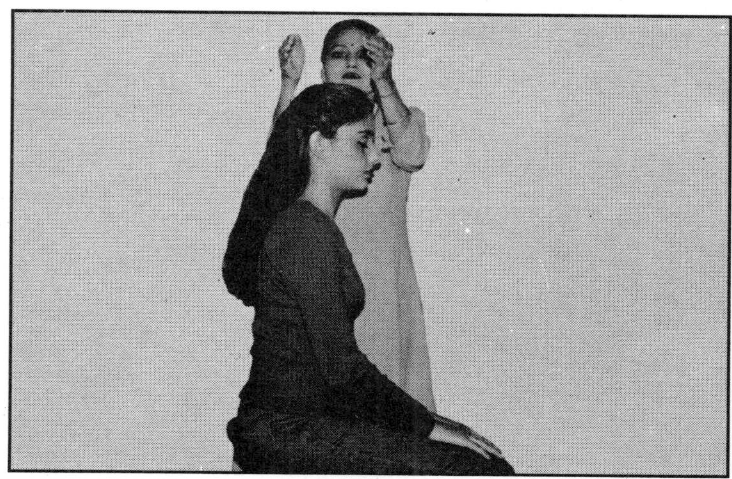

Step - 22
Practitioner releasing the Energy

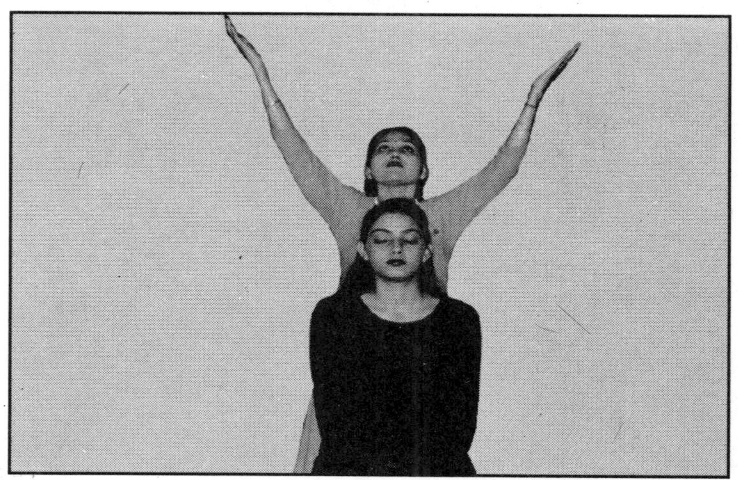

Step - 23

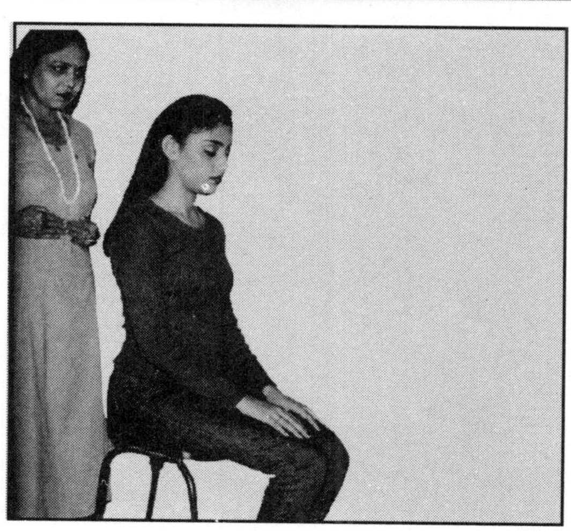

Step - 24
*Practitioner returning light and love to
the patient's vibral core.*

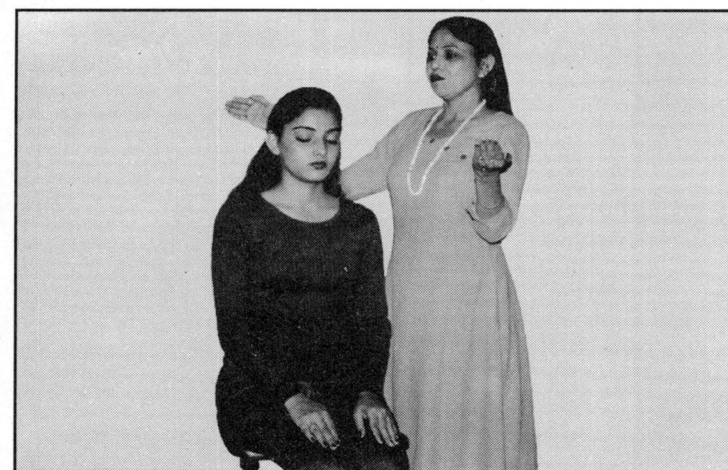

Step - 25

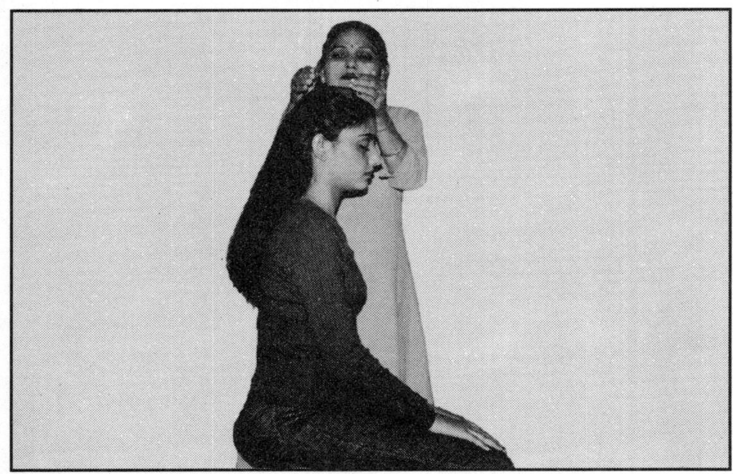

Step - 26

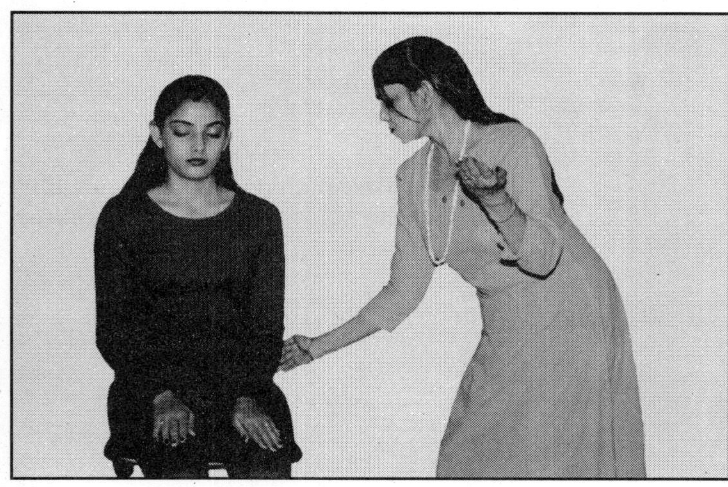

Step - 27

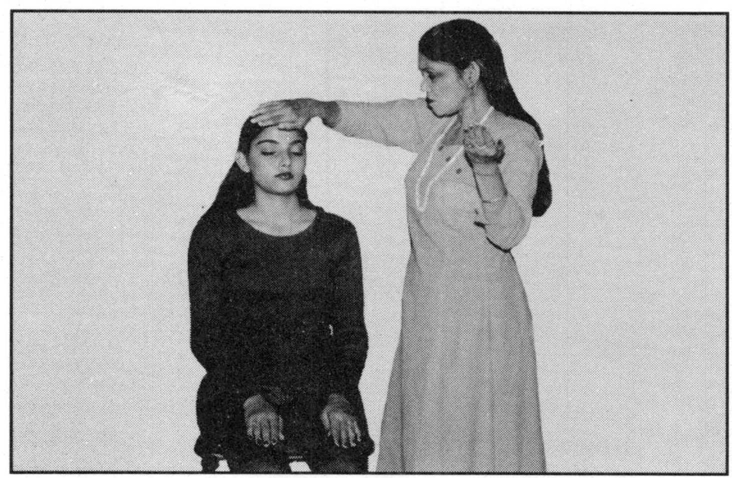

Step - 28

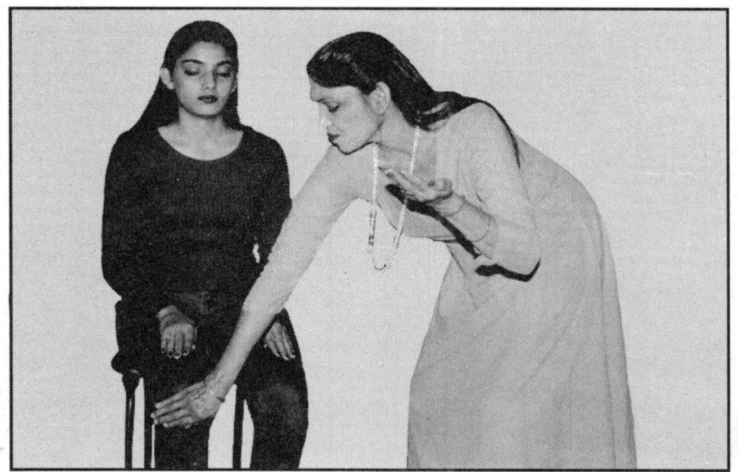

Step - 29

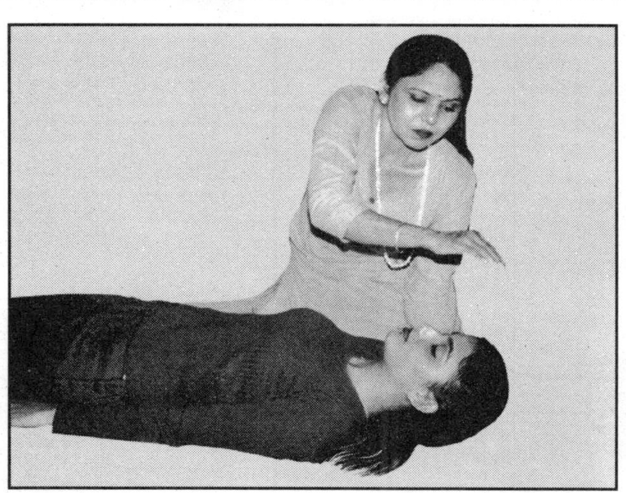

Complete treatment can also be taken this way in lying down position.

Step - 30
Initial assessment with the practitioner—left hand supporting the patient at the back of the neck.

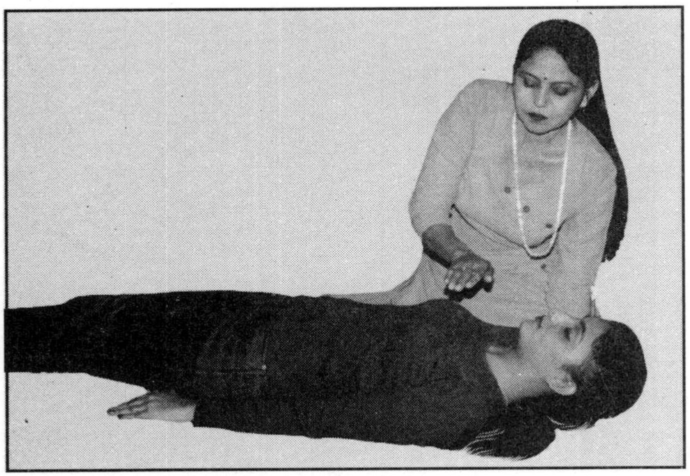

Step - 31

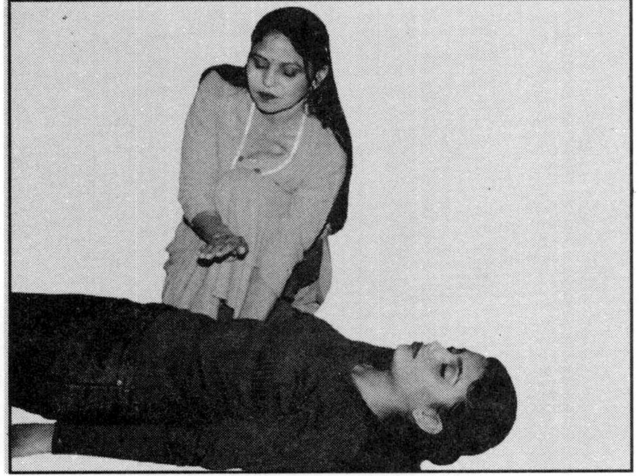

Step - 32

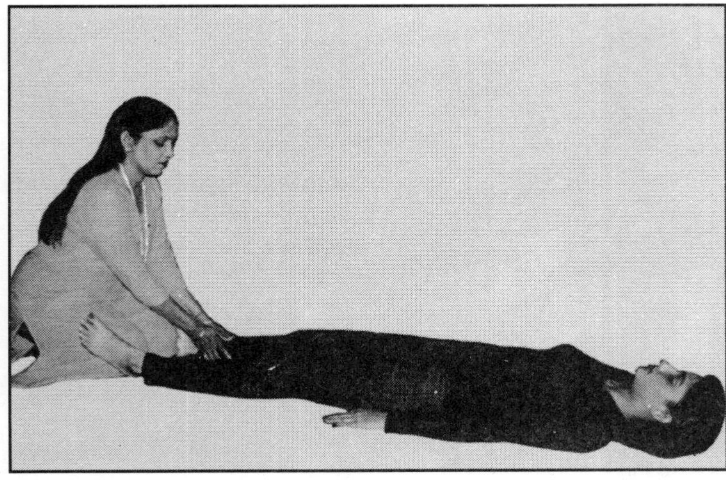

Step - 33
Practitioner pulling energy down leg.

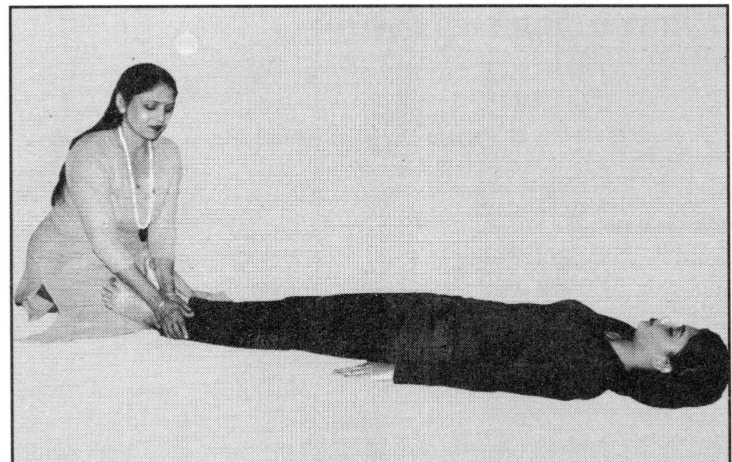

Step - 34

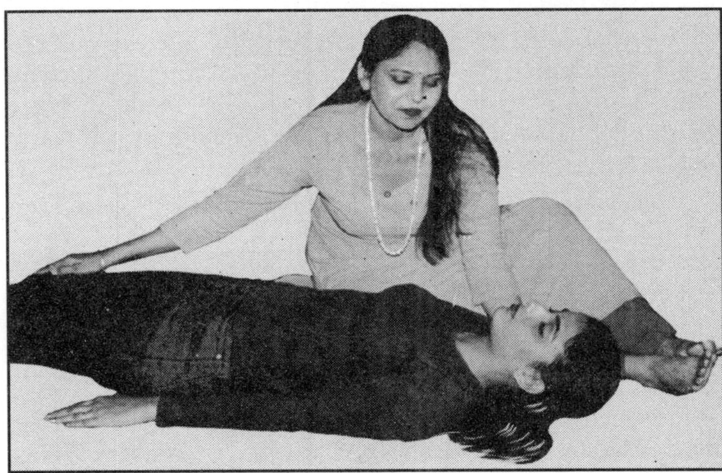

Step - 35

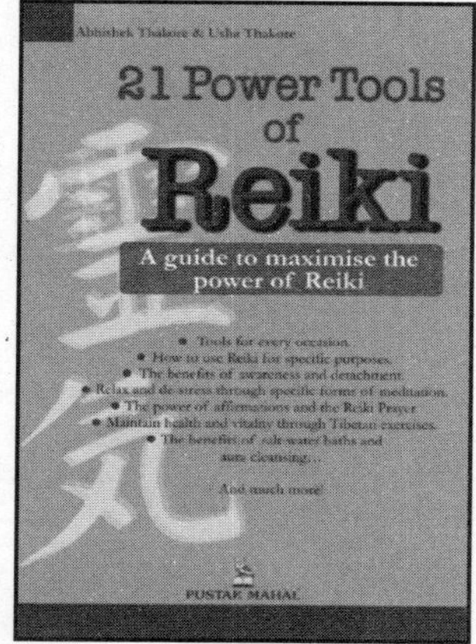

21 Power Tools of Reiki

—Abhishek Thakore & Usha Thakore

A guide to maximise the power of Reiki

The leading New Age therapy, although extremely popular, Reiki is generally taught at the very basic level. It can, however, do much more than simply heal diseases. Channelled properly, Reiki can be used for very specific purposes with astonishing results. Through the 21 power tools, this book teaches you just how, in a step-by-step manner.

The outcome of five years' research, **21 Power Tools of Reiki** is a collection of different methods and tools that make Reiki most effective by concentrating the flow of energy. The book outlines these 21 power tools that you could use for every occasion. Use these tools – and feel the difference!

This book includes: ❖ Tools for every occasion ❖ How to use Reiki for specific purpose ❖ The benefits of awareness and detachment ❖ Relax and de-stress through specific forms of meditation ❖ The power of affirmations and the Reiki Prayer ❖ Maintain health and vitality through Tibetan exercises ❖ The benefits of salt-water baths and aura cleansing… And much more!

Demy Size • Pages: 136 • Price: Rs. 88/- • Postage: Rs. 15/-

Healing Through Reiki

—M.K. Gupta

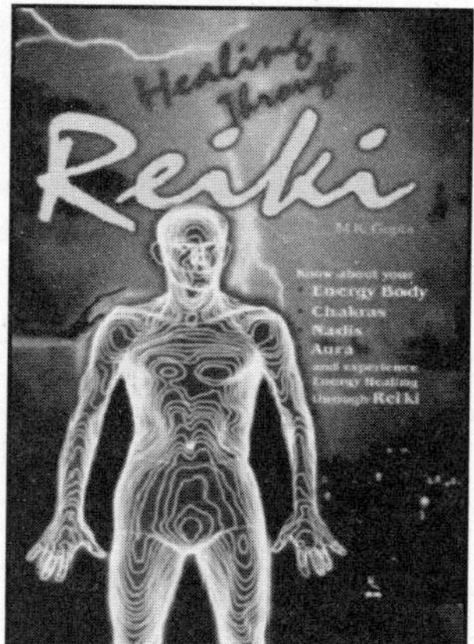

Contrary to what some people believe, Reiki is not a shady practice rooted in unfounded principles, but a systematic healing therapy based on the universal life force that pervades the entire cosmos. The Japanese refer to this invisible but universal energy as *Ki*, the Chinese as *Chi*, while Indians term it *prana*. This energy forms an invisible pranic form around our physical body. This pranic form provides energy to the physical body and any disturbance in the pranic form affects our physical body, causing various ailments. Reiki is the science of tapping this pranic energy and using it to heal and nourish the physical body. Correcting any energy imbalance in the pranic form automatically heals the corresponding physical body.

In this book, the author highlights the association between the Japanese-discovered Reiki and the Indian healing techniques based on chakras, nadis and Yoga. Besides detailing the basic principles of Reiki, the book also outlines Reiki attunement or the process of empowerment. With many photos and illustrations, the book reveals Reiki treatment for specific ailments.

Demy Size • Pages: 102 • Price: Rs. 80/- • Postage: Rs. 15/-

The Healing Touch of REIKI

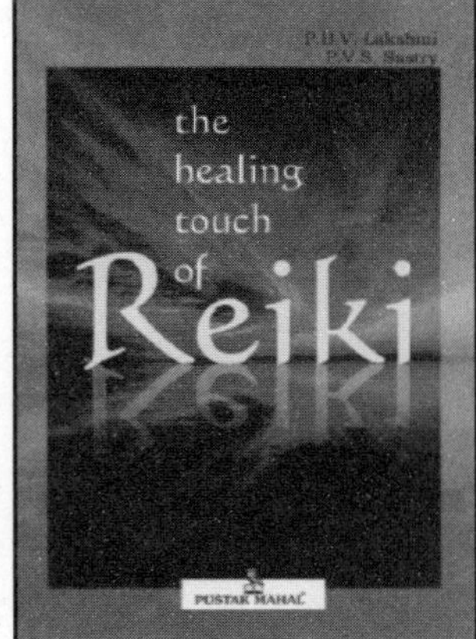

—P.B.V. Lakshmi, P.V.S. Sastry

A guide to maximise the power of Reiki

The authors offer their readers a meaningful understanding of the History of Reiki. The book gives a detailed account of endocrine system in depth, including its function. The authors firmly believe that faith in one's own inner self and the positive attitude prepare one to get healed. Open mindedness, unconditional love and total surrender can see to it that one can achieve higher levels of consciousness.

Though there are several techniques available in this world, Reiki is one of the holiest, simplest and easiest to practise by everyone at all times. As such, healing is an integrated process and the constant practice of Reiki which is a high level deep rooted Meditation by a practitioner, invokes cosmic energy through the 'Chakras' to enhance the energy levels at all the five levels i.e. Physical, Mental, Emotional, Intellectual and Spiritual. The authors want to emphasize that practice of Reiki can bring in enormous benefits such as it can enhance the Creativity, bring in Wisdom, reverse the Aging Process, amplify the Energy Level, and reduce the Basal Metabolic Rate (BMR).

Demy Size • Pages: 112 • Price: Rs. 80/- • Postage: Rs. 15/-

Master Approaches to New Age Alternative Therapies

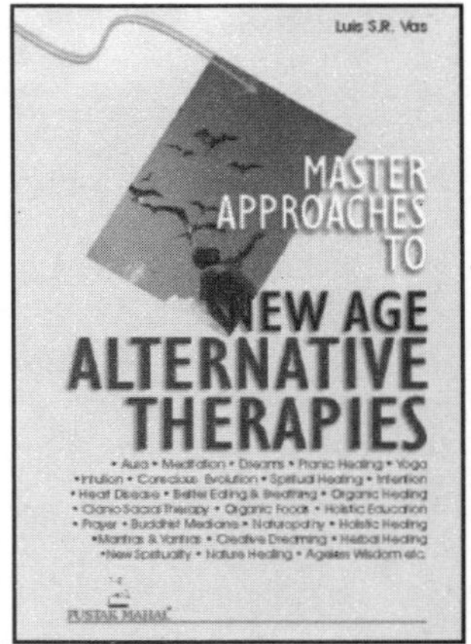

—Luis S.R. Vas

Physical health is closely linked to mental and spiritual health. In fact, very often a physical ailment is but a manifestation of a problem at the psychological level. As such, people down the ages have tried to explore this inextricable connection and come out with incredible solutions to a variety of ailments.

This book is a masterly volume providing an overview of the different approaches propounded by thinkers and researchers over time. For instance, Choa Kok Sui, a Filipino practising Pranic Healing (by dividing the body into the physical visible body and the invisible energy body) claiming to cure illnesses of eye, liver, kidney, heart in a few sessions through it. Barbara Brennan, an American and a former NASA physicist, bases her healing techniques "on the anatomy and physiology of the human energy field, or auric field". Dr. Benedict Lust (1872-1945), the father of Naturopathy believed that man could stay healthy and strong as long as he lived in accordance with Natural laws and Yogic practices, as given in an organised system by Maharshi Patanjali in the first century B.C. and known to be a miracle cure for a range of illnesses. Including these, the book brings the basic theories and practices of over 30 such masters from every part of the globe—ranging from Rosemary Gladstar (Herbal Healing), John Robbin (Healing through Organic Foods), and Lama Surya Das (Healing through Buddhist Spiritual Medicine) to Indian masters (Healing through Meditation) and Ancient masters (Healing through Natural Tantras).

Demy Size • Pages: 200 • Price: Rs. 80/- • Postage: Rs. 15/-